Managing Obstetric Emergencies and Trauma

D0588977

The MOET Course Manual

Edited by

Richard Johanson, Charles Cox,
Kate Grady and Charlotte Howell

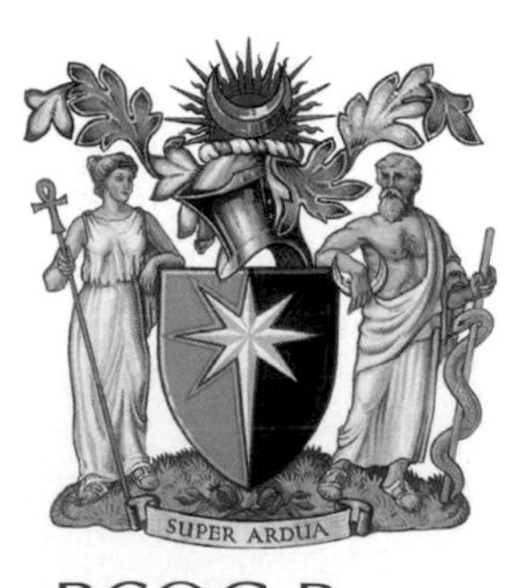

RCOG Press

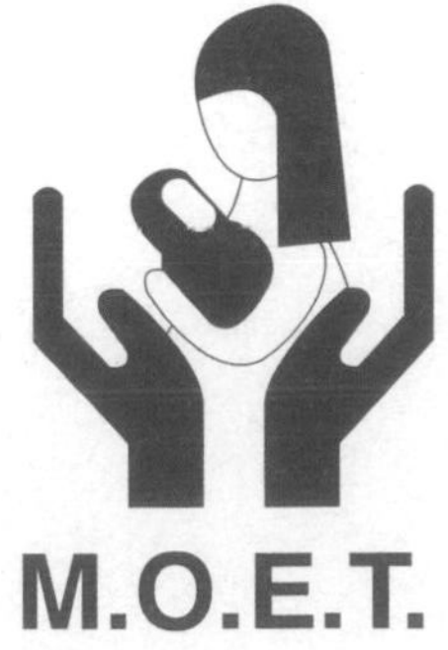

Published by the **RCOG Press** at the Royal College of Obstetricians and Gynaecologists, 27 Sussex Place, Regent's Park, London NW1 4RG

www.rcog.org.uk

Registered charity no. 213280

First published 2003

© 2003 Richard Johanson, Charles Cox, Kate Grady and Charlotte Howell

Apart from any fair dealing for the purposes of research or private study, criticism or review, as permitted under the Copyright, Designs and Patents Act, 1988, no part of this publication may be reproduced, stored or transmitted in any form or by any means, without the prior written permission of the publisher or, in the case of reprographic reproduction, in accordance with the terms of licences issued by the Copyright Licensing Agency in the UK. Enquiries concerning reproduction outside the terms stated here should be sent to the publisher at the UK address printed on this page.

The use of registered names, trademarks, etc. in this publication does not imply, even in the absence of a specific statement, that such names are exempt from the relevant laws and regulations and therefore for general use.

While every effort has been made to ensure the accuracy of the information contained within this publication, the publisher can give no guarantee for information about drug dosage and application thereof contained in this book. In every individual case the respective user must check current indications and accuracy by consulting other pharmaceutical literature and following the guidelines laid down by the manufacturers of specific products and the relevant authorities in the country in which they are practising.

The right of Richard Johanson, Charles Cox, Kate Grady and Charlotte Howell to be identified as Editors of this work has been asserted by them in accordance with the Copyright, Designs and Patents Act, 1988.

ISBN 1 900364 70 0

Photography: Sara Paterson-Brown
RCOG Press Editor: Jane Moody
Design/typesetting: Karl Harrington, FiSH Books
Printed by Cambrian Printers, Llanbadarn Road, Aberystwyth, Ceredigion SY23 3TN

Professor Richard Johanson 1957–2002

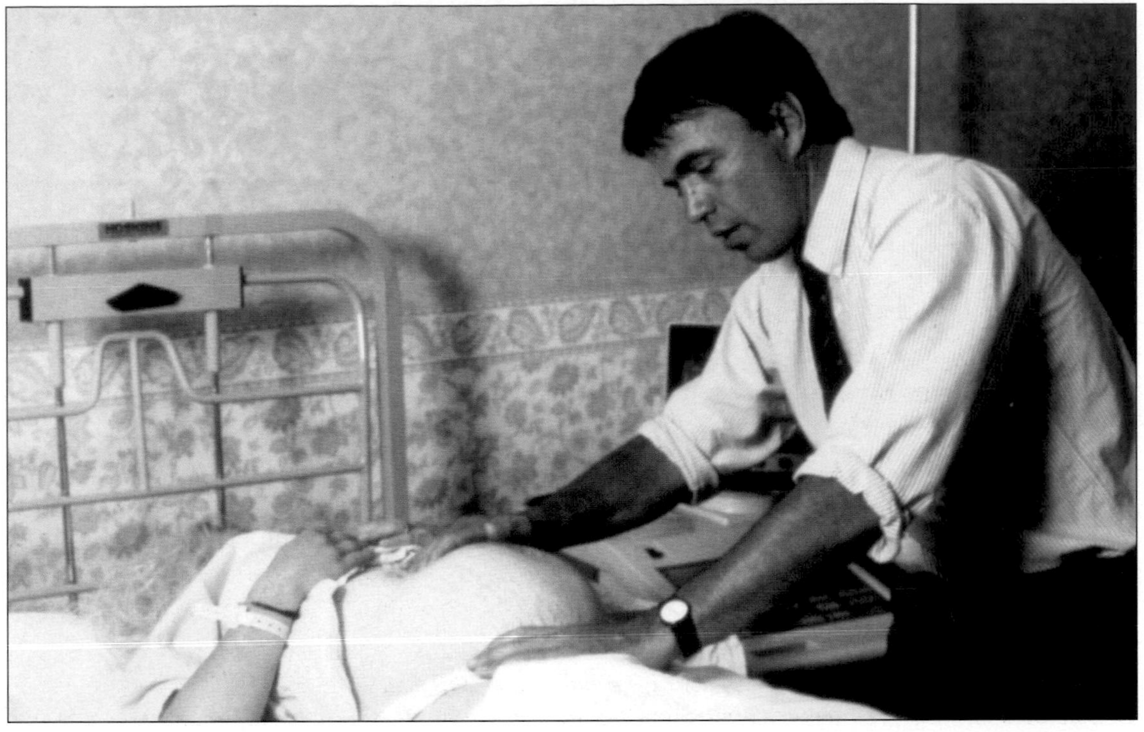

"It's never too late to be what you might have been"

George Eliot

This quotation had meaning for Richard – it was posted on his study wall.

Richard had two major aims in obstetrics – to avoid unnecessary intervention but to apply urgent skilled intervention when needed and he had a gift for both. He wanted interventions to be based on the best evidence available and for there to be good audit to check that the correct processes were being followed. His experience in Stoke and overseas had given him the skills to achieve these aims. His drive was for simple emergency protocols to save the lives of mothers and babies. This led to his leadership in practice and education in labour ward emergencies.

Initially he organised structured training for life-threatening obstetric emergencies in the West Midlands and in 1997 he and Charles Cox were the inspiration for developing the 'Managing Obstetric Emergencies and Trauma' (MOET) course, aimed at senior obstetricians and anaesthetists. A modified MOET course was taken overseas where he introduced ideas and protocols with tact and efficiency.

He worked closely with midwives in research and in the implementation of labour ward guidelines. He organised national meetings dealing with childbirth and worked with the National Childbirth Trust and Baby Lifeline, again to promote safer childbirth without over-medicalisation. The foundation of his research charity 'Childbirth without Fear' aims to continue to improve the care of women during childbirth.

Richard will be remembered by many, particularly by his trainees. His boundless enthusiasm and generosity with his time, ideas and academic work meant that there was a queue to work with him. The publication problem would be solved and the trainee would have a nationally respected mentor who continued to take an interest in their career.

Perhaps instinctively feeling that time was precious led him to achieve so much so quickly. Much of it was due to the intellectual sparking between him and his anaesthetist wife, Charlotte. They demonstrated the teamwork that is part of the philosophy of MOET.

"To see a human being reveal really exceptional qualities one must be able to observe his activities over many years. If these activities are completely unselfish; if the idea motivating them is unique in its magnanimity; if it quite certain that they have never looked for any reward; and if in addition they have left visible traces on the world – then one may say, without fear of error, that one is in the presence of an unforgettable character."

[Jean Giono, from a short story called *The Man Who Planted Trees*]

Contents

Contributors

The late Professor RB Johanson BSc MA MD MRCOG	
Mr C Cox FRCS (Ed) FRCOG	Consultant Obstetrician and Gynaecologist, Wolverhampton
Dr NA Coleman FRCA	Consultant in Anaesthesia and Intensive Care, Stoke-on-Trent
Dr K Goswami BSc MBBS MRCOG	Consultant Obstetrician and Gynaecologist, Coventry
Dr K Grady BSc FRCA	Consultant Anaesthetist, Manchester
Mr D Griffiths MRCOG	Consultant Obstetrician and Gynaecologist, Swindon
Mr K Hinshaw MBBS MRCOG	Consultant Obstetrician and Gynaecologist, Sunderland
Dr C Howell MB BChir FRCA	Consultant Anaesthetist, Stoke-on-Trent
Miss S Irani MD MRCOG	Consultant Obstetrician and Gynaecologist, Birmingham
Dr M Khadra MB BCh MRCOG	Specialist Registrar, Obstetrics, Stoke on Trent
Mrs G Masson MBChB MRCOG	Consultant Obstetrician, Stoke-on-Trent
Dr BGR Prasad MBBS FRCA FFARCSI	Consultant Anaesthetist, Birmingham
Dr H Sidhu MD MRCOG	Consultant Obstetrician and Gynaecologist, Craigavon
Dr GV Sunanda MBBS MRCOG	Consultant Obstetrician and Gynaecologist, Birmingham
Dr CB Wykes BSc MBBS MRCOG	Specialist Registrar Obstetrics and Gynaecology, Brighton
Mr PF Young MBChB MRCOG	Consultant Obstetrician and Gynaecologist, Stoke-on-Trent

Acknowledgements

The course owes much to two established courses and their organisations, BATLS – Battlefield Advanced Trauma Life Support – and ALSO – Advanced Life Support in Obstetrics.

We would like to thank Professor Peter Roberts and Professor James Ryan, present and past Professors of Military Surgery, for their help, advice and allowing access to their course material.

We would also like to thank Mr Kim Hinshaw and Dr Ann Ryall and other ALSO faculty members for their advice and support.

The obstetric emergency guidelines are based on those prepared initially by Richard Johanson and Charlotte Howell with Claire Rigby (Clinical Governance Support Officer, ASQUAM) for the Achieving Sustainable Quality in Maternity Programme in North Staffordshire. We are grateful to Claire for all her hard work in preparing the original guidelines and for her help in collating this manual. The Cochrane Database has provided a wealth of evidence.

The chapters on resuscitation have been informed by the new international guidelines produced by an evidence-based process from the collaboration of many international experts under the umbrella of the International Liaison Committee on Resuscitation (ILCOR).

We would also like to thank Advanced Life Support Group (ALSG), who gave permission for the reproduction of some of the material used in this text in particular from the books *Advanced Paediatric Life Support: The Practical Approach, BMJ Books* (ISBN 0-7279-1554-1) and *Safe Transfer and Retrieval: The Practical Approach, BMJ Books* (ISBN 0-7279-1583-5). We also thank Bios Scientific Publishers for permission to reproduce material from the book *Managing Obstetric Emergencies* 1999 (ISBN 1-85996-122-3).

We acknowledge and sincerely thank Sue Wieteska for her hard work in the final preparation of the manuscript. We thank her also for her tremendous support for our organisation. Our grateful appreciation goes to Jane Moody, for editing this text with vigour, flair and feeling.

A great many people have put a lot of hard work into the production of this book and the accompanying course. The editors would like to thank all the contributors for their efforts and all the MOET providers and instructors who took the time to send their comments during the development of the text and the course, in particular Sue Maurice and Derek Tufnell who spent considerable time helping us by scanning the text thoroughly and Nicky Osborne for her comments.

We would like to thank Angela Railton, who, at a time close to publication, has put enormous time and expertise into the proof-reading of this manuscript.

The photographs used throughout the text were taken at a MOET course held in London at the RCOG, by Sara Paterson-Brown.

Algorithm 23.1 was written by Poonam Pradhan.

Chapter 17 The management of shoulder dystocia was derived from the chapter on shoulder dystocia written by Onsy Louca and Richard Johanson for the *Yearbook of Obstetrics and Gynaecology* Volume 6.[100] We acknowledge comments from Barbara Franks.

Charles Cox
Kate Grady
Charlotte Howell
October 2002

Abbreviations

ABG	arterial blood gases
ACLS	Advanced Cardiac Life Support
AED	automated external defibrillator
AFE	amniotic fluid embolism
AFP	alphafetoprotein
ALS	advanced life support
ALSG	Advanced Life Support Group
ALSO	Advanced Life Support in Obstetrics
APCR	activated protein C resistance
APTT	activated partial thromboplastin time
ARDS	acute respiratory distress syndrome
ATLS	Advanced Trauma Life Support
BATLS	Battlefield Advanced Trauma Life Support
BNF	*British National Formulary*
BP	blood pressure
bpm	beats per minute
CEMD	Confidential Enquiries into Maternal Deaths
CJD	Creutzfedt–Jakob disease
CNS	central nervous system
CPP	cerebral perfusion pressure
CPR	cardiopulmonary resuscitation
CSE	combined spinal/epidural analgesia
CT	computed tomography
CTG	cardiotocography
CVA	cerebrovascular accident
CVP	central venous pressure
CXR	chest X-ray
DIC	disseminated intravascular coagulation
DVT	deep vein thrombosis
EACA	epsilon-aminocaproic acid
ECG	electrocardiograph(y)
ECV	external cephalic version
EDTA	ethylenediamine tetraacetic acid
EMD	electromechanical dissociation
FAST	focused abdominal sonography for trauma
FBC	full blood count
FDP	fibrin degradation products
FFP	fresh frozen plasma
FHR	fetal heart rate
GCS	Glasgow Coma Scale
GTN	glyceryl trinitrate
Hb	haemoglobin
hCG	human chorionic gonadotrophin
HDU	high dependency unit
HELLP	haemolysis, elevated liver enzymes and low platelet count
ICP	intracranial pressure
ICU	intensive care unit
IM	intramuscular
INR	international normalised ratio
IPPV	intermittent positive-pressure ventilation
IPV	internal podalic version

ITU	intensive therapy unit
IV	intravenous
IVU	intravenous urogram
LFT	liver function tests
LMA	laryngeal mask airway
LMWH	Low-molecular weight heparins
LVF	left ventricular failure
MAP	mean arterial pressure
$MgSO_4$	magnesium sulphate
MoM	multiples of the normal median
MSSU	midstream sample of urine
N	newton
NIBP	non-invasive blood pressure
PE	pulmonary embolism
PEA	pulseless electrical activity
PEEP	positive end expiratory pressure
PDPH	post-dural puncture headache
PGE_2	prostaglandin E_2
PGF_2	prostaglandin F_2
PIOPED	Prospective Investigation of Pulmonary Embolism Diagnosis
PR	per rectum
PV	per vaginam
RCOG	Royal College of Obstetricians and Gynaecologists
RCT	randomised controlled trial
Rh	rhesus
RSI	rapid sequence induction
SAG-M	saline-adenine-glucose-mannitol
SIRS	systemic inflammatory response syndrome
SpR	specialist registrar
U&Es	urea and electrolytes
UTI	urinary tract infection
VE	vaginal examination
VF	ventricular fibrillation
V/Q	ventilation/perfusion
VT	ventricular tachycardia
VTE	venous thromboembolism

Foreword

Managing any medical emergency requires a clear understanding of the principles involved and a systematic and logical progression through lifesaving and damage-limiting treatments. The difficulty we have in obstetrics is two-fold: firstly, being faced with very rare emergencies without much, if any, previous experience and, secondly, being exposed to fairly frequent but often unanticipated emergencies on the delivery suite. To keep a clear head, coordinate staff and resources and effectively deal with each situation as it arises forms much of the art of the acute obstetric clinician. Such an approach requires practice, either at the bedside, or increasingly by 'skills and drills' training, especially with the reduced experience that junior doctors' hours has imposed. No approach, however, is effective without core knowledge and solid understanding.

This manual is recommended reading prior to the Managing Obstetric Emergencies and Trauma (MOET) course, as it provides essential anatomical, physiological and pathological information, which the authors use to explain basic logical principles of resuscitation and treatment, which they describe clearly. Unfortunately, true clinical scenarios are not planned and are often unanticipated, and it is therefore even more important that practising clinicians are armed with this wealth of information. This manual contains essential knowledge for emergency obstetrics and trauma: it is based on sound principles, is easy to read and gives useful practical advice and management plans. I wouldn't be without it.

Sara Paterson-Brown

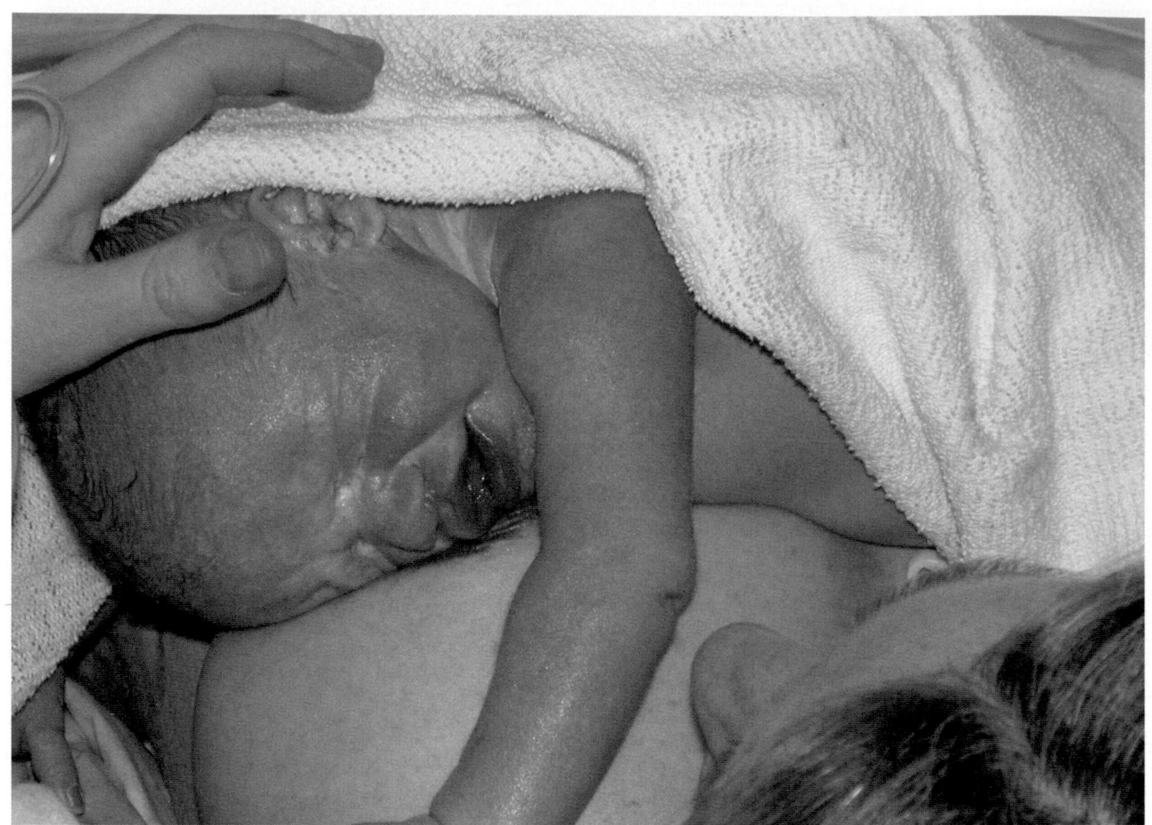

A successful outcome

Preface

This book is the core text for the Managing Obstetric Emergencies and Trauma (MOET) course. It is also useful as a stand-alone text.

Obstetricians should be able to advise on and be prepared to be involved with the care of all pregnant women, including those who have suffered trauma, either accidental or deliberate.

In the good (bad) old days trainee obstetricians were likely to have been exposed to a range of emergencies through working in accident and emergency, surgery and even anaesthetics. Those days are long gone!

Wide experience in a variety of specialties now invites the accusation of 'lack of focus' and indecisiveness.

It is unrealistic to expect trainees to have recent first-hand experience of uncommon emergencies such as cardiac arrest or trauma and even in their own specialty it is unlikely that they will have personally managed all of the major obstetric emergencies, despite the requirement to complete a logbook of experience.

Other disciplines have recognised that one way to achieve confidence and competence in dealing with the less common life-threatening emergencies is to run 'skills and drills' courses. Perhaps the most well known of these courses is the 'Advanced Trauma Life Support' (ATLS) course, sponsored by the American College of Surgeons.

It is worth remembering how the ATLS course came into being. In February 1976, a Nebraskan orthopaedic surgeon crashed in his plane, with his wife and four children aboard. His wife was killed, three children sustained critical injuries, the other child had minor injuries and he sustained serious injuries. The care he received at the primary healthcare centre led him to state 'When I can provide better care in the field with limited resources than what my children and I received at the primary care facility, there is something wrong with the system and the system has to be changed'(sic).

From this tragedy developed Advanced Trauma Life Support, which was intended for all medical practitioners to enable them to supply supportive treatment for the first hour after injury – 'the golden hour'.

In the United Kingdom, the Military introduced a course called Battlefield Advanced Trauma Life Support BATLS in advance of The College of Surgeons of England introducing ATLS to this country.

These principles of trauma life support included in BATLS are now taught to all members of the Defence Medical Services including doctors, nurses, vets, physiotherapists and combat medical technicians.

It was suggested that a course merging the broader concepts of advanced life support and managing obstetric emergencies should be developed as part of Calman implementation for obstetricians. So the Managing Obstetric Emergencies and Trauma (MOET) courses came to be. The course is interactive and aims to consolidate and share old knowledge and hopefully gain new insights from one's colleagues and very occasionally from the instructors!

Early on in the development of MOET, there was interaction with those leading the ALSO programme.[1] From the curricula and experiences of trainees, these two courses complement each other. MOET is aimed at the senior trainee and established specialist.

The anaesthetist is part of every emergency medical drill team known to hospital practice and outside. The concept of 'skills and drills' courses is not unfamiliar to the anaesthetist. Advanced Life Support courses (ALS – cardiopulmonary resuscitation) are 'core' in many region's training and anaesthetists train as ATLS, APLS (Advanced Paediatric Life Support) and ALSO or MOET providers at their own choice according to their subspecialty interests. Anaesthetists are aware of the universal demand for their resuscitation skills but equally aware that supportive resuscitation measures must be backed by definitive treatment of a medical and, more frequently in an emergency setting, a surgical nature. They are aware, from both their day-to-day practice, their experience of medical emergencies and their experience of drill-style courses, that they are part of a team and that the team requires surgical input. It is a principle of 'skills and drills' courses that every team member, regardless of specialty, should be able to provide immediate life support, to a life-saving level, and that every team member recognises the role of the specialist and when the specialist skills are required.

The realisation that life threats to the heavily pregnant patient, both obstetric and non-obstetric, require specific management has attracted anaesthetists to ALSO and MOET courses. With this in mind, MOET has developed an anaesthetic slant to its course and guarantees that a proportion of the faculty on each course will be anaesthetists.

Alongside this natural development of the team, an unsolicited interest has developed among accident and emergency doctors, who are most welcome to our organisation as they are likely to be the first to see obstetric patients who have suffered major trauma and cardiorespiratory arrest outside hospital.

The course comprises a first day devoted to basic and advanced life support, neonatal life support and trauma life support. This includes what the self-respecting first-aider should be able to achieve and should be immediately familiar to devotees of television's *ER* and *Casualty*! This part of the course is didactic and teaches an approach that is familiar to the emergency services around the world and may come in useful at rugby matches, equestrian events, on aeroplanes and by the side of the road. The philosophy is to develop an approach to the ill or traumatised patient that will carry over to the assessment and management of the pregnant patient.

The second day is not so didactic and deals with emergency obstetric conditions, both common and not so common, including conditions unfamiliar in countries with developed health systems.

The course is supported by midwives, who attend lectures and undertake skills training alongside their medical colleagues. Their presence and input is valued, not least for the emphasis towards a team approach. The course has been successfully evaluated.[2,3] Further follow-up studies are being undertaken. Modified versions of MOET have been run in Bangladesh and Armenia under the auspices of UNICEF and the Family Care charity, and in Russia and Estonia.

Richard Johanson

Charles Cox

Kate Grady

Charlotte Howell

SECTION 1
Introduction

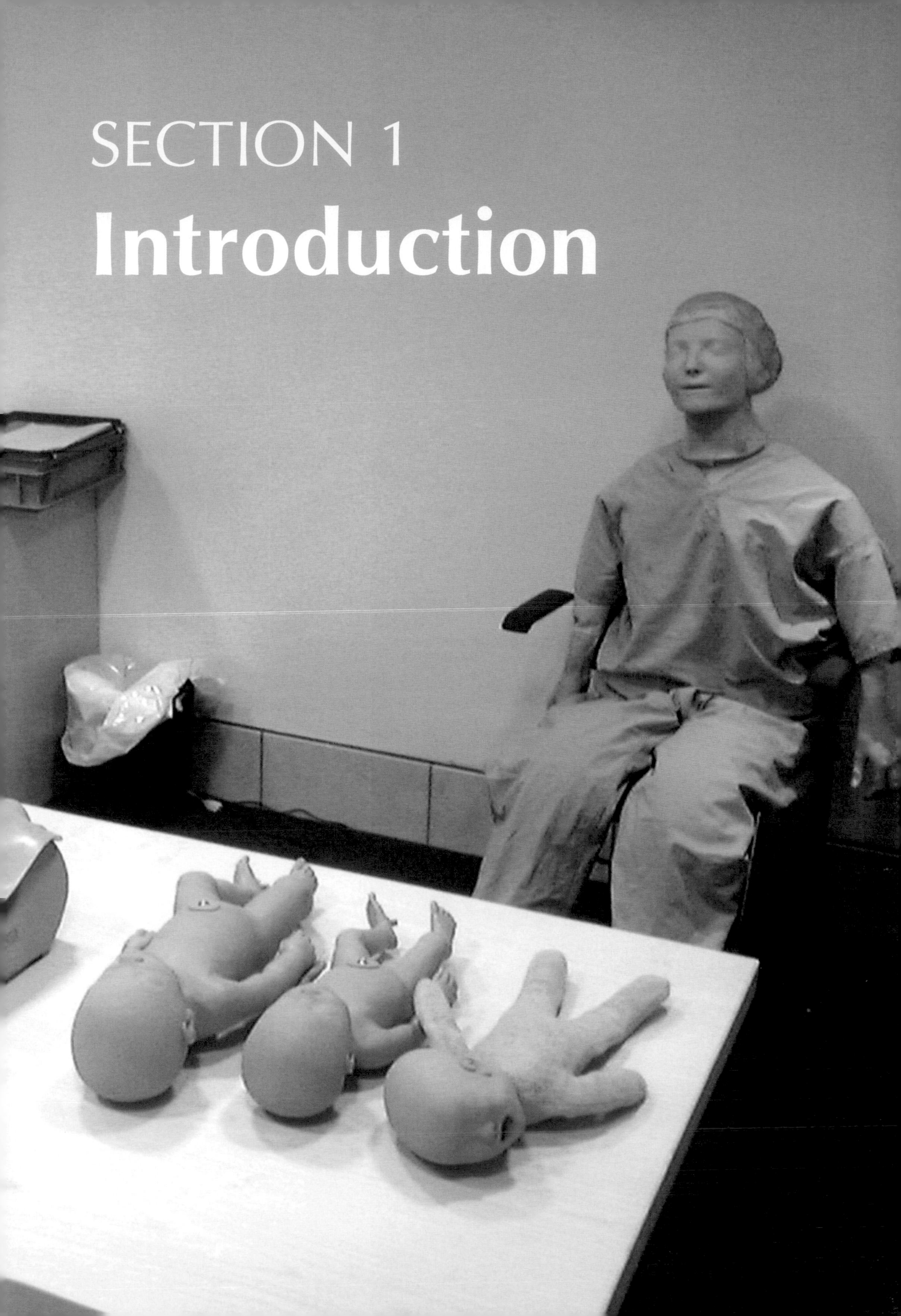

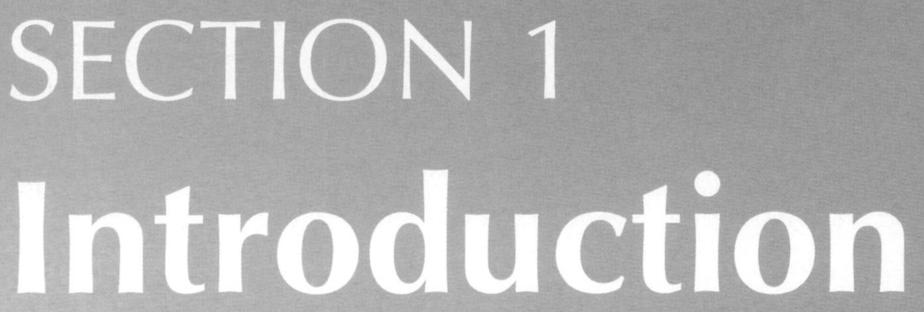

Chapter 1
Introduction

This course will provide you with a system for managing the sick and seriously injured. The system is designed to be simple and easy to remember when life-threatening emergencies arise. The system is known as the structured approach. The structured approach is the ABC of resuscitation and trauma life support and is practised throughout all walks of medicine and the emergency services. It is familiar to the lay public and is a concept known even to schoolchildren. The structured approach has led to the development of courses that attend to the needs of all patients, from neonates to children, adults and now for those with altered physiology and anatomy – pregnant women.

This course (and the manual) is divided into sections that provide a structured revision in resuscitation, trauma life support and obstetric emergencies for obstetricians, midwives, anaesthetists and accident and emergency (A&E) doctors. The structured approach is applied to resuscitation and is taught didactically as a 'skill and drill'. Subsequently, what has been learned is applied to the seriously injured patient. The management of the seriously injured patient follows the same principles as the management of a seriously ill patient. The seriously injured patient is a good model to teach these principles – providing hooks to which the practice can be applied.

Trauma management is not widely taught to obstetricians but trauma happens to their patients and those in other specialties will consider them the experts.

The 1997–99 Confidential Enquiries into Maternal Deaths in the United Kingdom[4] reported seven deaths as a result of road traffic accidents and eight cases of death due to domestic violence. An article in the *British Journal of Obstetrics and Gynaecology* draws attention to the fact that, in the capital of Mozambique, violent death accounts for as many deaths as pregnancy hypertension.[5]

The physiological adjustments of pregnancy affect the response of the mother to illness and injury. These changes mean that resuscitation should be tailored to the pregnant patient. This course teaches the application of resuscitation and trauma management to pregnancy.

The third section allows sound principles as learned in the foregoing two sections to be applied to life-threatening problems in obstetrics. This allows the doctor caring for the pregnant patient to practice the management of both common and rare emergencies until confidence has been achieved.

Chapter 2
Structured approach

The structured approach refers to the A,B,C,D,E approach to lifesaving, practised universally and widely. It is applied to the management of the seriously ill and the seriously injured. Assessment is carried out by primary survey and secondary survey. In short, A,B,C,D,E denote **A**irway, **B**reathing, **C**irculation, **D**isability (neurological status) and **E**xposure and environmental control, which are attended to in the primary survey. The primary survey uncovers immediately life-threatening problems by priority, i.e. the order in which they will most quickly kill. Problems are dealt with as they are found, so effectively there is a process of simultaneous evaluation and resuscitation. The secondary survey is a comprehensive assessment and uncovers problems that are not as immediately threatening.

Aim of the MOET course

The aim of the MOET course is to provide you with a system for assessment and management that is simple to remember, effective and unlikely to be forgotten in the heat of being faced with serious illness or injuries that you would otherwise have felt unable to manage.

Objectives

On successfully completing this topic, you will be able to:

- identify the correct sequence to be followed in assessing and managing seriously ill or seriously injured patients
- understand the concept of primary and secondary survey
- carry out an initial assessment and management survey on a trauma patient.

Approach to management

The approach to an apparently lifeless patient is the cardiopulmonary resuscitation (CPR) drill, which starts with assessment of airway, breathing, and circulation and action as necessary. See Chapter 3.

In the seriously injured patient who has signs of life the following approach is taken:

- As much history as possible should be sought, including mechanism of injury, speed, height of fall, pre-existing medical problems, medications and details of pregnancy where appropriate.
- Consider their management in four phases:
  - Primary survey — Identify life-threatening problems
  - Resuscitation — Deal with these problems as you find them
  - Secondary survey — Top to toe, back to front examination
  - Definitive care — Specific management

- In the pregnant patient the sequence should be as follows:
  - Primary survey — Identify life-threatening problems
  - Resuscitation — Deal with these problems as you find them
  - Assess fetal well-being and viability — Dependent on maternal resuscitation, but may require delivery
  - Secondary survey — Top to toe, back to front examination
  - Definitive care — Specific management
- Continuous re-evaluation

Primary survey

Same for all, adults, children, elderly, pregnant

The system follows a simple 'ABC' approach, with resuscitation taking place as problems with **A**irway, then **B**reathing, then **C**irculation, then **D**isability (neurological status) are identified. The medical logic in the ABC approach is that an **A**irway problem will kill the patient more quickly than a **B**reathing (ventilation) problem, which in turn will kill a patient more quickly than a **C**irculation (bleeding) problem, which in turn will kill a patient more quickly than a **D**isability (neurological) problem.

Manoeuvres to secure the patient's airway should not cause harm or further harm to the cervical spine. Therefore, in caring for the airway, the cervical spine must be protected.

A B C D E

- **A**irway (with cervical spine protection if appropriate)
- **B**reathing and ventilation
- **C**irculation with aggressive volume replacement and haemorrhage control
- **D**isability or neurological status
- **E**xposure and environmental control (full exposure to assess, and keep warm)

Speak to the patient at the very beginning. The response gives you several pieces of clinical information – to be able to speak, the patient must:

- have circulating oxygenated blood
- have a reasonably patent airway
- have a reasonable tidal volume to phonate
- have reasonable cerebral perfusion to comprehend and answer.

If the patient does not respond and appears lifeless, open airway, assess for breathing by watching chest, listening and feeling and if necessary give two rescue breaths and assess for signs of circulation (swallowing and breathing movements and carotid pulse).

If no circulation, start chest compressions as CPR drill (see Chapter 3).

Do the primary survey as follows:

Airway (with cervical spine control if appropriate)

Do not be distracted by other injuries; the airway **must** take priority. Assess by patient response to "Hello, how are you, Mrs Tilt", looking for chest movement, listening and feeling for air movement. Carry out simple manoeuvres to correct the problem and consider endotracheal intubation or a surgical airway if necessary.

The integrity of the cervical spine must be considered. It is always safer to assume a cervical spine fracture in patients with multiple injuries, especially if there is a blunt injury above the level of the clavicle or in an unconscious patient. If a cervical spine injury is suspected, the cervical spine must be immobilised either manually or by a hard collar, blocks on a backboard and straps to secure the blocks alongside the neck. The use of a long spine board is recommended.

You will learn how to size and apply hard collars, blocks and straps or tapes in moulage (practice drills on actors who are made up to look like patients).

Then consider:

Breathing and ventilation

Look at the neck to see if the trachea is deviated or the neck veins engorged. Look at the chest for obvious injury. Look and feel to see if it is expanding equally, percuss and auscultate. If there is a restriction to ventilation consider the reason (which you will learn from Chapter 8 Thoracic emergencies, and the thoracic trauma lecture) and do something about it!

Of those who die from chest injuries, 25% die unnecessarily and 85% of these could be saved without surgery.

Then consider:

Circulation and haemorrhage control

The most common cause of hypotension in obstetric practice and in trauma is hypovolaemia but remember that hypotension is a very late sign, developing only when significant blood loss has occurred. Have a low threshold of suspicion for bleeding and fluid replacement.

Signs of hypovolaemia are:

- increase in heart rate
- cold, pale skin
- fall in urine output
- altered level of consciousness
- narrowed pulse pressure
- hypotension (late sign).

Signs of hypovolaemia are late to show in the pregnant patient, as she compensates by shutting down bloodflow to the fetoplacental unit.

Disability or neurological status

The mini-neurological examination assesses: pupillary function and level of consciousness by AVPU (see below). It serves to determine the severity of the brain injury and the likelihood of a surgically treatable lesion. Intracranial haematomas cause reduced level of consciousness, dilated pupil on the side of the injury and weakness of the arm or leg on the opposite side. When applied repeatedly the examination can be used to determine objectively any neurological deterioration. It is supplemented by CT scanning.

AVPU assessment of the patient's level of consciousness

Alert
Voice responsive
Pain responsive
Unresponsive

Remember that the level of consciousness not only reflects the neurological status but can also be influenced by hypovolaemia and hypoperfusion.

A dilated pupil and weakness on the opposite side may be significant of a focal lesion, which is operable but must be acted on early.

Remember that, in the pregnant patient, fits may be due to eclampsia.

Exposure

Adequately expose the patient to make a full assessment, taking care to avoid cooling and potential hypothermia.

Monitoring

Pulse oximetry should be used as early as possible to detect inadequate saturation of haemoglobin with oxygen secondary to airway, breathing or circulation problems. Heart rate should be noted by ECG and pulse oximetry. Non-invasive (or invasive) blood pressure monitoring is mandatory. End tidal CO_2 monitoring may be appropriate.

The pulse oximeter measures the saturation of haemoglobin with oxygen. It works on the principle of differential absorption of light of a particular wavelength by oxygenated and deoxygenated haemoglobin. Depending on the absorption levels, a ratio of oxygenated to deoxygenated blood is determined. Its limitations are that the patient must be well perfused to get a reading and ambient light and dyes such as nail polish or methaemoglobin in the blood cause erroneous readings. A fall in oxygen saturation is a late sign of an airway, breathing or even a circulation problem.

Adjuncts to assessment

Consider urinary catheter (contraindicated in the male until a urethral rupture has been excluded) and nasogastric tube (contraindicated if there is a suspected fracture of the base of the skull).

Essential X-rays during the primary survey and resuscitation are chest, pelvis and lateral cervical spine.

Resuscitation

The resuscitation phase is carried out **simultaneously** with the primary survey.

Life-threatening conditions are managed as they are identified. Do not move on to the next stage of the primary survey until a problem found has been corrected.

If patient's condition seems unsatisfactory, go back and reassess, starting again with ABC.

Airway with cervical spine protection

An airway problem is identified if the breathing is noisy (gurgling, sonorous). There may be an airway problem if you are not able to hear or feel breathing.

If an airway problem is identified, open/clear the airway (taking care not to cause movement of the cervical spine) by chin lift, jaw thrust or suctioning. Consider an oropharyngeal airway to keep patent and tracheal intubation or cricothyroidotomy if necessary.

Remember that in an unconscious patient the airway will need to be protected from gastric contents or soiling from above, so call an anaesthetist early. All trauma patients are likely to have a full stomach. The pregnant patient is more prone to regurgitation because she has a mechanical obstruction to gastric emptying, reduced gastro-oesophageal tone and, if aspirated, the gastric contents cause a more serious chemical pneumonitis because gastric pH is lower in the pregnant patient.

The 'gold standard' in airway opening, maintenance and protection is intubation.

If possible, wait for the arrival of the anaesthetist to intubate the patient. It is difficult and unpleasant to intubate a patient who is awake. It is inadvisable to intubate an unconscious patient without drugs.

Drugs should only be used to intubate by those with adequate anaesthetic training.

Pregnant patients are often more difficult to intubate than non-pregnant patients and attention has to be paid to the increased risks of gastric regurgitation and aspiration. If possible, wait for an anaesthetist who will carry out a 'rapid sequence induction' ('crash' induction – pre-oxygenation, cricoid pressure, rapid unconsciousness by the administration of drugs followed by rapid placement of the endotracheal tube in the trachea).

If the airway cannot be maintained by manoeuvres and oropharyngeal and nasal airways, consider intubation or surgical airway, but only as a last resort.

Administer supplementary oxygen to all trauma patients through a tight-fitting face-mask with reservoir bag at a flow of 12–15 l/minute (fully on at the wall rotameter).

If you have made manoeuvres to clear the airway and still there is no return of spontaneous respiration, this may be because the airway is still obstructed or because there is no breathing. Establish the nature of the problem by administering breaths to the patient. If the chest does not move, there is still an airway problem. If it does, the airway is clear but there is a breathing problem.

Breathing and ventilation

Assist ventilation if necessary by mouth to pocket mask, self-inflating bag to pocket mask, facemask and self-inflating bag or by tracheal intubation and self-inflating bag . Always remember to attach the system to supplemental oxygen.

Tension pneumothorax is a quickly remedied but life-threatening injury. The signs of a tension pneumothorax are:

- distension of the neck veins
- deviation of the trachea away from the affected side
- hyperresonant percussion note on affected side
- reduced breath sounds on the affected side.

Decompress immediately by inserting a cannula through the second intercostal space in the mid-clavicular line on the affected side. This must be followed by placement of a chest drain.

Other life-threatening chest injuries are open pneumothorax, massive haemothorax, flail chest with pulmonary contusion and cardiac tamponade.

Treat an open pneumothorax by placing a dressing over the injury and seal the dressing on three sides only to create a one-way valve or by Asherman seal.

Life threatening things in the chest!

- **A**irway
- **T**ension pneumothorax
- **O**pen pneumothorax
- **M**assive haemothorax
- **F**lail chest
- **C**ardiac tamponade

ATOM FC!

Circulation with aggressive volume replacement and haemorrhage control

Establish and maintain a minimum of two large-calibre intravenous lines; 16-gauge is the smallest adequate size.

Take blood for full blood count, urea and electrolytes, crossmatch, coagulation screen, amylase, glucose and pregnancy test. Remember that the blood group of a pregnant patient will probably be known, so you will be able to order type-specific blood (which is available within ten minutes) as well as fully crossmatched blood. Decide on amounts of type-specific and fully crossmatched blood to be requested.

If there is a suspicion of blood loss, replace with warmed crystalloid, synthetic colloid or blood and blood products.

Continually assess response to fluid replacement in:

- heart rate
- skin colour
- urine output
- level of consciousness
- pulse pressure
- blood pressure.

Have a low threshold for suspected bleeding, especially in the heavily gravid patient. Consider CVP monitoring early. Be aware of potential fluid overload in pre-eclampsia/eclampsia.

The pregnant patient will compensate for blood loss by reducing perfusion to the fetoplacental unit.

Pregnant women can lose up to 35% of their circulating blood volume before maternal signs of hypovolaemia develop. The fetus may be inadequately perfused although the mother's vital signs are normal.

The earliest sign of hypovolaemia may be fetal distress. Think: 'Is the fetoplacental unit being perfused?' Successful outcome depends on the early recognition of shock, restoration of volume and control of haemorrhage.

Examples of blood loss

• fractured pelvis	3 litres
• closed femoral fracture	1.5 litres
• closed tibial fracture	500 ml

Stop the bleeding

Haemorrhage must be arrested as soon as possible and the circulating volume restored. Put pressure on an obvious compressible source of bleeding. Uncontrolled (non-compressible) haemorrhage, i.e. to abdomen, chest, pelvis or fractures, requires urgent surgical intervention.

Consider the source of bleeding and call the appropriate surgeon.

Maternal resuscitation may be compromised unless the pregnancy is interrupted. There may also be fetal reasons to interrupt the pregnancy but these should not take priority over maternal resuscitation.

Indications for caesarean section are:

- maternal cardiac arrest
- inadequate exposure during laparotomy for other abdominal trauma
- unstable pelvic or lumbosacral fracture with the patient in labour
- uterine rupture
- placental abruption.

Perimortem caesarean section

CPR is ineffective unless left-sided tilt is instituted and maintained. Even with tilt, aortocaval compression can compromise resuscitation. Emergency caesarean section allows improvement in the venous return and should be performed if correctly positioned CPR is unsuccessful after five minutes. Caesarean section also reduces maternal oxygen consumption, makes ventilation easier and allows CPR to be carried out in the supine position.

Open cardiac massage and defibrillation could be considered as the caesarean section is taking place.

Maternal resuscitation should be continued throughout the caesarean section, as there are reports of late maternal survival.

Fetal prognosis after delivery at perimortem caesarean section is very poor.

Disability

Consider the presence of a neurological injury. A head injury has the potential to compromise the airway and breathing. Subdural and extradural haematomata are surgically treatable and extradurals have a good prognosis if treated early.

Assess fetal wellbeing and viability

Adequately resuscitate the mother for this to be optimised.

Use ultrasound:

- to detect fetal heart and check rate
- to ascertain the number of babies and their positions
- to locate the position of the placenta and the amount of liquor
- to look for retroplacental bleeding and haematoma
- to detect an abnormal position of the fetus and free fluid in the abdominal cavity suggesting rupture of the uterus
- to detect damage to other structures
- to check for free fluid and blood.

Secondary survey

You can carry out the secondary survey once the patient is stable. The secondary survey may not take place until after surgery, if surgery has been necessary as part of the resuscitation phase.

This is a top-to-toe process as follows:

- scalp and vault of skull
- face and base of skull
- neck and cervical spine
- chest
- abdomen
- pelvis
- remainder of spine and limbs
- neurological examination
- PR and VE if indicated
- examination of holes caused by injury.

A repeat mini-neurological examination and Glasgow Coma Scale scoring should be performed during the secondary survey (see Chapter 11).

Definitive care

This takes place under the supervision of the relevant specialists. It is of utmost importance to the patient's continued quality of life.

The mismanaged minor injury may be the only residual effect of a life-threatening series of injuries but it is that with which the patient has to live for the rest of her life.

Summary

Primary survey	Identify life-threatening problems A B C D E • Airway with cervical spine protection • Breathing and ventilation • Circulation with aggressive volume replacement and haemorrhage control • Disability or neurological status • Exposure depending on environment
Resuscitation	Deal with these problems as you find them
Assess fetal wellbeing and viability	Dependent on maternal resuscitation, but may require delivery
Secondary survey	Top to toe, back to front examination
Definitive care	Specific management
Continuous re-evaluation	

SECTION 2
Resuscitation

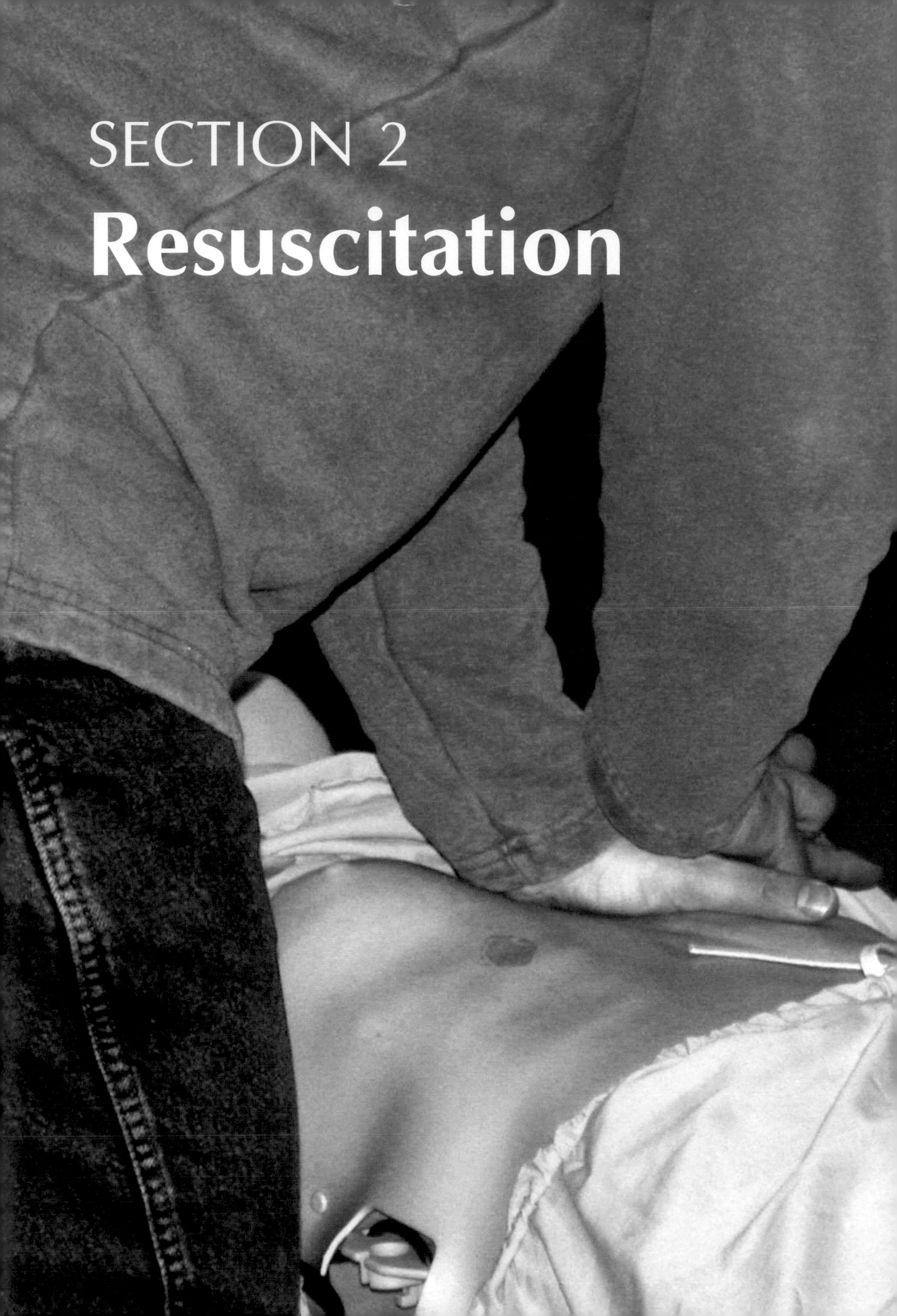

Algorithm 3.1. Cardiopulmonary resuscitation key points

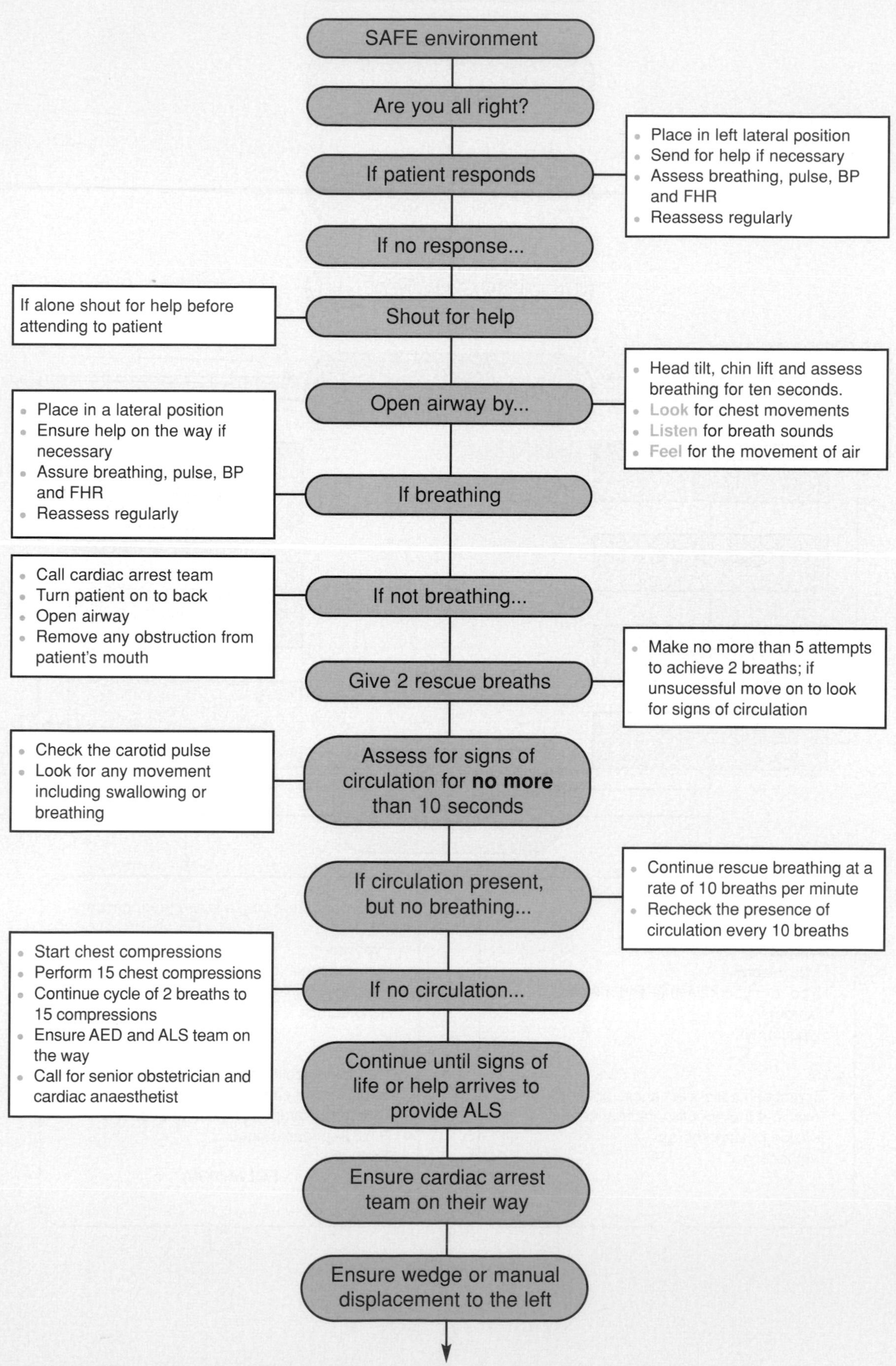

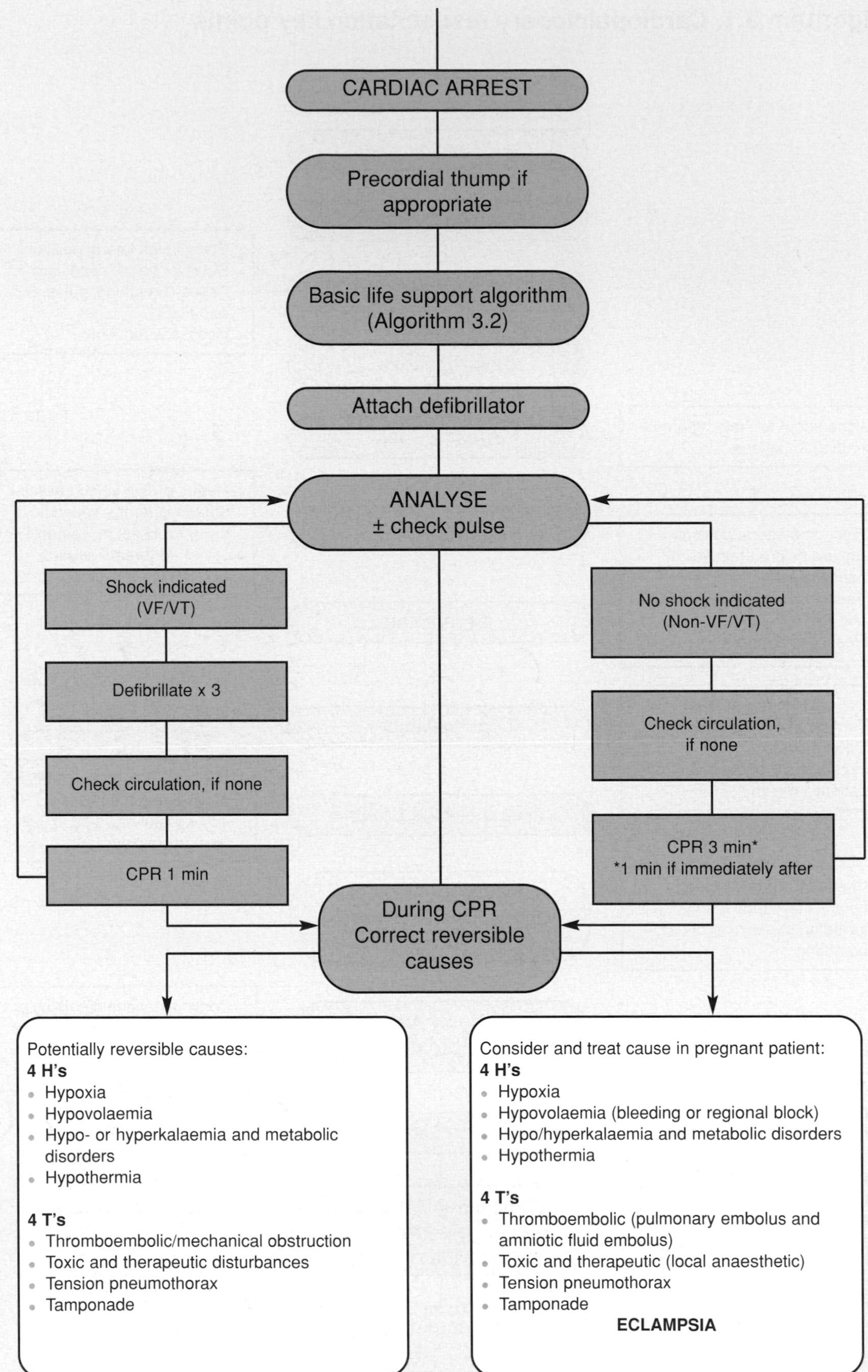
CARDIAC ARREST
Precordial thump if appropriate
Basic life support algorithm (Algorithm 3.2)
Attach defibrillator
ANALYSE
± check pulse
Shock indicated (VF/VT)
Defibrillate x 3
Check circulation, if none
CPR 1 min
No shock indicated (Non-VF/VT)
Check circulation, if none
CPR 3 min*
*1 min if immediately after
During CPR
Correct reversible causes
Potentially reversible causes:
4 H's
Hypoxia
Hypovolaemia
Hypo- or hyperkalaemia and metabolic disorders
Hypothermia
4 T's
Thromboembolic/mechanical obstruction
Toxic and therapeutic disturbances
Tension pneumothorax
Tamponade
Consider and treat cause in pregnant patient:
4 H's
Hypoxia
Hypovolaemia (bleeding or regional block)
Hypo/hyperkalaemia and metabolic disorders
Hypothermia
4 T's
Thromboembolic (pulmonary embolus and amniotic fluid embolus)
Toxic and therapeutic (local anaesthetic)
Tension pneumothorax
Tamponade
ECLAMPSIA

Chapter 3

Cardiopulmonary resuscitation in the non-pregnant and pregnant patient

Objectives

On successfully completing this topic, you will be able to:

- understand and perform basic and advanced life support
- understand the importance of early defibrillation where appropriate
- understand the adaptations of CPR in the pregnant patient.

Introduction and incidence

Although cardiac arrest is fortunately a rare event in pregnancy, it is estimated to occur in every 30 000 deliveries.[6] In the Confidential Enquiry into Maternal Deaths (CEMD) report for the last triennium (1997–99)[4] the most common *Direct* cause of maternal death was thromboembolism, which results in cardiac arrest. It is important that the healthcare teams know the appropriate actions to take in such an event, to promote positive outcomes for both the mother and the child.

Management

The rescuer must ensure a safe environment, shake the patient and shout. If no response, call for assistance and then return to the patient.

To open airway

Place your hand on the patient's forehead and gently tilt head back (not if cervical spine injury is suspected). At the same time with your fingertips under the point of the patient's chin, lift the chin to open the airway. A jaw thrust may be required to open the airway. Do this by placing fingers behind the angle of the jaw and moving jaw anteriorly to displace tongue from the pharynx.

If you have any difficulty, turn the patient on to her back with a slight tilt to the left and then open the airway as described. Try to avoid head tilt if injury to the neck is suspected.

Further detailed information on airway management and ventilation is given in Chapter 6.

Assess breathing

Assess breathing for ten seconds by looking for chest movements, listening for breath sounds and feeling for the movement of air. If no breathing, put out a cardiac arrest call and give two rescue breaths.

Royal Cornwall Hospitals

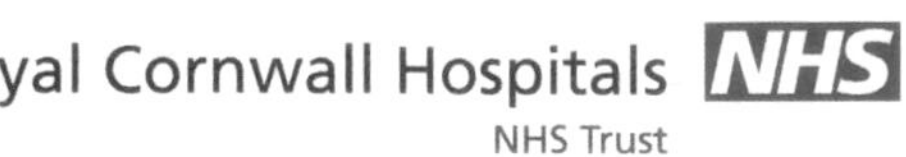

NHS Trust

Infant Resuscitation

Airway

Check for response

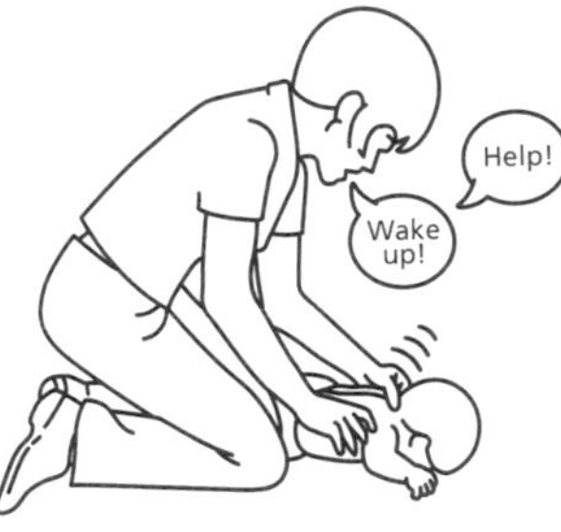

- If **unconscious**, open the airway

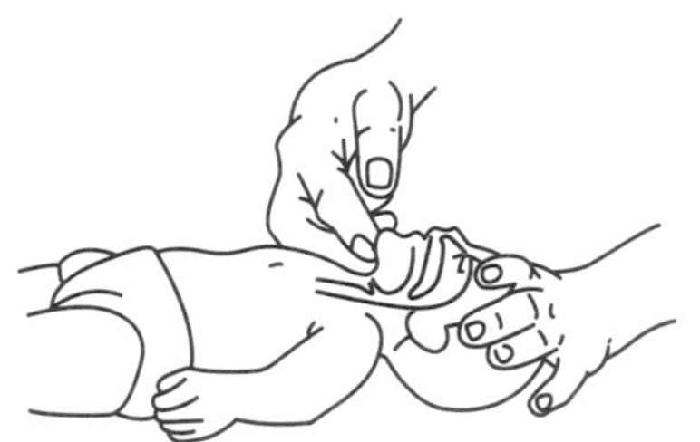

Breathing

Check for breathing

Look
Listen
Feel

- If **breathing**, continue to watch breathing and pulse
- If **no breathing**, blow gently into lungs ~~twice~~ 5 times

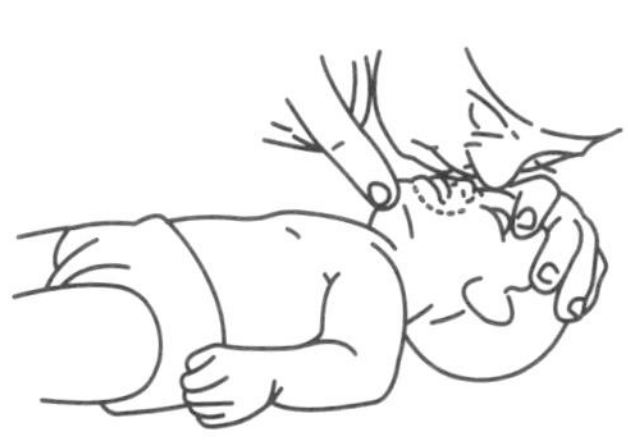

Circulation

Check for signs of circulation

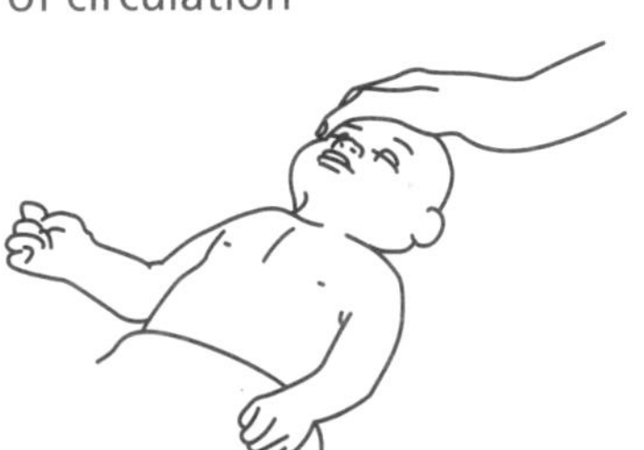

- If **signs of life**, continue rescue breathing (as above)
- If **no signs of change**, start chest compressions and blow ~~once~~ twice every ~~five~~ 15 compressions

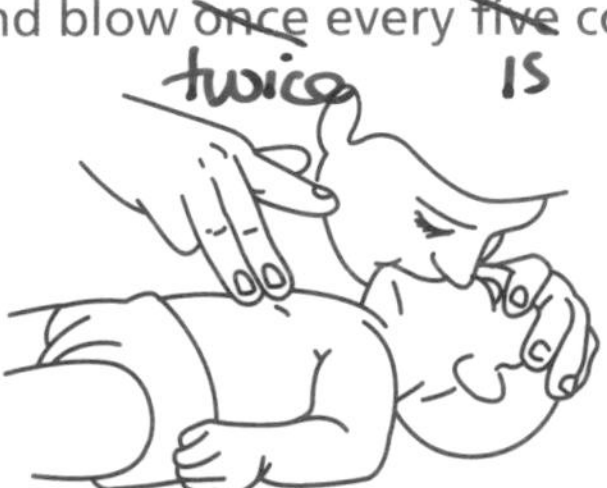

Algorithm 3.2. Basic life support

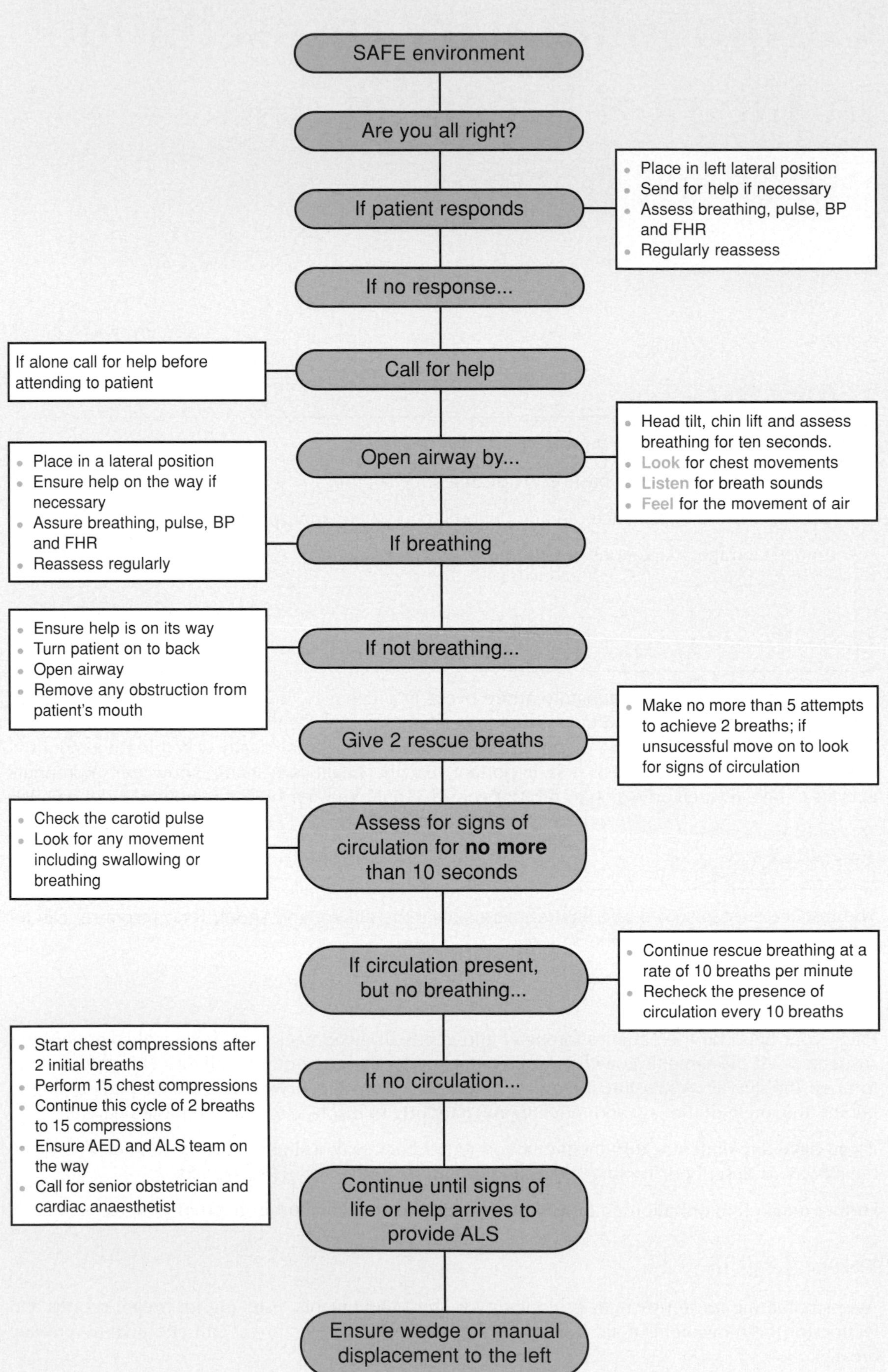

Give two rescue breaths

Do this by ensuring head tilt and chin lift and closing the soft part of the patient's nose with your thumb and index finger, with the palm of your hand on the patient's forehead. Open her mouth a little but maintain chin lift. Take a breath and place your lips around her mouth, making sure that you have a good seal. Blow steadily into her mouth over 1.5–2.0 seconds, watching for her chest to rise. The target tidal volume is 400–500 ml. Maintaining head tilt and chin lift, take your mouth away from the patient and watch for her chest to fall as the air comes out. Take another breath and repeat the sequence to give another effective breath, recheck the patient's mouth for an obstruction and ensure that head tilt and chin lift are adequate.

If circulation present but no breathing continue rescue breathing at a rate of ten breaths/minute

Recheck the circulation every ten breaths, taking no more than ten seconds each time. If the patient starts to breathe on her own but remains unconscious, turn her into the recovery position and apply oxygen 15 litres/minute. Check her condition and be ready to turn her back to start rescue breathing if she stops breathing.

If no circulation (or you are at all unsure) start chest compressions after two initial breaths

With the patient tilted to the left, locate the lower half of the sternum:

- using your index and middle fingers identify the lower rib margins
- keeping your fingers together slide them up to the point where the ribs join the sternum
- with your middle finger on this point place your index finger on the sternum
- slide the heel of your other hand down the sternum until it reaches your index finger; this should be the middle of the lower half of the sternum.

Place the heel of one hand there, with the other hand on top of the first.

Interlock the fingers of both hands and lift them to ensure that pressure is not applied over the patient's ribs. Do not apply any pressure over the top of the abdomen or bottom tip of the sternum.

Position yourself above the patient's chest and with your arms straight press down on the sternum to depress it 4–5 cm.

To combine rescue breathing and compression, after 15 compressions tilt the head, lift the chin and give two effective breaths. Return your hands immediately to the correct position and give 15 further compressions continuing the cycle of two breaths to 15 compressions.

Two-person CPR is preferred if there are two rescuers, maintaining a ratio of two breaths to 15 compressions.

Basic life support (two breaths to 15 compressions) should continue until the AED arrives, when the AED algorithm (Algorithm 3.3) should be followed, or until advanced life support arrives, when the ALS algorithm (Algorithm 3.4) should be followed.

Automated external defibrillator

If an automated external defibrillator (AED) is available, attach, analyse rhythm and defibrillate as indicated in Algorithm 3.3. AEDs are increasingly available in public places.

The most frequent initial rhythm in cardiac arrest is ventricular fibrillation (VF). Successful defibrillation diminishes with time. The AED allows for early defibrillation by lesser-trained personnel, as it performs rhythm analysis, gives information by voice or visual display and the delivery of the shock is then activated manually. After the first three shocks give uninterrupted CPR for one minute. If defibrillation is not indicated CPR should be continued for three minutes, at which stage the AED will prompt further analysis of rhythm.

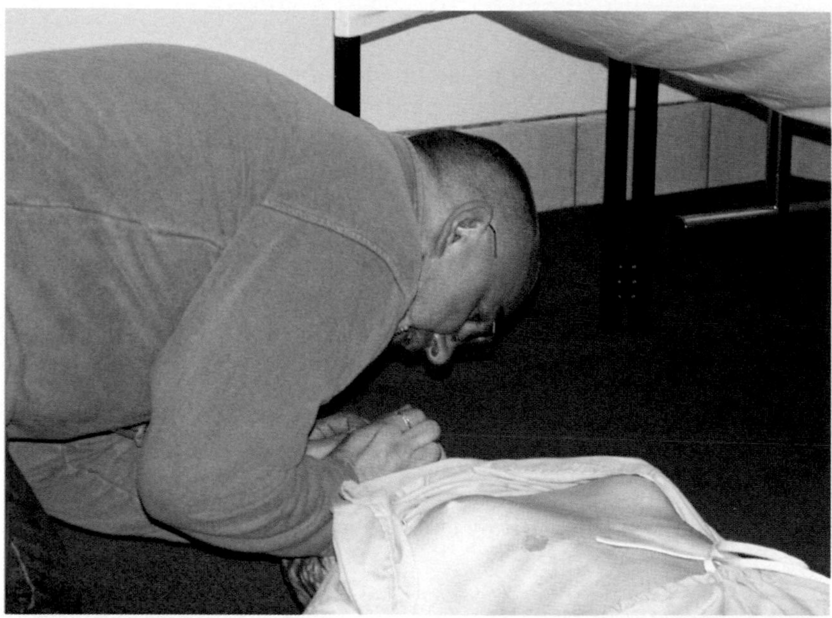

Assess breathing: Look, listen and feel

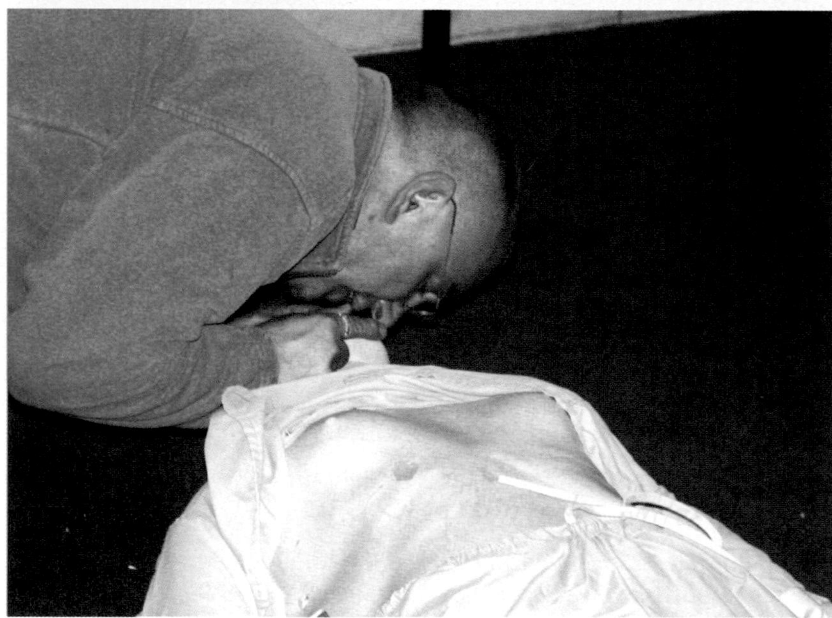

Give two rescue breaths

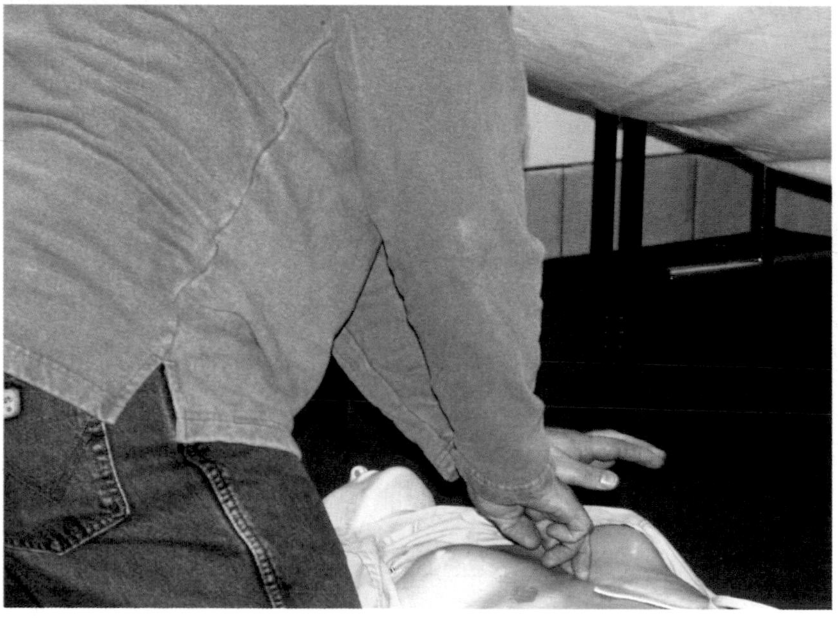

Locate the lower half of the sternum

Algorithm 3.3. Automated external defibrillator

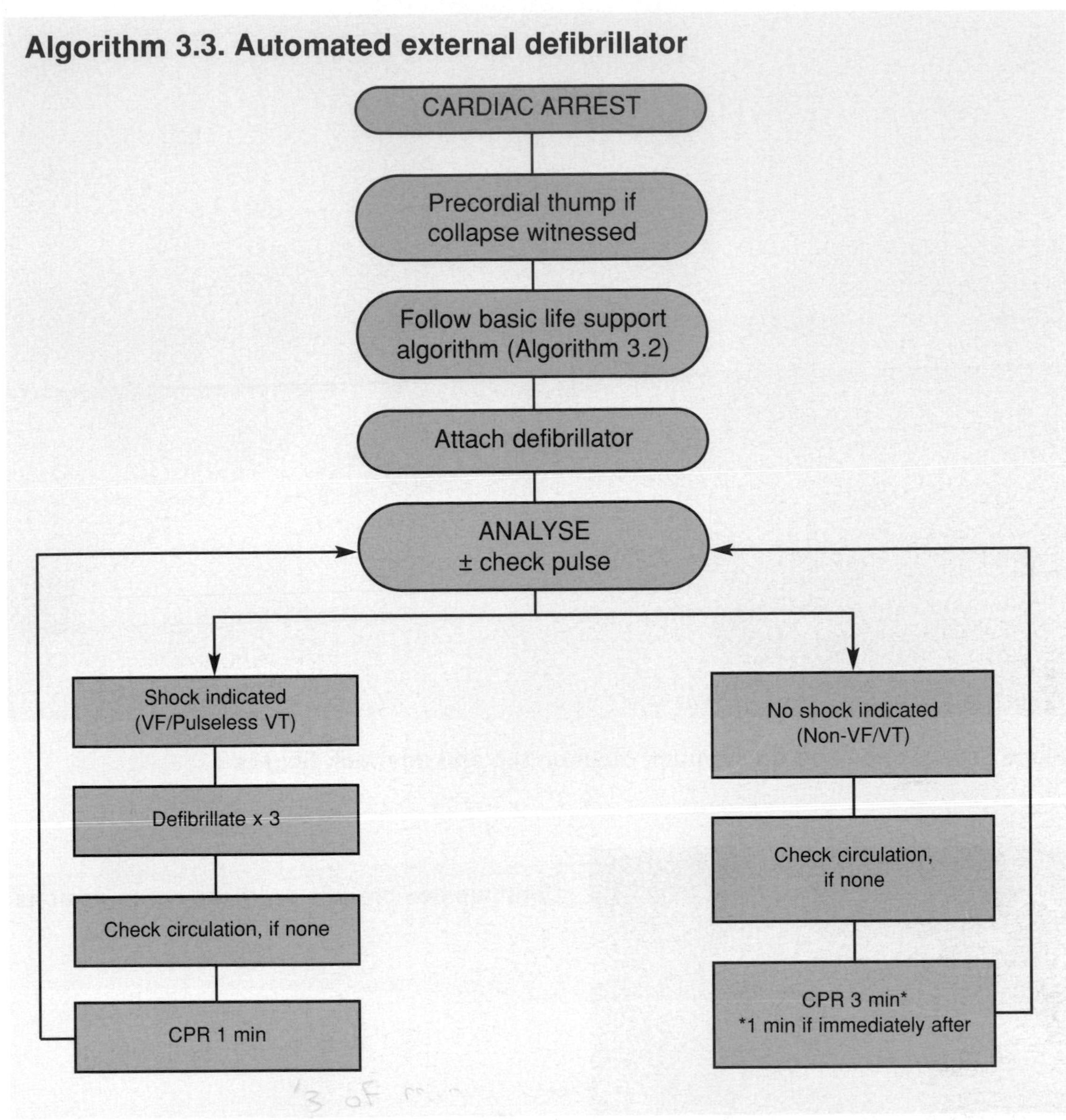

Attach defibrillator/monitor and assess cardiac rhythm

If using a manual defibrillator, place defibrillator gel pads on patient's chest, one below the right clavicle and one over the cardiac apex, taking care to avoid breast tissue. Place defibrillator paddles firmly on gel pads.

Turn immediately to advanced life support algorithm (Algorithm 3.4)

When advanced life support arrives, the rhythm is assessed and defibrillation is instituted (200J, 200J, 360J) or biphasic equivalent for a shockable rhythm. IV access should be carried out and the airway secured with intubation. Once intubated, the patient is ventilated at 12–14 breaths per minute and chest compressions are performed at 100/minute. Epinephrine (adrenaline) 1mg IV is given every three minutes. Reversible causes of cardiac arrest are considered and treated as necessary.

If the patient remains in VF, a successful outcome relies on continued defibrillation (360J, 360J, 360J) or biphasic equivalent and correction of causes or contributing factors. Anti-arrhythmic agents may be needed. Sodium bicarbonate should only be given to patients with severe acidosis pH less than 7.1; base excess less than –10.

If VF/VT can be positively excluded, defibrillation is not indicated. The patient is in asystole or pulseless electrical activity (PEA). The causes of cardiac arrest are:

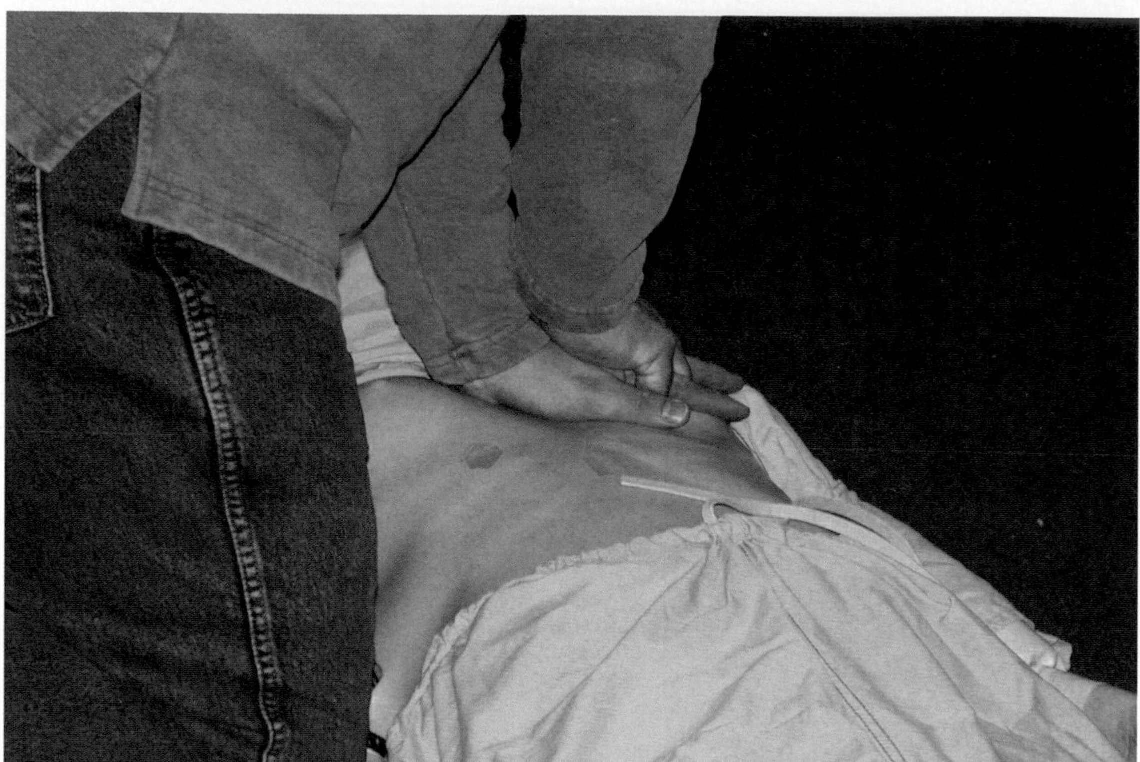

Place heel of one hand on sternum, other on top and interlock fingers

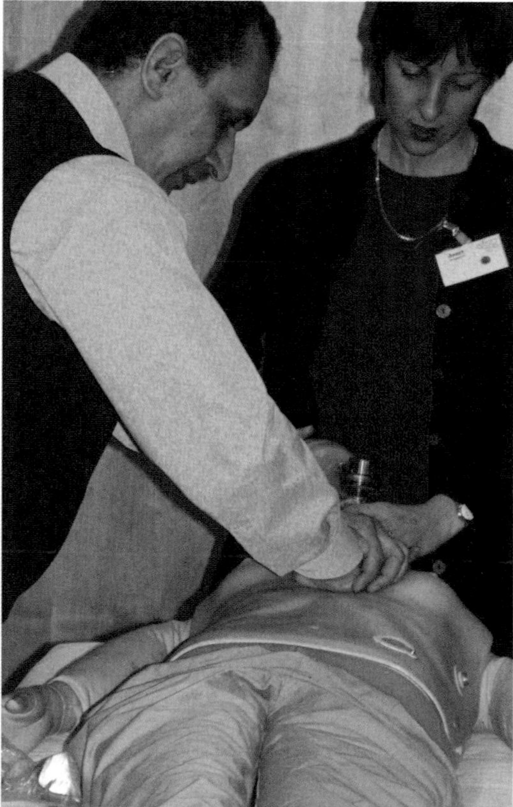

Continue two breaths to fifteen compressions

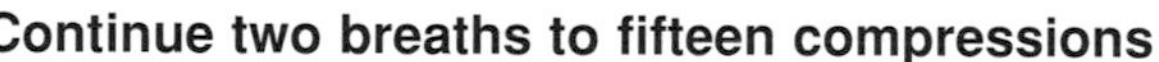

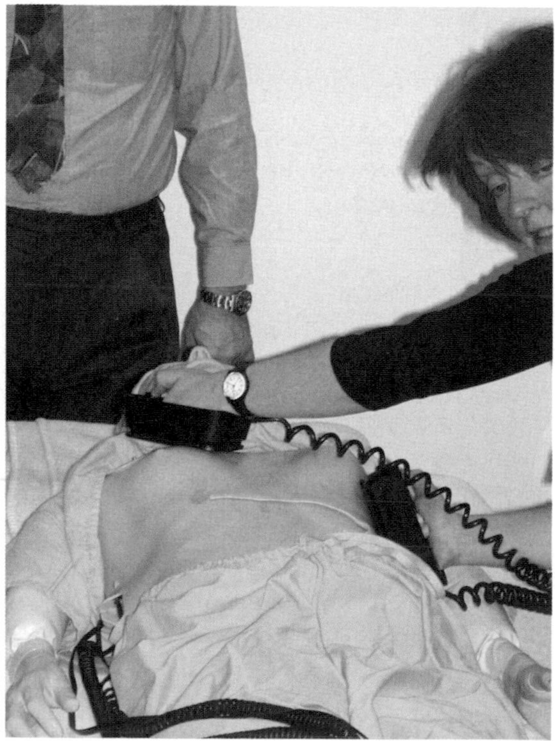

Defibrillation "Oxygen away – stand clear!"

Algorithm 3.4. Advanced life support

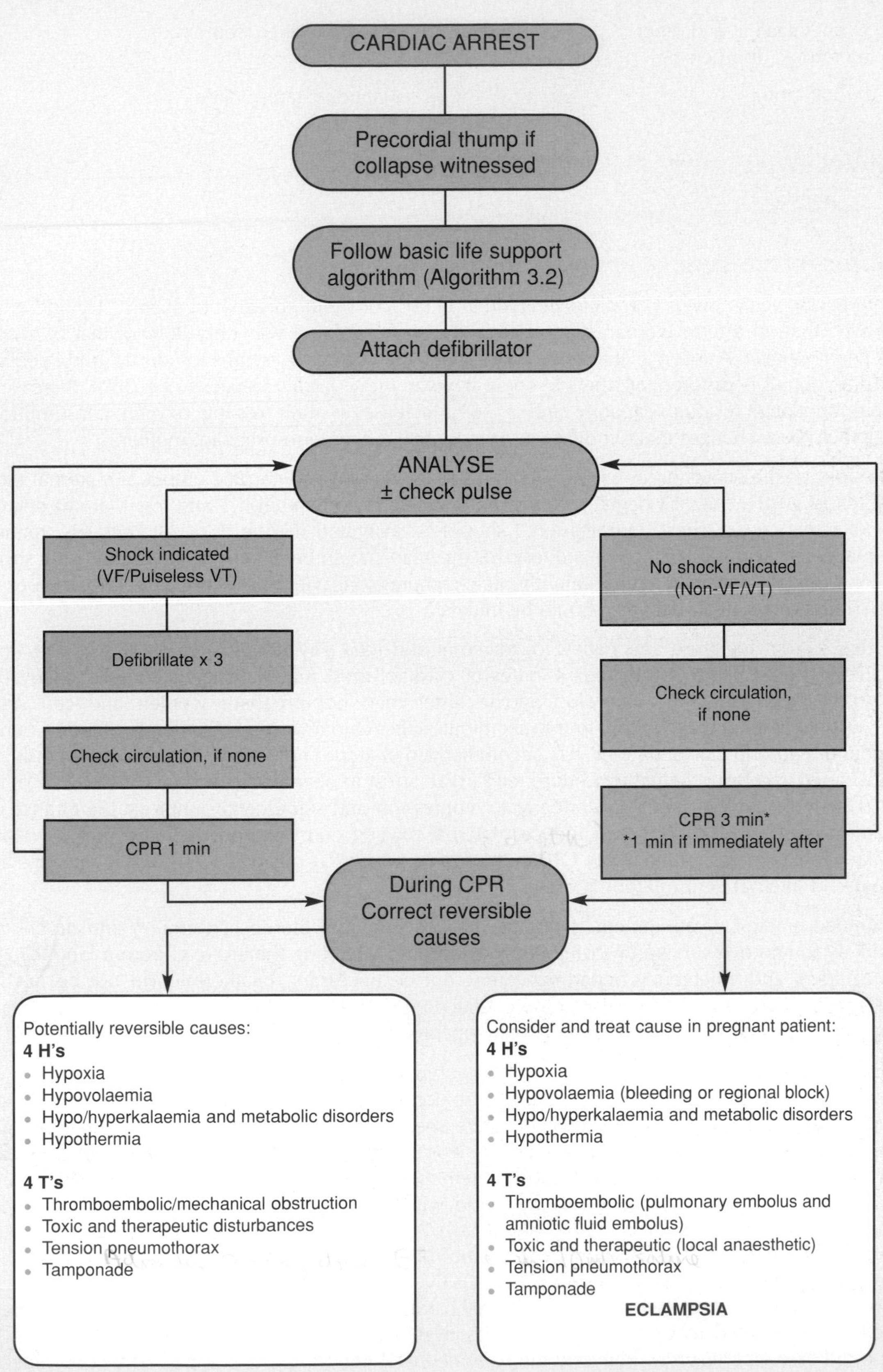

Four Hs:

- hypoxia
- hypovolaemia
- hyperkalaemia and other metabolic disorders
- hypothermia

Four Ts:

- thromboembolism
- toxicity
- tension pneumothorax
- cardiac tamponade

and, with particular reference to pregnancy

- eclampsia.

Perform emergency caesarean section

At term, the vena cava is completely occluded in 90% of supine pregnant patients.[7] Ueland *et al.*[8] showed that, in a term woman lying supine, the stroke volume was only 30% of that of a non-pregnant woman. As soon as the infant is delivered, the vena cava returns to normal[7] and adequate cardiac output is restored. Mothers become hypoxic more readily because of a 20% decrease in their functional residual capacity and a 20% increase in their resting oxygen consumption.[9] Together, these changes make it difficult to resuscitate a near-term pregnant mother.

To minimise the effects of the gravid uterus on venous return and cardiac output, a maternal tilt to the left of greater than 15 degrees, to prevent aortocaval compression,[10] and less than 30 degrees for effective closed chest compression,[11] should be instituted (Figure 3.1). Alternatively, manual displacement of uterus to the left and towards the head should be effective (Figure 3.2).[12] If a strong pulse cannot be obtained after several thoracic compressions with this manoeuvre, preparations for a peri-arrest caesarean delivery should be initiated.

Evidence from literature and review of maternal and fetal physiology suggests that a caesarean delivery should begin within four minutes of cardiac arrest and delivery accomplished by five minutes. Pregnant women develop anoxia faster than non-pregnant women and can suffer irreversible brain damage within four to six minutes after cardiac arrest.[13] The Resuscitation Council guidelines for special situations has recommended that prompt caesarean delivery should be considered as a resuscitative procedure for cardiac arrest in near-term pregnancy.[14] Delivery of the fetus will obviate the effects of aortocaval compression and significantly improve the chance for maternal resuscitation. This will reduce maternal oxygen consumption, increase venous return, make ventilation easier and allow CPR in the supine position. Consider open cardiac massage and the use of internal defibrillator paddles.

A limited amount of equipment is required in this situation. Sterile preparation and drapes are unlikely to improve survival. Moving the mother to an operating theatre (e.g. from a labour room or accident and emergency department) may not be necessary. Diathermy will not be needed initially, as there is little blood loss if no cardiac output. If the mother is successfully resuscitated, she can be moved to theatre to complete the operation.

Timing of delivery is also important for the survival of the infant and its normal neurological development. From discussion so far, there is no doubt that uterine evacuation is an important step during maternal resuscitation. However, there seems to be reluctance among obstetricians to perform peri-arrest sections. Concerns include worries about neurological damage to the delivered infant. In a comprehensive review of postmortem caesarean deliveries between 1900 and 1985 by Katz *et al.*,[10] 70% (42/61) of infants delivered within five minutes survived and all developed normally. However, only 13% (8/61) and 12% (7/61) of infants survived delivery at 10 and 15 minutes post-cardiac arrest and only one infant in both groups had neurological sequelae. While the optimal interval between arrest to delivery is five minutes, there are case reports of intact infant survival after more than 20 minutes of maternal cardiac arrest.[15–17] Review of postmortem caesarean section, as reported in Confidential Enquiries over the past 25 years, shows that there was no reported case where survival beyond the early neonatal period was accompanied by neurological disability.[18] Evidence suggests that if the fetus survives the neonatal period then the chances of normal development are good.

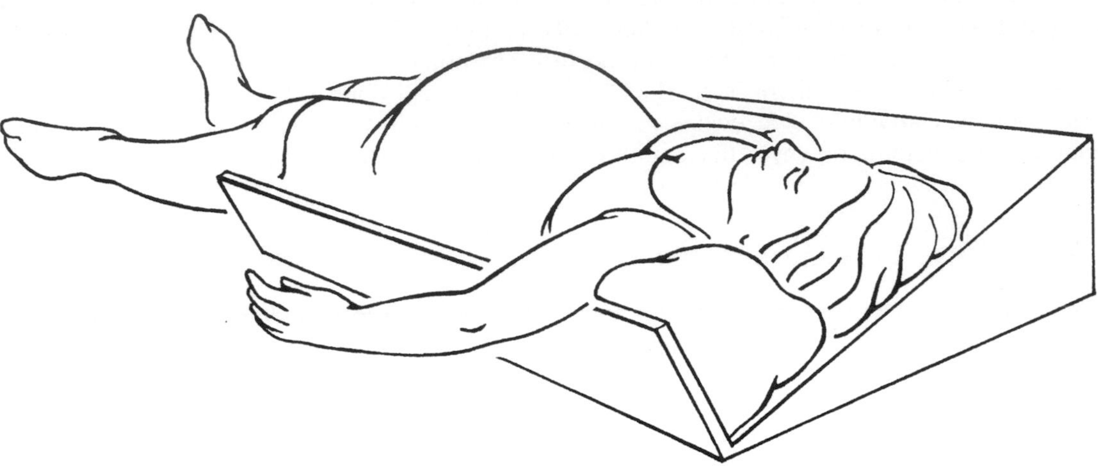

Figure 3.1 Left-lateral tilt

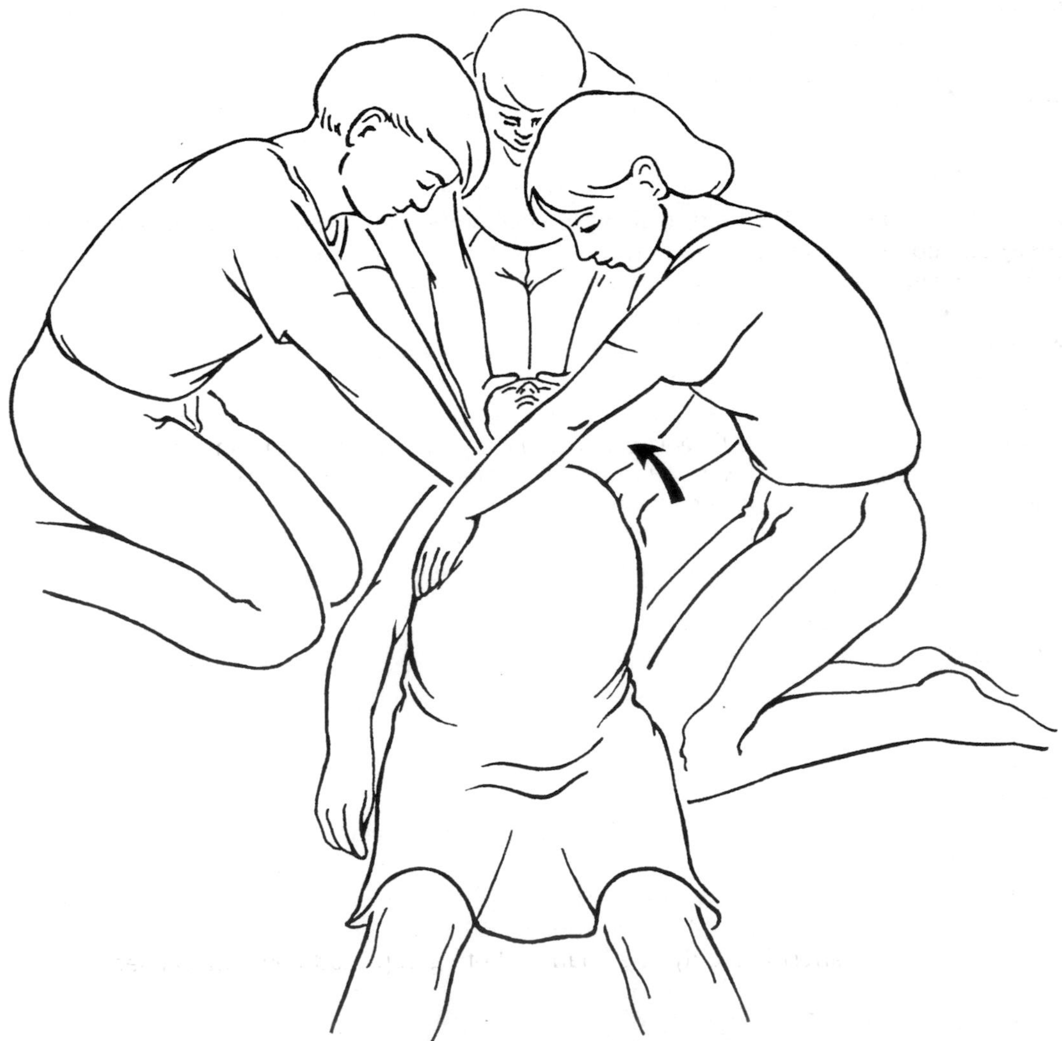

Figure 3.2 Manual displacement of the uterus to the left and towards the head

When a mother in the second half of her pregnancy suffers a cardiac arrest, immediate resuscitation should commence. Should immediate resuscitation fail, every attempt should be made to start the caesarean section by four minutes and deliver the infant by five minutes. CPR must be continued throughout the caesarean section and afterwards, as this increases the chances of a successful neonatal and maternal outcome. There are no recommendations regarding the surgical approach for caesarean section but there is no doubt that the classical approach is aided by the natural diastasis of recti abdomini that occurs in late pregnancy[14] and a bloodless field in this clinical situation. It is accepted, however, that operators should use the technique with which they are most comfortable.

Make decision to abandon CPR if unsuccessful

Do not abandon CPR if rhythm continues as VF/VT. A decision to abandon CPR should only be made after discussion with the consultant obstetrician and senior clinicians.

Medico-legal issues

No doctor has been found liable for performing a postmortem caesarean section. Theoretically, liability may concern either criminal or civil wrongdoing. Operating without consent may be argued as battery if the mother is successfully resuscitated. However, the doctrine of emergency exception would be applied because a delay in treatment could cause harm. The second criminal offence could be 'mutilation of corpse'. An operation performed to save the infant would not be wrongful, because there would be no criminal intent. The unanimous consensus of the literature is that a civil suit for performing perimortem caesarean section, regardless of the outcome, would not result in a judgement against the surgeon.[10]

Few instruments (a scalpel and a pair of artery forceps) are needed to perform a perimortem caesarean section, as there is no effective circulation. Time is of the essence and it should not be wasted in obtaining a sterile field, waiting for elaborate equipment (e.g. cautery, section trays) waiting for the consultant to come from home or transferring to theatre. It is important that an anaesthetist is in attendance at the earliest opportunity. Should resuscitation be successful and the mother regains consciousness, a general anaesthetic needs to be administered. If resuscitation is successful mother can be moved to a theatre to complete the operation.

Communication and teamwork

Wherever possible, have senior input from the obstetric, anaesthetic and midwifery professions. Ensure that the family is looked after and kept informed. Document timings and interventions accurately. If the mother dies, you will need to inform the coroner and the GP.

Logistics

Recruit as many staff as possible. You will need an individual responsible for each of the following:

- recording events and management
- communication
- runner/porter/transport.

Algorithm 4.1 Amniotic fluid embolism key points

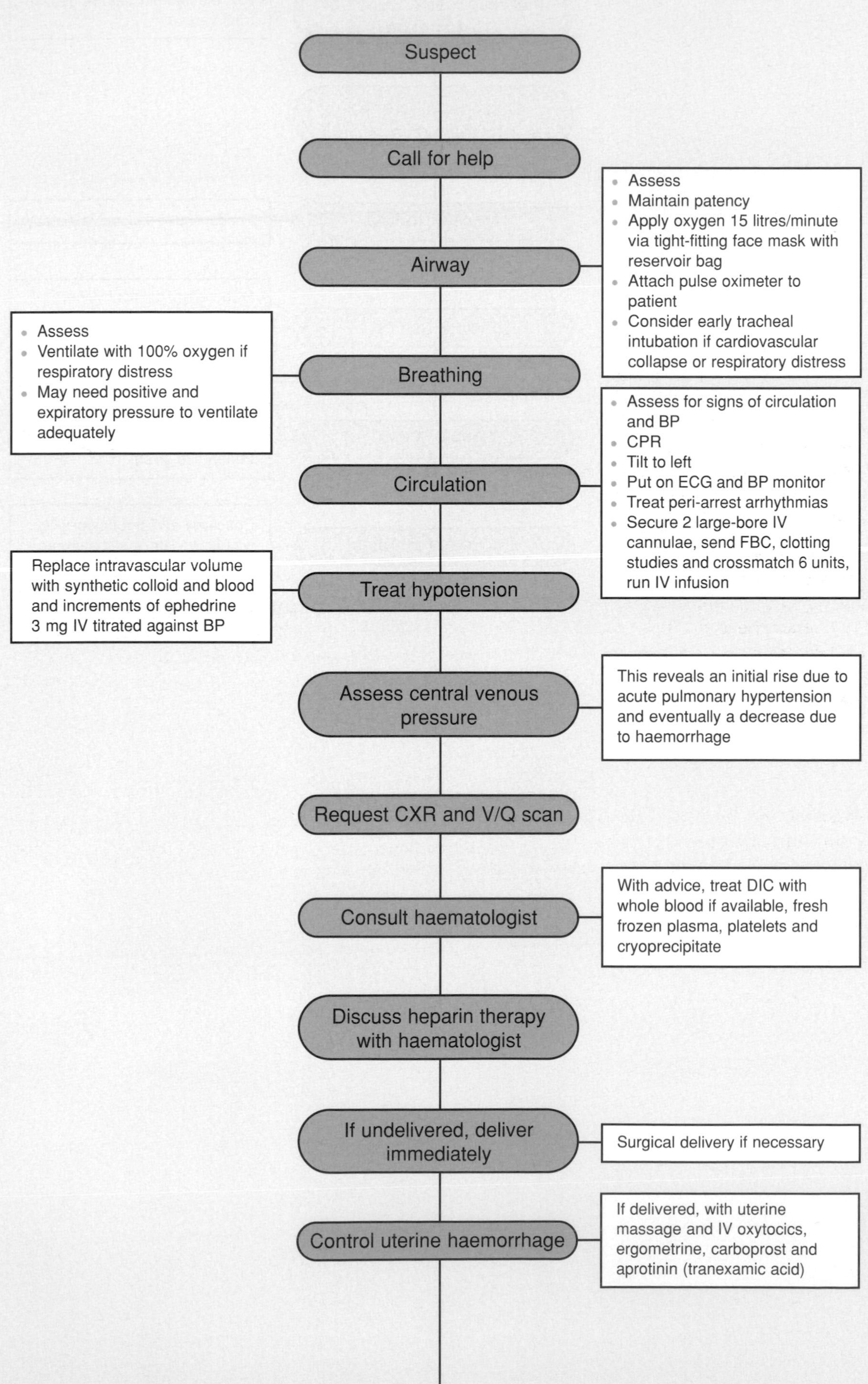

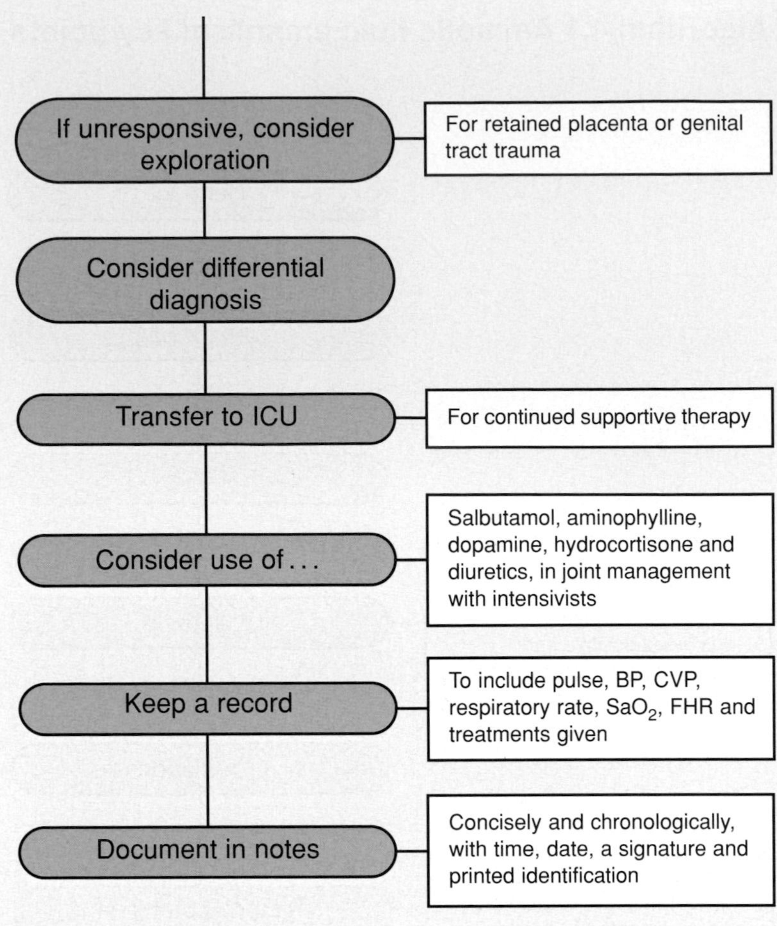
If unresponsive, consider exploration
For retained placenta or genital tract trauma
Consider differential diagnosis
Transfer to ICU
For continued supportive therapy
Consider use of . . .
Salbutamol, aminophylline, dopamine, hydrocortisone and diuretics, in joint management with intensivists
Keep a record
To include pulse, BP, CVP, respiratory rate, SaO_2, FHR and treatments given
Document in notes
Concisely and chronologically, with time, date, a signature and printed identification

Chapter 4
Amniotic fluid embolism

Objectives

On successfully completing this topic, you will be able to:

- recognise the features of amniotic fluid embolism and suspect the diagnosis early
- describe the treatment of suspected amniotic fluid embolism.

Introduction

This rare occurrence has sudden and dramatic presentation and often has devastating consequences.

Much of the evidence for these guidelines is derived from two major published retrospective series[15,16] and from the Confidential Enquiries into Maternal Deaths in the UK.[4] The evidence for the pathophysiology of the condition is circumstantial and suggested treatment is based upon the experience of the authors. There is no evidence from randomised trials to guide us, nor is there ever likely to be any.

Incidence

The estimated incidence is between 1 in 8000 and 1 in 80 000 pregnancies. Deaths due to amniotic fluid embolism (AFE) had reduced by half in the 1997–99 Confidential Enquiry compared with the 1994–96 report. AFE is the fifth leading cause of *Direct* death. The 1997–99 CEMD suggested that some women are now surviving what was a previously fatal condition and it was the third leading cause of *Direct* deaths.[4] The most recent population-based study[16] had a population frequency of one case per 20 646 deliveries.

Suspect

Clark,[15] in his registry of amniotic fluid embolism required the following features to be present for the diagnosis to be made:

- acute hypotension or cardiac arrest
- acute hypoxia (dyspnoea, cyanosis or respiratory arrest)
- coagulopathy – laboratory evidence of disseminated intravascular coagulation (DIC) or fibrinolysis or severe clinical haemorrhage*
- onset of the above during labour, caesarean section, evacuation of the uterus or within 30 minutes postpartum
- absence of other confounding conditions or explanations for the signs and symptoms observed.

* Coagulopathy is only necessary to make the clinical diagnosis if the patient survives long enough for DIC to become established (more than 30 minutes)

Symptoms and signs of amniotic fluid embolism

The following were noted in Clark's series (n = 43):[15]

Hypotension	100%
Fetal distress (of those *in utero* at onset)	100%
Pulmonary oedema or ARDS	93%
Cardiopulmonary arrest	87%
Cyanosis	83%
Coagulopathy (the remainder did not live long enough)	83%
Dyspnoea	49%
Seizure	48%
Uterine atony	23%
Bronchospasm	15%
Transient hypertension	11%
Cough	7%
Headache	7%
Chest pain	2%

Clearly the most common features are very severe. The lesser symptoms are often prodromal. Seizures relate to profound cerebral hypoxia and permanent neurological sequelae in survivors are not uncommon.

The condition is essentially characterised by cardiovascular collapse, profound hypoxia and subsequent coagulopathy.

Suspect amniotic fluid embolism if:

- Respiratory collapse: Cyanosis, dyspnoea, hypoxia, falling oxygen saturation, pulmonary oedema, respiratory arrest
- Cardiovascular collapse: Hypotension, tachycardia, arrythmias, cardiac arrest
- Coagulopathy (DIC): Will usually develop within 30 minutes if patient survives
- Other symptoms: Fetal distress, convulsions, uterine atony, cough, shivering, sweating, and anxiety

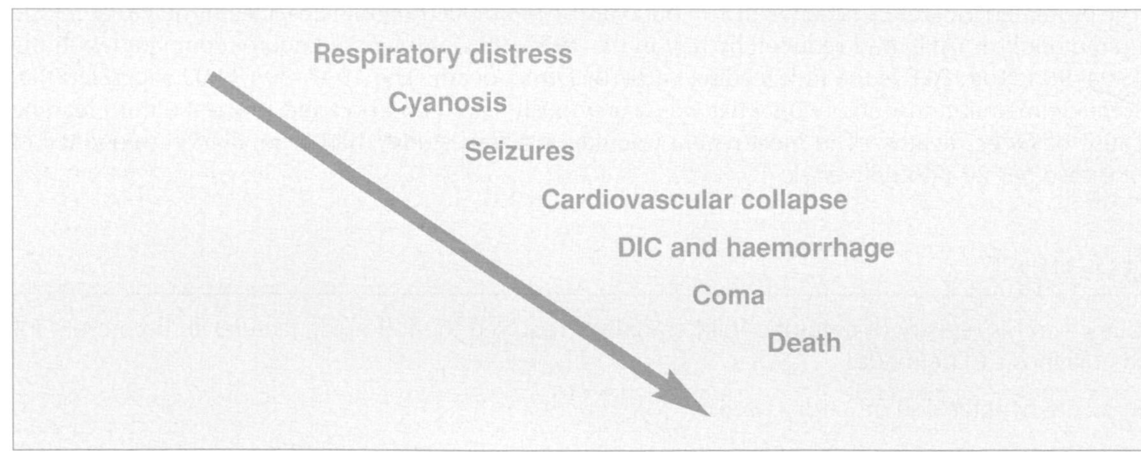

Logistics

- Recruit as many staff as possible
- Need individual responsible for each of the following:
  - recording events and management
  - communication
  - runner/porter/transport.

Mortality rates are high. Early appreciation of the diagnosis and prompt correction of hypoxia and circulatory insufficiency are likely to be the key to successful management.

Timing

AFE may occur during labour (70%), during caesarean section (19%) or immediately postpartum (11%). AFE has also been reported during first-trimester surgical termination of pregnancy, second-trimester termination, abdominal trauma and amniocentesis.[4]

Labour characteristics

Uterine hyperstimulation has commonly been believed to be a factor in the aetiology of AFE. The finding has varied in the various Confidential Enquiries and was not believed to be a factor by Clark[15] in his series or by Morgan[18] in a review of 272 published cases. Furthermore, no correlation was found between AFE and length of labour or oxytocin use in Clark's series. It is noted, however, that uterine tetany appear to develop after the onset of the symptoms of the event.

Of the women included in the national registry, 78% had ruptured membranes. In 13% of cases, maternal collapse occurred within three minutes of amniotomy or insertion of intrauterine pressure catheter.

There was coexistent placental abruption in 13% of cases and this may be a triggering event. Uterine tetany often occurs concomitantly and this is more likely to be a response to profound tissue hypoxia rather than the cause of entry of amniotic fluid into the maternal bloodstream.

Pathophysiology

It is believed that entry into the maternal circulation of amniotic fluid and associated debris is the initiating event. However, it has been shown that fetal squames can be detected in the maternal circulation in normal labour without the catastrophic events of AFE developing. The reason for this is not clear. There may be abnormal factors present in amniotic fluid in cases that develop AFE. One hypothesis is that the condition is an anaphylactoid reaction[15,19,20] because of the resemblance to septic shock. This is, at present, speculative but animal models suggest that the syndrome may be abolished by administering a leukotriene blocking agent, lending some credence to the argument. It has been suggested that estimation of tryptase levels (indicative of mast-cell degranulation) may clarify the issue. In one case(personal experience of the authors), tryptase levels were normal, as were all other markers of immune activation (methyl histamine, complement). There has been no published positive evidence as yet.

The physiological disturbance responsible for the extreme hypoxia is not well characterised but may be an initial and transient pulmonary vasospasm. Hankins *et al.*[21] demonstrated an initial and transient rise in pulmonary and systemic vascular resistance along with myocardial depression.

Systemic hypotension is the most prominent haemodynamic alteration documented in humans and results principally from left-sided heart failure. Proposed mechanisms include a direct depressant effect of amniotic fluid elements on the myocardium and myocardial ischaemia resulting from coronary artery vasospasm or global hypoxia.

The aetiological mechanism of the coagulopathy is obscure. It may be similar to that proposed for the coagulopathy related to severe placental abruption. In this model, the maternal immune system recognises fetal antigens and exerts potent thromboplastin-like effects, initiating the extrinsic pathway of the clotting cascade. Amniotic fluid contains procoagulants that may be capable of initiating intravascular clotting.

Diagnosis

Essentially, the diagnosis is a clinical one, with the triad of sudden cardiovascular and respiratory collapse, together with the development of a coagulopathy (as outlined above). Confirmation may be obtained at post mortem by the finding of fetal squames in the maternal pulmonary circulation. In the living, fetal squames or lanugo may be found in central venous blood[22] or maternal sputum.[23] Distinguishing between maternal and fetal squames is not straightforward, however, and there is a possibility of both false positive and negative results.

Chest X-ray may show evidence of pulmonary oedema, acute respiratory distress syndrome (ARDS) or right atrial enlargement and prominent pulmonary artery. The electrocardiograph may show a tachycardia and right-ventricular strain pattern. Arterial blood gases will show reduced P_aO_2 and metabolic acidosis. Clotting studies may show thrombocytopenia and elevated fibrin degradation products or D-dimers. In interpreting clotting results in pregnancy, remember the normal values are altered (e.g. fibrinogen levels are elevated in pregnancy and therefore a 'normal fibrinogen' may not be normal at all – discuss with haematologist).

Differential diagnosis

Pulmonary embolus	Infrequently peripartum, often accompanied by chest pain. Will not develop coagulopathy
Air embolism	May follow ruptured uterus, pressurised intravenous infusion or caesarean section. Distinguishing feature is precordial waterwheel murmur.
Septic shock	Evidence of preceding infection such as a urinary tract infection, pyrexia
Anaphylactic shock	
Eclampsia	Usually preceded or accompanied by hypertension
Toxic reaction to anaesthetic or local anaesthetic agents	
Acute left-ventricular fusion	Usually more insidious onset. Will not develop coagulopathy
CVA: No cyanosis or hypotension	
Massive obstetric haemorrhage	History may help. Beware concealed abruption; uterine tetany may be a feature of both. Central cyanosis should be less pronounced than in AFE
Aspiration of gastric contents	Usually in unconscious patient or during induction of, or emergence from, general anaesthesia.

Management

There is no specific treatment of the condition. Management is supportive and is essentially directed towards the hypoxia, cardiovascular support, correcting the coagulopathy and management of the massive obstetric haemorrhage that may ensue.

Treatment should be multidisciplinary, with early involvement of the consultant obstetrician, anaesthetist and haematologist. It is important to nominate an individual to record event times and drugs, volumes of fluid given, etc. If possible, there should be an individual responsible for communicating with the laboratory, other medical staff, intensive care unit, etc. Given the geographical location of the blood bank, a dedicated porter or transport driver is desirable.

Resuscitation and monitoring

Initial management should be aimed at providing maximal oxygenation and vital organ perfusion. High-flow oxygen should be administered and oxygen saturation and blood gases monitored. In unconscious patients, endotracheal intubation and mechanical ventilation with 100% oxygen and positive end expiratory pressure (PEEP) is required. If improved oxygenation results (arterial blood gases and pulse oximetry) lower levels of PEEP may be attainable. High PEEP may depress cardiac output by increasing intrathoracic pressure diminishing venous return.

Two large-bore cannulae should be sited. Blood should be sent for crossmatching and at least six units of group-specific blood with retrospective crossmatching should be ordered. Communication with the blood bank and haematology consultant, stressing the immediacy of need, is essential. It is wise to request clotting factors and platelets on suspicion of the condition, as DIC may take 30 minutes to develop. Blood needs to be sent for full blood count, clotting, fibrinogen and fibrin degradation product levels immediately and frequent repeat estimation of haematological parameters is required.

Cardiac arrest may occur and management is via respiratory support as above and standard ALS protocols (see Chapter 3).

If the woman is in labour, immediate delivery is required, by caesarean section if not deliverable immediately by operative vaginal delivery. General anaesthesia clearly is the method of choice. In the case of cardiac arrest, if electrical and mechanical output cannot be restored immediately, cardiac massage and ventilation should continue and caesarean section performed.

Circulatory support will depend on the reason for decreased cardiac output. Placement of a pulmonary artery flotation catheter or central venous line (this may be best achieved through the antecubital fossa due to coagulopathy) will help to distinguish the causes of shock. Available haemodynamic data[24] indicate that high left-heart filling pressures, reflecting a failing left ventricle, are a feature of the condition. In patients who survive the initial haemodynamic collapse, there is a high risk of secondary pulmonary oedema (70%). A small series (five patients) all of whom received inotropic therapy guided by invasive monitoring demonstrated 100% survival. In massive obstetric haemorrhage complicating AFE, large volumes of blood and blood products may be required. Monitoring filling pressures may help to prevent fluid overload and pulmonary oedema, which would be a very real danger with a poorly functioning left heart. This would clearly exacerbate the condition.

Placement of an arterial line aids haemodynamic assessment and allows frequent arterial blood gas analysis.

The coagulopathy will need to be corrected with platelets, fresh frozen plasma and cryoprecipitate (rich in fibrinogen). Consultant haematological involvement is essential.

Massive haemorrhage may be due not only to the coagulopathy but also to coexistent uterine atony. Uterine atony may be partly due to profound hypoxia and also to the presence of high levels of fibrin degradation products. There is thus a vicious circle in effect. Clearance of FDP may be enhanced by the administration of cryoprecipitate rich in fibrinogen. Oxytocic drugs will be needed (e.g. ergometrine, oxytocin, carboprost). Hot packs and uterine tamponade with a Rusch catheter[25] may reduce blood loss while the coagulopathy is corrected. Tranexamic acid may have a place. Volume replacement is most accurately guided by invasive monitoring.

Although the case for an anaphylactoid syndrome is not yet proven, in unresponsive cases it may be worth using sympathetic system augmentation as a therapy for AFE. Clark *et al.*[1] recommend giving 500 mg hydrocortisone sodium succinate intravenously every six hours until improvement of the patient or death occurs. Adrenaline may also be given.

Successful treatment of a moribund patient with AFE by cardiopulmonary bypass and thromboembolectomy has been reported.[26]

Patients who survive the initial insult are at high risk for heart failure, ARDS and DIC. If a patient with AFE sustains a cardiac arrest, her chance of neurologically intact survival is poor. As in other pregnancy cardiac arrests, delivery may actually improve the likelihood of success of the resuscitation.

Risk of recurrence

It is impossible to give an estimate of the risk of recurrence in future pregnancies of survivors, due to the small numbers involved. There are, however, reports of successful subsequent pregnancies[27] in the literature. There is no evidence to recommend mode of delivery. Both caesarean section and vaginal delivery have been reported.

Outcome

Maternal mortality rates are high. The true mortality rate is difficult to estimate as there may be under-reporting of the true incidence of the condition. In Clark's series[1] the maternal mortality rate was 61%, with neurologically intact survival in only 15%. Most died within one hour of the event. In Gilbert's population-based study,[2] maternal mortality was 26.4%. Gilbert's series[2] was later and the difference may reflect advances in care and more widespread provision of intensive care for sick obstetric patients, or it may reflect a difference in the reporting of cases, as the diagnostic criteria are not stated.

Perinatal mortality also is high. In Clark's series,[1] of the babies *in utero* at the time of the event, 79% survived, with half of the survivors being neurologically normal.

Conclusion

Fortunately, AFE is rare. From the similarities of AFE to septic and anaphylactic shock, a theory has been proposed that the clinical syndrome of AFE results when fetal antigens breach a maternal immunological barrier in susceptible mothers. This subsequently triggers the release of endogenous mediators that are responsible for dramatic physiological disturbances.

Most cases of AFE are associated with dismal maternal and fetal outcomes, regardless of the quality of care rendered. Improved understanding of the molecular pathophysiology of AFE may lead to the development of preventive measures and more effective and specific treatment. In the meantime, its occurrence remains unpredictable and unpreventable and its effects, for most part, untreatable.

Algorithm 5.1 Pulmonary embolism (PE) key points

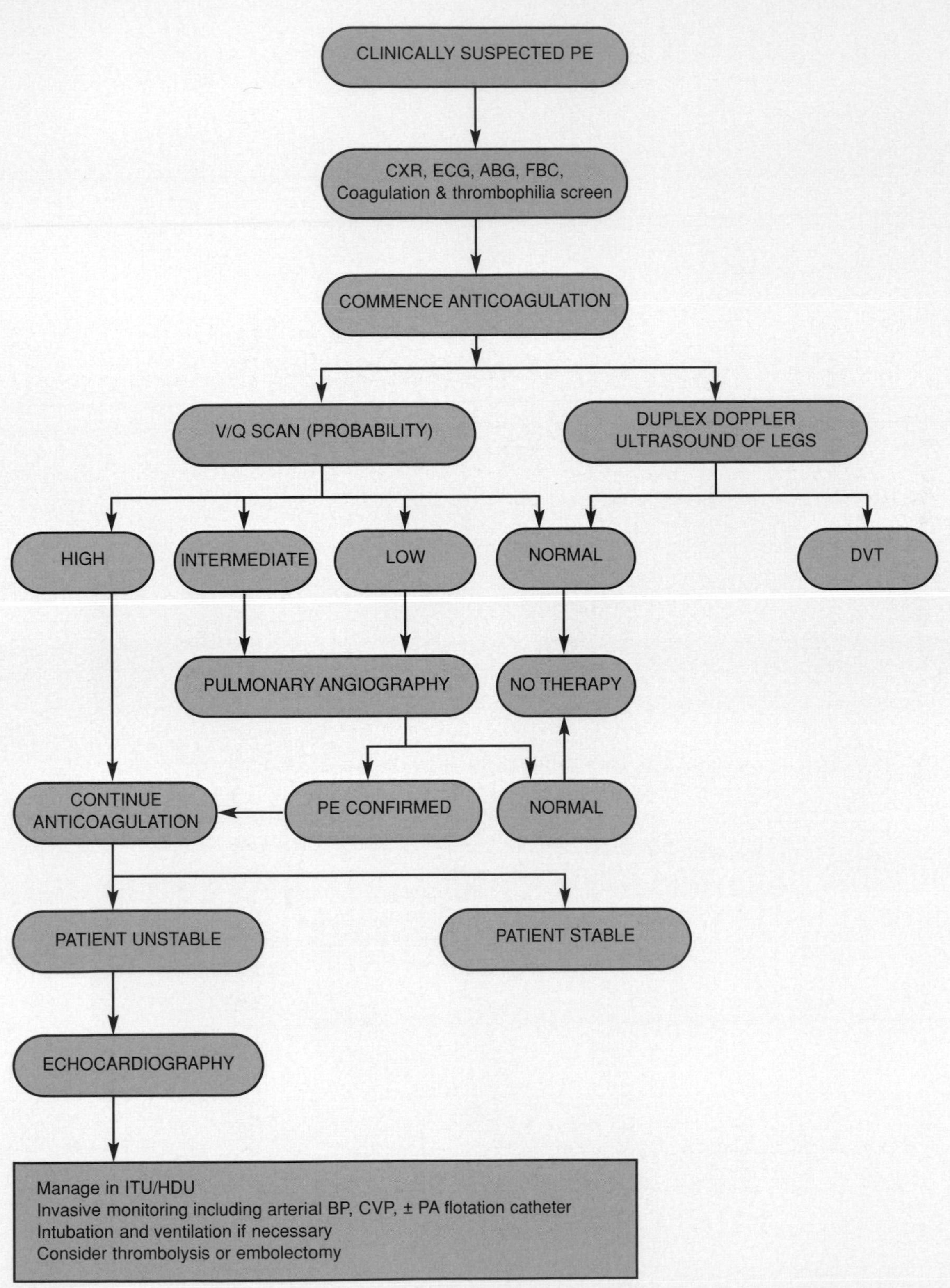

Chapter 5
Pulmonary embolism

Objectives

On successfully completing this topic, you will be able to:

- recognise the features of pulmonary embolism and suspect the diagnosis early
- describe the treatment of suspected pulmonary embolism.

Introduction and incidence

The latest triennial report of the Confidential Enquiries into Maternal Deaths (CEMD) in the UK shows thrombosis and thromboembolism to account for 33% of all direct maternal deaths.[4] The incidence of pulmonary embolism (PE) in pregnancy varies between one per 1000 and one per 3000 deliveries.[28] This depends upon whether deep venous thrombosis (DVT) has been treated adequately. Untreated, as many as 24% of patients with DVT will have PE, resulting in approximately 15% mortality. When patients are treated with anticoagulants, PE occurs in only 4.5% and mortality is reduced to less than 1%. The importance of timely diagnosis and treatment is therefore apparent.[29]

Deaths are as common in the antenatal period as in the postnatal period. Areas of substandard care include lack of appreciation of the risk factors for VTE, failure to obtain objective diagnosis and failure to provide adequate treatment and prophylaxis. The 1997–99 CEMD report shows a rise in the numbers of deaths in those in whom the diagnosis was missed or in whom risk factors were ignored.

Pregnancy is a thrombogenic state with a five- to six-fold increase in the risk of PE. The majority of DVT in pregnancy are ileofemoral, which are more likely to embolise.

Additional risk factors include:

- Operative delivery
  Caesarean section increases the risk of PE two- to eight-fold.[30] The risk is greater after an emergency procedure. The risk is also increased after prolonged labour and instrumental vaginal delivery. In the 1997–99 CEMD report the number of deaths from thromboembolism following caesarean section has fallen dramatically.
- Age
  The mortality from PE is nearly 100 times greater in pregnant women aged over 40 years compared with those aged 20–25 years.[28] Increasing parity is a further risk factor.
- Obesity
  The risk of PE is due to poor mobility and higher likelihood of venous stasis.
- Congenital and acquired thrombophilia
  Patients with congenital thrombophilia (antithrombin-3 deficiency, protein C and S deficiency, activated protein C resistance) and acquired thrombophilia (lupus anticoagulant and antiphospholipid antibody) are at increased risk of PE. It is difficult to estimate the risk for each thrombophilia. Family or past history of thromboembolism should warrant a search for these factors.

- Surgical procedures in pregnancy or puerperium
  Surgical procedures such as ovarian cystectomy and caesarean hysterectomy further increase the risk of PE. The other risk factors are restricted activity, hypertensive problems, dehydration, excessive blood loss and homocystinuria.

Clinical presentation

Common symptoms of PE are dyspnoea, tachypnoea and pleuritic chest pain. The other symptoms are cough, haemoptysis and leg pain. Massive PE may be associated with cyanosis, circulatory collapse with hypotension, syncope or convulsions and central chest pain.

Signs and symptoms of pulmonary embolism[29]

Findings	Patients with proven PE (%)
Tachypnoea	89
Dyspnoea	81
Pleuritic pain	72
Apprehension	59
Cough	54
Tachycardia	43
Haemoptysis	34
Temperature > 37°C	34

Tachycardia and few atelectatic râles may be the only findings on physical examination. Massive PE may produce right-sided heart failure with jugular venous distension, an enlarged liver, a left parasternal heave and fixed splitting of the second heart sound.

Clinical evidence of DVT is rarely found in patients with PE. In the Prospective Investigation of Pulmonary Embolism Diagnosis (PIOPED) study, only 15% of patients with PE had clinical evidence of DVT.[31]

In summary, symptoms and physical findings must be interpreted with caution during pregnancy, because dyspnoea, tachypnoea and leg discomfort occurs commonly as pregnancy progresses.

Management

1. Remember the risk factors for thromboembolism.
2. Suspect PE in all patients presenting with sudden onset of shortness of breath, chest pain, unexplained tachycardia or cardiovascular collapse.
3. Involve the senior obstetrician, anaesthetist and medical team.
4. Assess and ensure adequate airway, breathing and circulation.
5. Transfer the patient to the high-dependency area when appropriate and commence monitoring: non-invasive BP, pulse oximetry, ECG, urine output.
6. Send FBC, clotting studies, U&Es, LFT and thrombophilia screen.
7. Request ECG, ABG and CXR.

These investigations do not confirm or refute the diagnosis of PE.

ECG

This is non-specific for diagnosis of PE. The changes in electrical axis that occur in normal pregnancy make the ECG findings in PE even less specific. Sinus tachycardia is the most common abnormality. Right-axis deviation and right-ventricular strain pattern may be present with a large PE. S1, Q3, T3 pattern is very rare.

Chest X-ray

This will help to exclude pneumothorax and pneumonia.[32] The non-specific radiological changes in PE include segmental collapse, a raised hemidiaphragm, consolidation and unilateral pleural effusion.[33] Wedge-shaped infarction is a rare finding. CXR is necessary for the accurate interpretation of ventilation/perfusion scans. The radiation exposure to the fetus is small (less than 10 μGy) and therefore should not be withheld.

Arterial blood gases

These should be monitored in the upright position to avoid a false low PaO_2. ABG in PE may reveal a reduced PaO_2 and a normal or low $PaCO_2$. With smaller emboli, normal values may be found.[32] If the patient is unstable, radial artery cannulation is of benefit both for repeated ABG and haemodynamic monitoring.

8. Commence anticoagulation.
   Treat clinically suspected PE while awaiting confirmation from objective tests. The aim of treatment is to prevent further thromboembolic complications and extension of the existing thrombus.

   Intravenous unfractionated heparin is the mainstay of treatment. Initiate treatment with IV bolus of 5000 iu heparin given over five minutes. Follow this with heparin infusion of 1000–2000 iu per hour and adjust the dose to maintain APTT at 1.5–2.5 times the patient's control (heparin level at 0.2 to 0.4 u/ml). Repeat APTT every six hours during the first 24 hours of therapy. Thereafter monitor the APTT daily unless outside the therapeutic range.[33]

   Additional options for patients in shock include thrombolytic therapy using streptokinase, pulmonary embolectomy and transvenous catheter fragmentation of the clot. Expert advice should be sought, where appropriate, in the management of these patients.

   Patients in shock should be managed on the intensive care unit. These patients will need arterial BP and CVP monitoring. They will also need haemodynamic support with adequate fluid management and inotropic agents in order to ensure maximal right-heart filling. They may need intubation and ventilation, measurement of pulmonary artery pressure, wedge pressure and cardiac output using pulmonary artery floatation catheters.

9. Perform ventilation/perfusion (V/Q) scan and duplex Doppler leg ultrasound scan.
   V/Q scanning is the most useful initial test in patients with suspected PE and should be organised urgently. V/Q scans are interpreted using standardised criteria (PIOPED).[31] Based on the extent of ventilation–perfusion mismatches, the scan is interpreted as normal, low probability, intermediate probability or high probability for PE. A normal scan reliably excludes PE and a high-probability V/Q scan is considered sufficient evidence for diagnosing PE in a patient with a high clinical suspicion. Treatment should be continued when ultrasound scan reports an intermediate or high probability of PE.

   The radiation dose from V/Q scan is considered to pose negligible risk to the fetus.[34] Perfusion scan alone can be performed with a ventilation scan being performed only if the perfusion scan is abnormal.

Probability of pulmonary thromboembolism based on V/Q scan report

Scan category	Probability (%)
High probability	87
Intermediate probability	30
Low probability	14
Normal	4

Duplex Doppler ultrasound scan of the legs

Bilateral Doppler ultrasound leg studies should be performed in all cases of suspected PE. A positive scan study for DVT is considered sufficient to justify the use of anticoagulation therapy.[35]

10. Perform pulmonary angiography.
Pulmonary angiography is the gold standard for diagnosing PE. It is indicated following intermediate or low probability results on V/Q scan[36] with a high clinical suspicion of PE, even if Doppler ultrasound of the legs is negative. It should be considered if the clinical probability of PE is high, even if the V/Q scan shows low probability and the Doppler ultrasound examination of the leg is negative. It should also be considered if cardiovascular collapse or hypotension is present and where other investigations have failed to give a firm diagnosis.[28,32]

    This is an invasive test with high radiation exposure.[34] It may be associated with reactions to intravenous contrast agents.

Additional tests

Non-invasive imaging techniques such as spiral-computed tomography and magnetic resonance imaging have been used for diagnosing PE. These modalities allow direct visualisation of the thrombus within the pulmonary artery. These techniques have not been fully evaluated in pregnancy.[32]

Echocardiography

Experience with use of this technique in pregnancy is limited. It can show well-defined abnormalities with a large central pulmonary embolus. It may also help to eliminate other causes of central chest pain, collapse and hypotension such as myocardial infarction, pericardial tamponade and aortic dissection. Its usefulness lies in the fact that it is a bedside test and can be done in patients who are too unstable to be transported for pulmonary angiography.

Additional information

Anticoagulation

Anticoagulation following pulmonary embolism should be continued throughout pregnancy and at least six weeks postpartum or until a three month course of anticoagulation therapy is completed.

Heparin is the anticoagulation of choice in pregnancy, since it does not cross the placenta. There are no randomised controlled studies for the treatment of PE in pregnancy. However, rapid and prolonged anticoagulation prevents extension of the thrombus and its recurrence. Acute therapy is with IV unfractionated heparin in doses mentioned above for five to ten days, the dose adjusted to maintain APTT at 1.5–2.5 times the control.

Treatment thereafter may be continued with subcutaneous heparin in a dose of 10 000 iu twice daily.[28] Maintaining mid-interval APTT in the therapeutic range (1.5–2.5 times the control) following subcutaneous heparin may be problematic and lead to under or over anticoagulation. Assessment of anti-Xa level may then be helpful in preventing such complications.[32]

Complications of heparin therapy are allergy, thrombocytopenia and osteoporosis. Platelet count should be monitored on a monthly basis in patients on long-term heparin therapy.

Low-molecular weight heparins (LMWH) are being increasingly used in pregnancy. They have been shown to be effective, safe and associated with fewer adverse effects when compared with unfractionated heparin in non-pregnant patients.

LMWH have higher bioavailability following subcutaneous administration (85% versus 10% for unfractionated heparin). The half-life is two to four times (18 hours) that of unfractionated heparin, allowing once daily administration. Anticoagulation using enoxaparin (Clexane®, Rhône-Poulenc Rorer) 1 mg/kg subcutaneously, based on the early pregnancy weight, every 12 hours for the acute treatment of PE has been reported in the immediate treatment of DVT and PE in pregnancy.[37]

Frequent monitoring does not appear to be necessary. The platelet count should be rechecked seven to nine days after commencing treatment.

Following acute therapy, the dose of LMWH could be reduced to prophylactic levels, i.e., 40 mg enoxaparin once a day or 5000 iu deltaparin once a day. Monitoring is by measuring anti-Xa activity, therapeutic range being 0.4–1.0 units/ml three hours post-injection. Enoxaparin is available in syringes of 40 mg, 60 mg, 80 mg and 100 mg. The dose closest to the patients weight should be employed.

Warfarin crosses the placenta and is associated with a characteristic embryopathy in the first trimester. Major fetal CNS abnormalities such as microcephaly and optic atrophy are seen with warfarin use in the second and third trimesters. In addition, there is a higher risk of intracerebral bleeds from the trauma of delivery and a higher risk of bleeding complications during labour and delivery. For all these reasons, warfarin is not preferred in the antenatal period. However, warfarin can be initiated in the postpartum period and overlapped with heparin until INR is maintained at 2.0–3.0.

Vena caval filters are indicated when there is recurrent PE despite adequate anticoagulation, contraindication to anticoagulation and complication of anticoagulation such as heparin-induced thrombocytopenia. Suprarenal placement is recommended in pregnancy.[33]

Audit standard

All high- and medium-risk women should use anti-embolism stockings and subcutaneous heparin until fully mobile: heparin 5000 iu (20 mg enoxaparin) 12-hourly if medium-risk or eight-hourly if high-risk.

Chapter 6

Airway management and ventilation

Objectives

On successfully completing this topic, you will be able to:

- understand the importance of patency, maintenance and protection
- identify the circumstances in which airway compromise may occur
- understand the assessment and management of airway and ventilation.

Introduction

An obstructed airway and/or inadequate ventilation results in tissue hypoxia within minutes, and this can lead to organ failure and death. Some organs are more sensitive to hypoxia than others. For example, cerebral hypoxia, even for a short period of time, will cause agitation, then a decreased level of consciousness and eventually, irreversible or fatal brain damage.

Because obstruction to the airway can quickly result in hypoxia, with damage or death, management of the airway is the first concern.[38] The next presenting threat to life results from inadequate ventilation (breathing) so attention to this is given next priority.

Carbon dioxide is produced by cellular metabolism and carried in the blood to the lungs to be exhaled. If there is airway obstruction, there is a build up of carbon dioxide in the blood (hypercarbia), which causes drowsiness, acidosis and a rise in intracranial pressure.

Supplementary oxygen must be administered to all seriously injured and ill patients through a tight-fitting facemask attached to a reservoir bag at a flow of 12–15 l/minute (full on at the wall rotameter).

A before B before C before D

Importance of patency, maintenance and protection of airway

The airway must be open, maintained and protected if there is risk of regurgitation and aspiration (which there is in the heavily pregnant patient). The gold standard for this is intubation. If there is a **B** problem, ventilatory support may be necessary once you have established a patent airway.

Circumstances in which an airway problem is likely to occur

Suspect airway problem in:

- head injury with decreased level of consciousness (because there is reduced muscle tone and the tongue is likely to slip back into the pharynx)
- other causes of decreased level of consciousness:
  - hypoxia
  - hypovolaemia
  - eclampsia
  - poisoning
  - alcohol.
- maxillofacial injuries:
  - mid-face fractures can move backwards and block the airway
  - mandible fractures can allow the tongue to fall backwards
  - bleeding and secretions caused by these injuries can block the airway.
- open injuries to the neck:
  - direct trauma to the larynx and supporting structures
  - bleeding inside the neck compressing the hypopharynx or trachea
- burns to the face and neck:
  - swelling of the upper and lower airway due to direct burns or inhaling hot smoke, gases or steam, will cause airway obstruction.

Airway problems may be:

- immediate (block the airway quickly) or
- delayed (come on after a time delay – minutes or hours) or
- deteriorate with time – this is often insidious because of its slow progression and is easily overlooked (as with burns to the upper airway – consider the potential for deterioration during transfer and if a risk secure a definitive airway before transfer).

An airway that has been cleared may obstruct again:

- if the patient's level of consciousness decreases
- if there is further bleeding into the airway
- if there is increasing swelling in or around the airway.

Assessment of airway

Talk to the patient. Failure to respond implies an obstructed airway, a breathing problem with inability to exhale enough air to phonate and/or an altered level of consciousness with the potential for airway compromise. A positive, appropriate reply in a normal voice indicates that the airway is patent, breathing normal and brain perfusion adequate.

Look to see if the patient is agitated, drowsy or cyanosed. The absence of cyanosis does not mean the patient is adequately oxygenated. Look for use of accessory muscles of respiration.

Remember that a patient who refuses to lie down quietly may be trying to sit up in an attempt to keep his airway open and/or his breathing adequate. The abusive patient may be hypoxic and should not be presumed to be merely aggressive or intoxicated.

Listen for abnormal sounds. Snoring, gurgling and gargling sounds are associated with partial obstruction of the pharynx. Hoarseness implies laryngeal injury. Total obstruction equals total silence!

Feel for air movement on expiration and check if the trachea is in the midline.

Assessment of ventilation

To make the airway patent is the first step but only the first step. A patent airway allows oxygen to pass to the lungs but this will only happen with adequate ventilation. Ventilation may be compromised by airway obstruction, altered ventilatory mechanics or by central nervous system depression. If breathing is not improved by clearing the airway attempt to ventilate by facemask. If ventilation is possible the airway is patent but there is a problem with spontaneous ventilation. If ventilation is not possible this suggests that the airway continues to be obstructed. If there is a problem with spontaneous ventilation look for a cause within the chest or an intracranial or spinal injury as a cause and assist ventilation.

- **Inspect**
  Look for chest movement and obvious injuries.
- **Palpate**
  Palpate for chest movement and palpate the back of the patient's chest for injuries. Palpate the trachea, checking it is in the mid line.
- **Percuss**
  Percussion should be resonant and equal bilaterally.
- **Auscultate**
  Air entry should be equal bilaterally.

Airway management (as a problem is found)

Management comprises:

- clearing the obstructed airway
- maintaining the intact airway
- recognising and protecting the airway at risk.
  (Remember that the airway is at risk from aspiration in any patient with reduced level of consciousness, but in the pregnant patient regurgitation is more likely so the potential for aspiration is increased.)

Techniques for clearing, maintaining and protecting the airway need to be modified in the trauma patient in whom cervical spine injury is suspected or present.

Cervical spine injury is suspected

Cervical spine immobilisation should be instituted wherever there is suspicion of injury either by manual in-line immobilisation or by semi-rigid cervical collar, head blocks and backboard and straps.

Clearing the obstructed airway

In the patient with suspected cervical spine injury, manual inline immobilisation of the cervical spine and airway clearance are carried out together. In a patient with an altered level of consciousness, the tongue falls backwards and obstructs the pharynx. This can be readily corrected by chin lift or jaw thrust manoeuvres and blood and debris cleared by suction.

Chin lift

- Place the fingers of one hand under the chin and gently lift it upwards to bring the chin anteriorly.
- To open the mouth, use the thumb of the same hand to depress the lower lip slightly.
- The thumb may also be placed behind the lower incisors and, simultaneously, the chin gently lifted.
- This will open the upper airway in 70–80% of patients.

This manoeuvre will be practised in the skill station. See Figure 6.1.

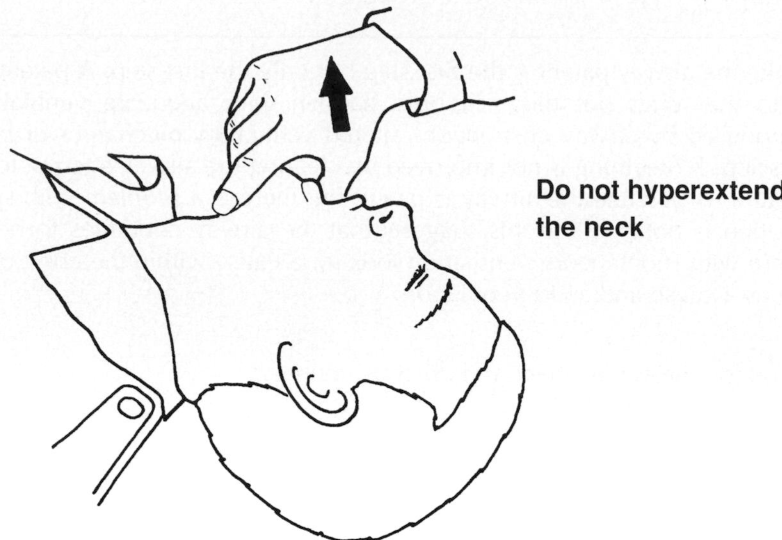

Figure 6.1 Chin lift

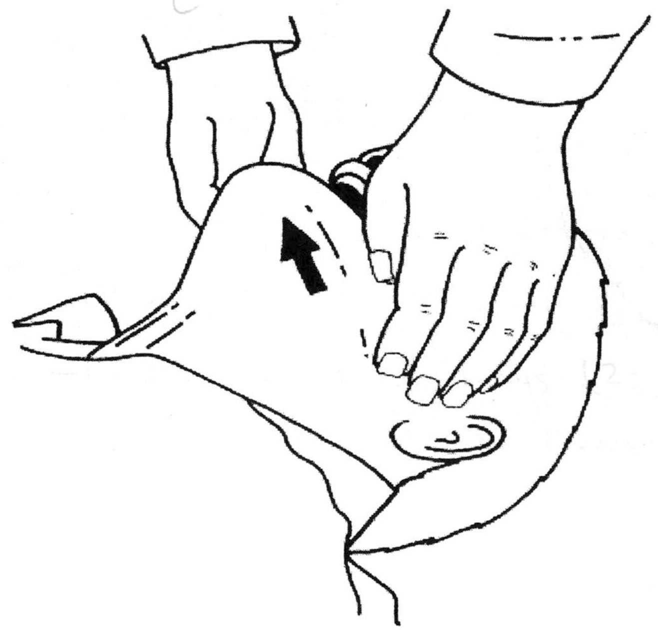

Figure 6.2 Jaw thrust

Jaw-thrust

- Grasp the angles of the mandible, one hand on each side and move the mandible forward.

The jaw-thrust is used for the injured patient because it does not destabilise a possible cervical spine fracture and risk converting a fracture without spinal cord injury to one with spinal cord injury.

This manoeuvre will open 95% of obstructed upper airways. It will be practised in the skill stations. See Figure 6.2.

Suction

Remove blood and secretions from the oropharynx with a rigid suction devise (for example, a Yankauer suction catheter). If there is bleeding at the external nares clear this with suction. A patient with facial injuries may also have a cribiform plate fracture – this means that suction catheters should not be inserted through the nose, as they could enter the skull and injure the brain.

If attempts to clear the airway do not result in the restoration of spontaneous breathing this may be because the airway is still not patent or because the airway is patent but there is no breathing. The only way to distinguish these two situations is to put either a pocket mask or facemask over the face and give breaths (either mouth-to-pocket-mask or self-inflating bag to either mask).

If the chest rises, this is not an airway problem but a breathing problem. If you are unable make the chest rise, this is an airway problem.

Decide what else you must do to secure a patent airway – the next step is tracheal intubation, either endotracheal or surgical airway. If this is a breathing problem you must continue to ventilate through the airway that you have. Prolonged ventilation is carried out through an endotracheal/tracheostomy tube.

Clearing the airway may result in improvement in level of consciousness and the patient being able to maintain his own airway.

If the patient cannot maintain his own airway you (or an assistant) need to continue with the jaw-thrust or chin-lift or try using an oropharyngeal airway.

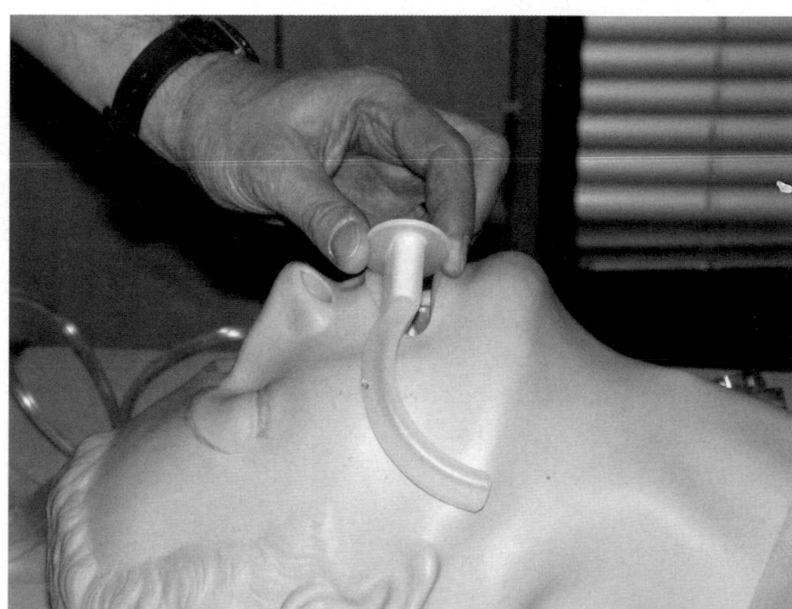

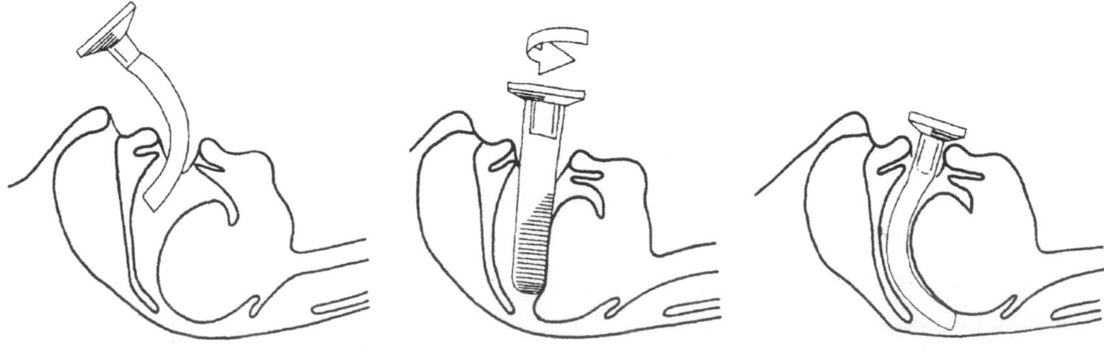

Figure 6.3 Oropharyngeal airway

Oropharyngeal airway

- The oropharyngeal airway (Guedel type) is inserted into the mouth over the tongue. It stops the tongue falling back and provides a clear passage for airflow.
- The preferred method is to insert the airway concavity upwards until the tip reaches the soft palate and then rotate it 180 degrees, slipping it into place over the tongue.
- Make sure that the oropharyngeal airway does not push the tongue backwards as this will block rather than open the patient's airway.
- A patient with a gag reflex may not tolerate the oral airway.

This procedure will be practised in the skill station. See Figure 6.3.

Nasopharyngeal airway

A nasopharyngeal airway can be used when there is oral injury, a fractured mandible or massetter spasm. It is better tolerated than the oropharyngeal airway by the more responsive patient.

A suspected fractured base of skull is a contraindication for use of this airway.

Be aware of the potential for this airway to cause bleeding, which may soil the lungs of a patient with obtunded laryngeal or pharyngeal reflexes (the unconscious or hypotensive patient). It should only be used if there is an airway problem, an oropharyngeal airway is not tolerated and an anaesthetist is unavailable.

BE VERY RELUCTANT TO USE.

Nasal airways do not have a large part to play in contemporary UK anaesthetic practice because of their potential to cause bleeding. Their use is limited to intensive care units where they might be placed by physiotherapists or anaesthetists to facilitate suctioning of chest secretions.

Lubricate the airway and insert it through either nostril, straight backwards – not upwards – so that its tip enters the hypopharynx.

A safety pin should be applied across the proximal end before insertion to prevent the tube disappearing into the airway.

Gentle insertion, good lubrication and using an airway that passes easily into the nose will decrease the incidence of bleeding.

The oropharyngeal and nasopharyngeal devices **maintain** the airway but do **not protect** it from aspiration.

Advanced airway techniques

Advanced airway techniques may be required:

- when the above techniques fail
- to maintain an airway over the longer term
- to protect an airway
- to allow accurate control of oxygenation and ventilation
- when there is the potential for airway obstruction
- to control carbon dioxide levels in the patient with a head injury, as a way of minimising the rise in intracranial pressure.

Advanced airway techniques are:

- endotracheal intubation
- surgical cricothyroidotomy
- surgical tracheostomy.

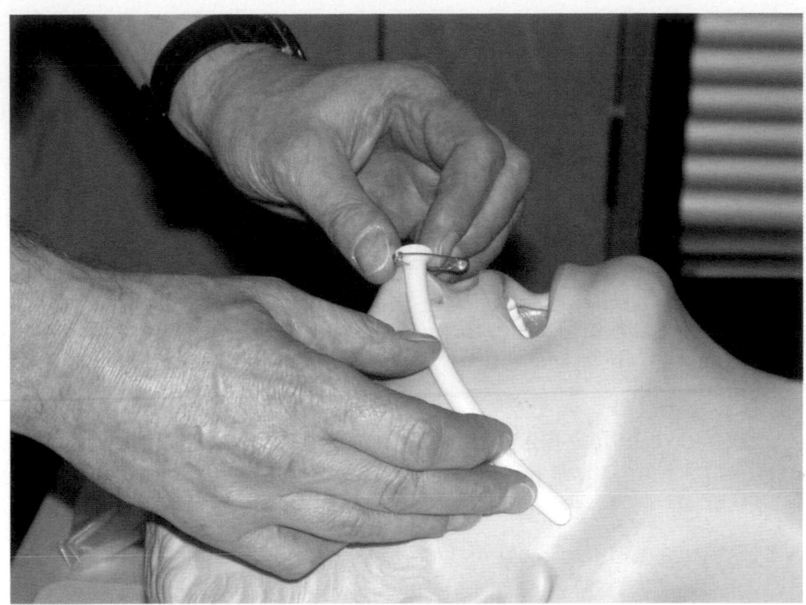

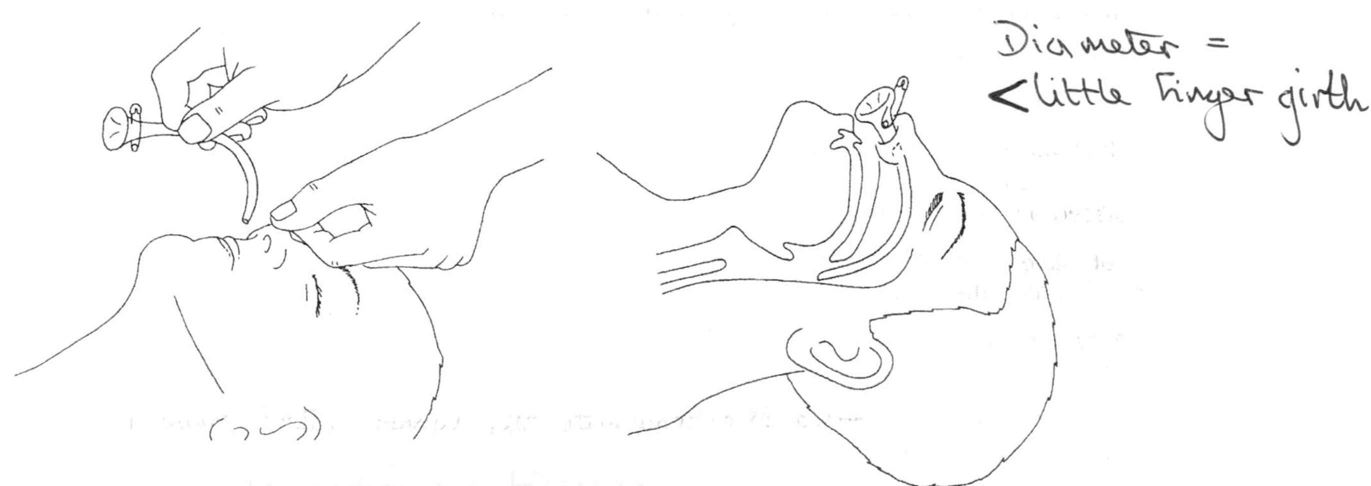

Figure 6.4 Nasopharyngeal airway

Definitive airway is a gold standard for opening, maintaining and protecting the airway. It means that there is a cuffed tube in the trachea. These advanced airway techniques provide a definitive airway.

Note: The pregnant patient is at increased risk of gastric regurgitation because she has a mechanical obstruction to gastric emptying and reduced lower oesophageal barrier as a result of hormonal effects on the smooth muscle. Trauma patients are also at increased risk of regurgitation because of reduced gastric emptying. Consequently, the pregnant patient (± trauma) without adequate pharyngeal and laryngeal reflexes (unconscious or hypotensive) is at increased risk of pulmonary aspiration. The chemical pneumonitis suffered when a pregnant patient aspirates is more severe than in a non-pregnant patient, as the gastric aspirate is more acidic in pregnancy. Consider early definitive airway.

Endotracheal intubation

This technique uses a laryngoscope to visualise the vocal cords. A cuffed endotracheal tube is placed through the vocal cords into the trachea. This skill will be practised in the skill station.

Tracheal intubation is not possible unless the patient is unconscious. If the patient is unconscious, intracranial pathology is implied and intubation without anaesthetic and muscle relaxation drugs will cause increases in blood pressure and intracranial pressure, which will exacerbate the intracranial condition. Intubation is therefore always a threat to patient wellbeing unless drugs are used.

In a patient with airway or respiratory compromise, the primary aim is to oxygenate the patient and this can initially be successfully achieved by positioning, use of oropharyngeal airways or use of facemask and self-inflating bag.

If this cannot be achieved, intubation is needed. It should only be carried out without drugs where there is an urgent need for intubation, i.e. in the case of complete airway obstruction or a respiratory arrest, where the airway cannot be otherwise maintained.

Intubation assisted by drugs (induction agents and muscle relaxants) should only ever be carried out by an anaesthetist or by somebody with suitable anaesthetic experience and confidence in the technique.

Tracheal intubation is taught on the MOET course (as it is on ATLS and similar courses) because MOET wishes to furnish the delegate with skills for rare emergencies, i.e. so that the obstetrician would have some skills in the case of complete airway obstruction or respiratory arrest where the airway could not be maintained by facemask and self-inflating bag technique.

It should be emphasised that heavily pregnant patients are in the main more difficult to intubate because of weight gain during pregnancy and the potential for large breasts falling back into the intubator's working space.

A surgical airway may be the preferred option.

Where anaesthetic skills and drugs are available, endotracheal intubation is the preferred method of securing a definitive airway. This technique should comprise:

- rapid sequence induction (RSI) of anaesthesia ('crash induction')
    - pre-oxygenation
    - application of cricoid pressure
    - rapid unconsciousness using drugs
    - no 'bagging'
    - rapid placement of endotracheal tube in trachea
    - inflation of cuff before removal of cricoid pressure
- maintenance of cervical spine immobilisation when indicated.

Endotracheal intubation is often more difficult in the pregnant patient.

Intermittent oxygenation during difficult intubation

Inability to intubate will not kill. Inability to oxygenate will.

If you can oxygenate by bag and mask, this will keep the patient alive.

Intubation of the hypoventilating or apnoeic patient may require several attempts and even then may not be successful. You must avoid prolonged efforts to intubate without intermittently oxygenating and ventilating. You should practise taking a deep breath when starting an attempt at intubation. If you have to take a further breath before successfully intubating the patient, abort the attempt and reoxygenate using the bag and mask technique.

Correct placement of the endotracheal tube

The main points are:

- See if the endotracheal tube has passed between the vocal cords.

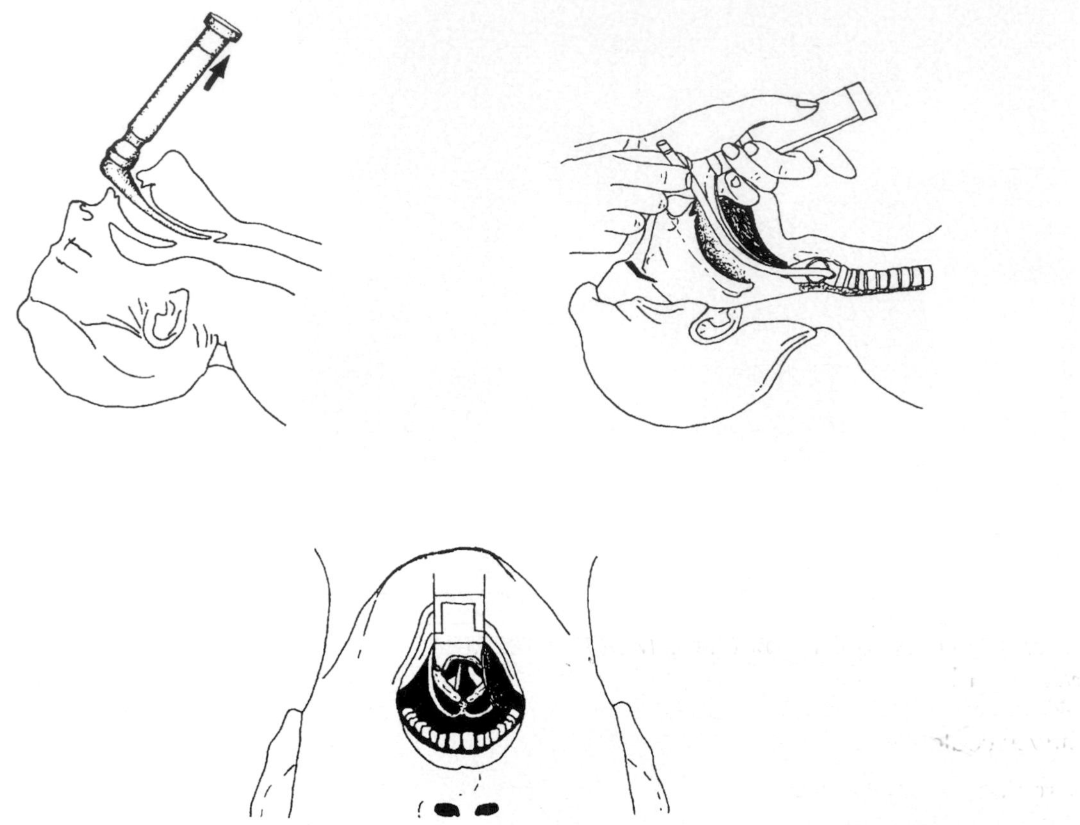

Figure 6.5 Endotracheal intubation

- Listen on both sides in the mid-axillary line for equal breath sounds.
- Listen over the stomach for gurgling sounds during assisted ventilation for evidence of oesophageal intubation.
- Monitor end-tidal carbon dioxide levels if equipment is available.
- If in doubt about the position of the endotracheal tube, take it out and oxygenate the patient by another method, bag and mask or surgical airway.

Note: Other methods for maintaining the airways:

- Both the laryngeal mask airway (LMA) and combitubes (devices that enter both) are used to make an airway patent and to maintain it. They do not have a place in the conventional management of the trauma or obstetric patient, at high risk of aspiration, as they do not protect the airway. They would be used only in a dire emergency where the airway could not be opened or maintained by other methods. Manually ventilating via a laryngeal mask can cause further problems in that the stomach can become inflated, further predisposing to regurgitation.
- Fibre optic intubation is an alternative if a suitably skilled anaesthetist is available.

Surgical airway

This should not be undertaken lightly.

A surgical airway is used when:

- a patient needing a definitive airway for resuscitation is too awake to tolerate endotracheal intubation without the use of anaesthetic drugs and there is no anaesthetist available in the time span in which the definitive airway is required

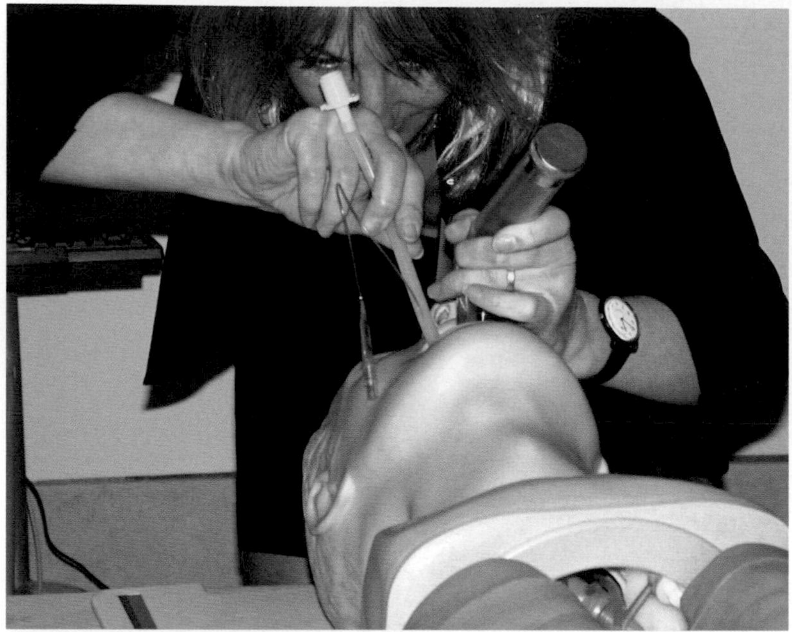

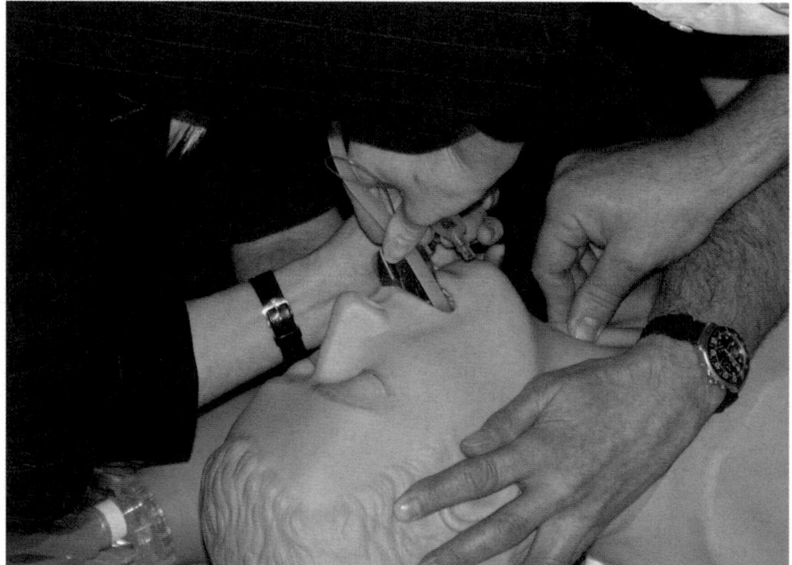

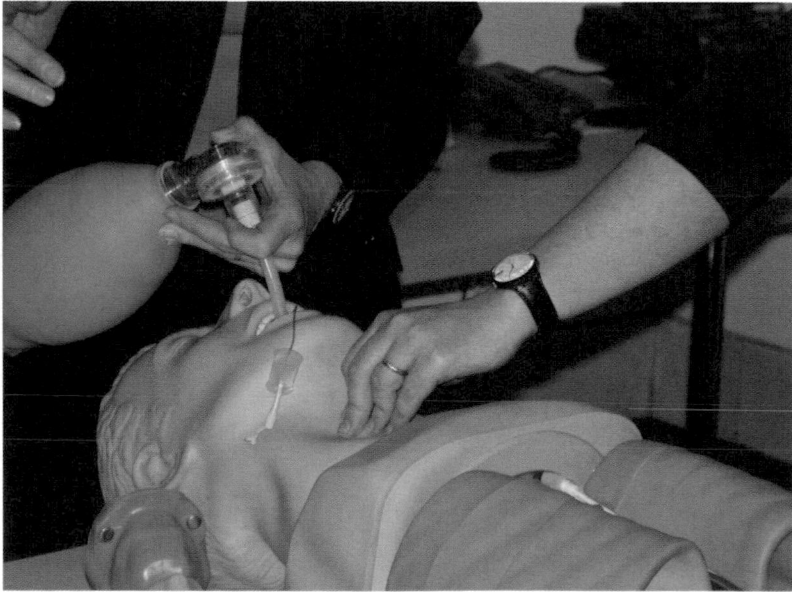

Intubation: maintained and protected airway

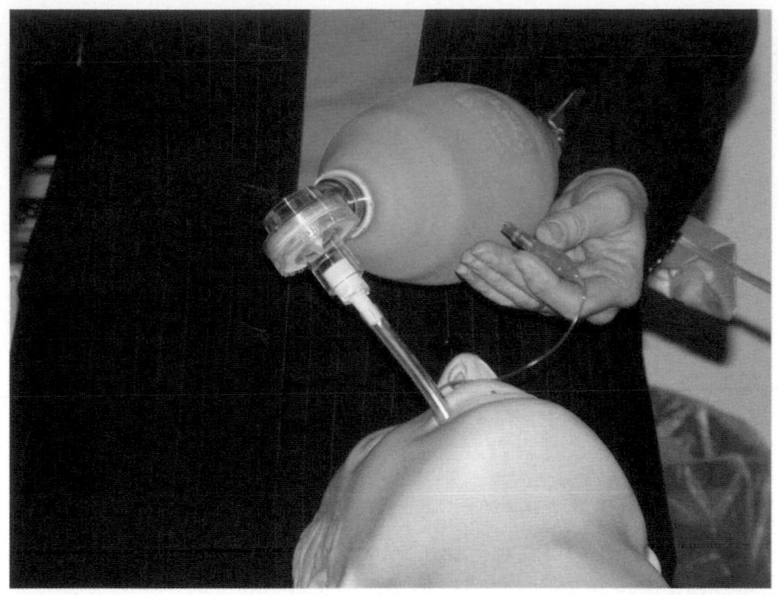

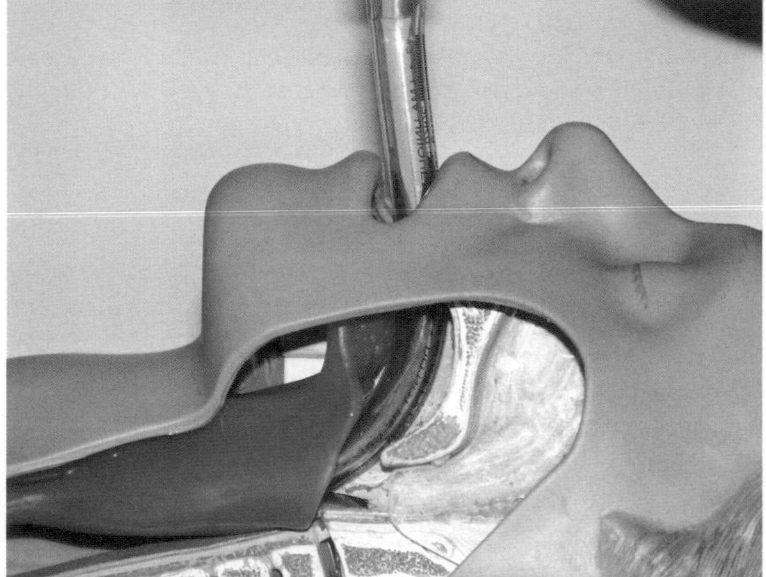

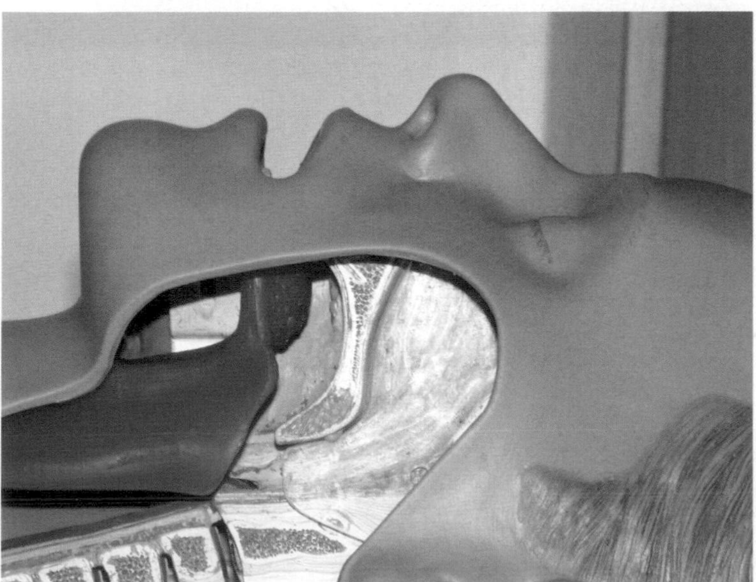

Intubation: maintained and protected airway

- trauma to the face and neck makes endotracheal intubation impossible
- a patient with face and neck burns requires airway protection to pre-empt delayed obstruction but expert anaesthetic help is unavailable to carry out endotracheal intubation.

Surgical cricothyroidotomy

Surgical cricothyroidotomy places a tube into the trachea via the cricothyroid membrane. A small tracheostomy tube (5–7 mm) is suitable. During the procedure, appropriate cervical spine protection must be maintained when indicated. There are also commercially available cricothyroidotomy sets. A cricothyroidotomy can be replaced by a formal tracheostomy (if needed) at a later time.

A needle cricothyroidotomy is a technique used to oxygenate in an emergency but it is not a definitive airway. A cannula-over-needle device is inserted to the cricothyroid membrane and attached to a flow of oxygen through oxygen tubing, which is intermittently interrupted by occluding the open lumen of a three-way tap at the patient end of the oxygen tubing.

This technique is of limited use in patients with high intrathoracic pressures (such as the heavily pregnant patient) or chest injuries and it does not allow exhalation of CO_2 so it can only be used for 30–40 minutes. It may buy time for skilled personnel capable of providing a definitive airway to arrive.

Cricothyroidotomy kits, which are superior to the intravenous cannula that was used in the past are available now. Most difficult-intubation trollies would carry one; familiarise yourself with the one in your own unit. This skill will be practised in the skill station.

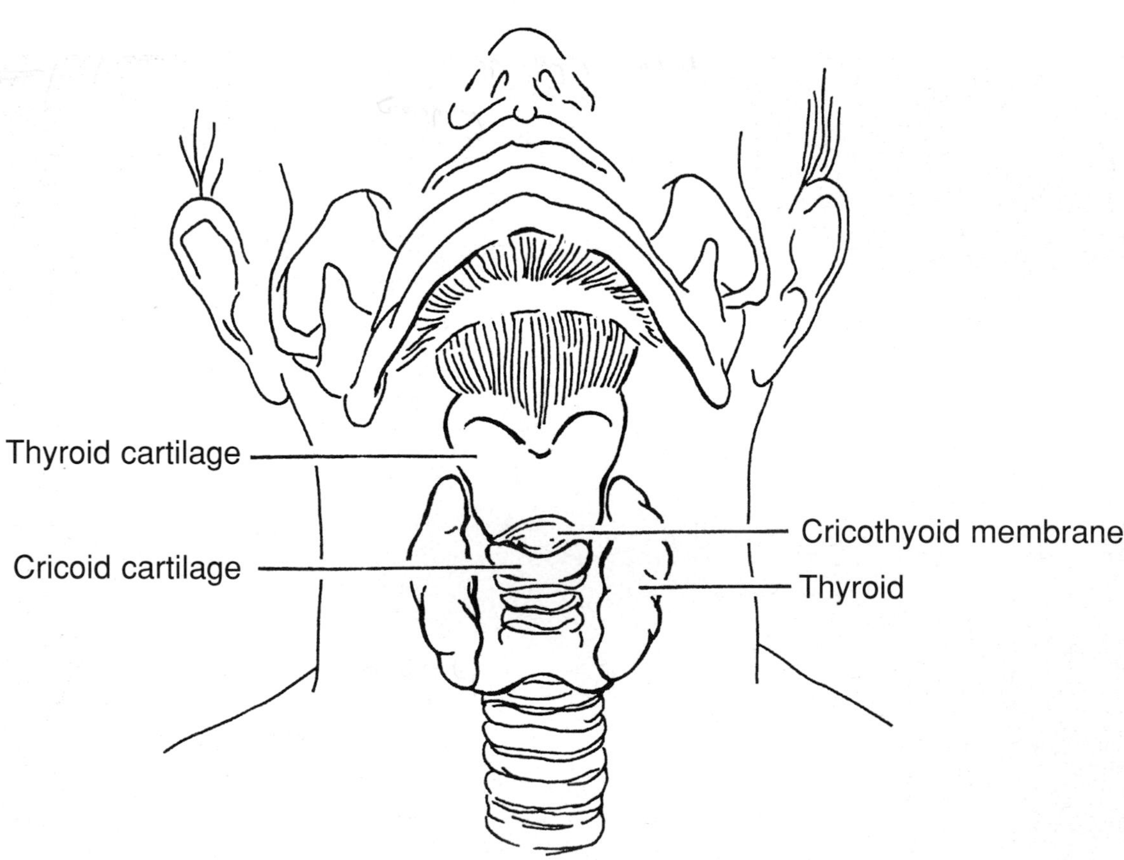

Figure 6.6 Anatomical landmarks for surgical airway

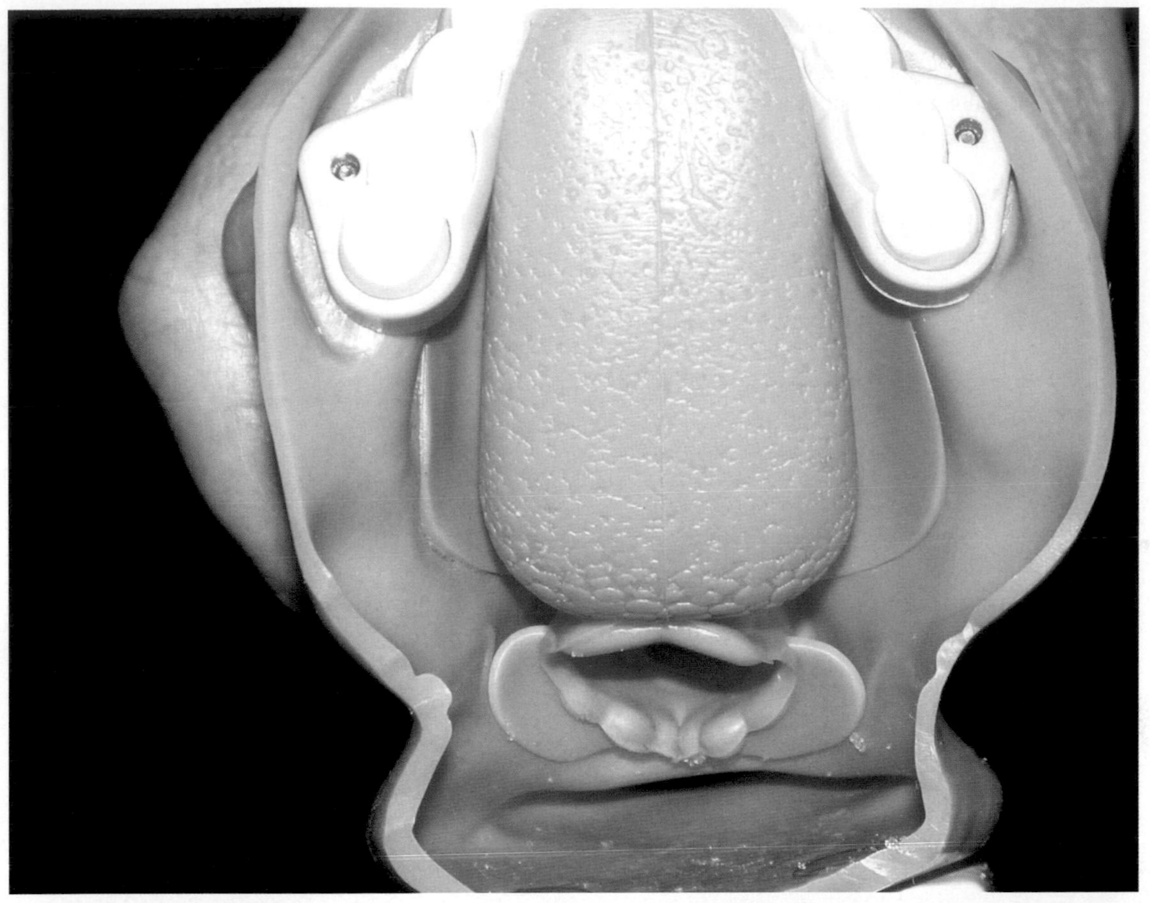

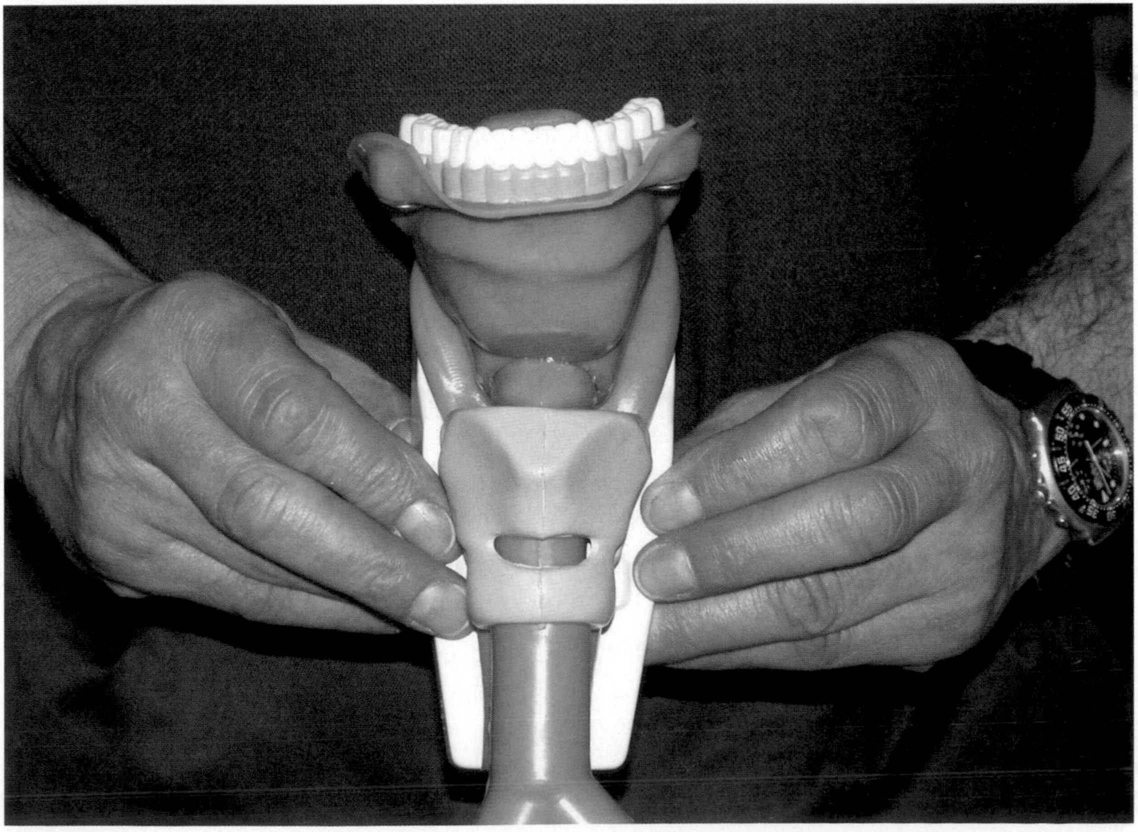

Anatomy of airway

Emergency tracheostomy

A formal surgical tracheostomy takes longer and is more difficult than a surgical cricothyroidotomy. Commercial sets are available for rapid tracheostomy using a Seldinger (guidewire) technique. This will be discussed in the skill station.

Oxygenation

The primary goal in providing supplementary oxygen is to maximise the delivery of oxygen to the cells. This is done by providing the highest possible oxygen concentration to the lungs, using high flow oxygen at 10–15 litres per minute. A pocket mask with an oxygen flow can deliver up to 55% oxygen. A correctly fitting bag-valve-mask system with a reservoir can be used to deliver up to 100% oxygen to the lungs.

Ventilation

Spontaneous ventilation (self-ventilation) means the same as breathing. Assisted (artificial) ventilation means the patient is receiving help with breathing. The aim is to improve gaseous exchange in the lungs and to breathe for the patient if spontaneous ventilation has stopped or is inadequate. The indication for assisted ventilation is when ventilation is inadequate as in:

- chest injury
- respiratory depression due to drugs (such as opiates)
- head injury.

Assisted ventilation can be achieved by the following techniques:

- mouth-to-mouth (or nose) – unlikely in hospital
- mouth to pocket-mask
- self-inflating bag to pocket mask or facemask
- self-inflating bag to endotracheal tube or tracheostomy tube
- automatic ventilation via endotracheal tube or tracheostomy tube.

These techniques will be practised in the skill stations.

Summary

- Talk, look, listen, feel
- Try simple manoeuvres, i.e. chin lift, jaw thrust, suction
- Try simple adjuncts, namely the oropharyngeal airway
- Tracheal intubation, endotracheal or surgical airway is gold standard because this makes the airway patent, maintains patency and protects airway
- Beware of cervical spine injury during airway management.

Algorithm 7.1 Neonatal resuscitation key points

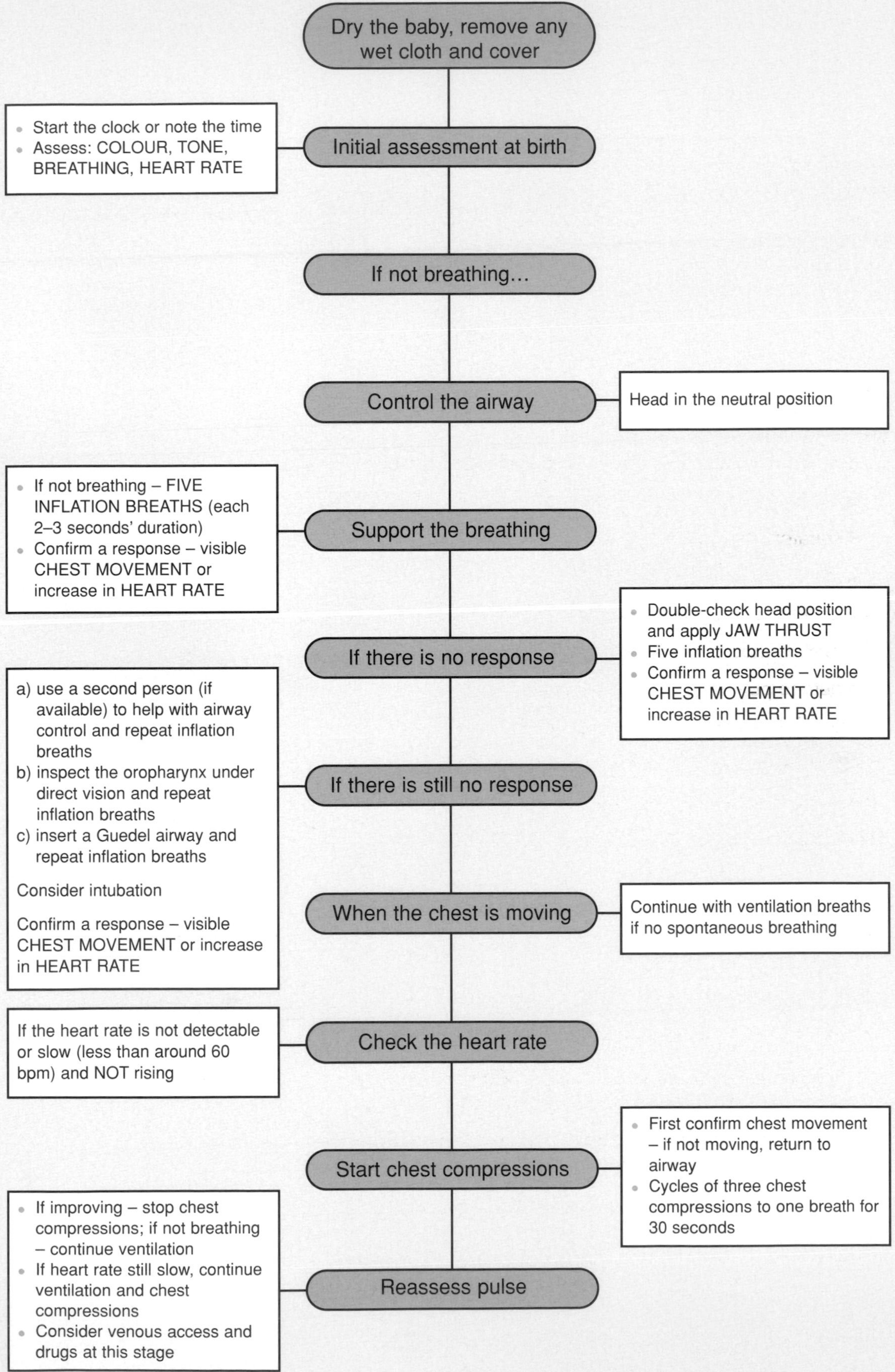

AT ALL STAGES, ASK... DO YOU NEED HELP?

Chapter 7

Neonatal resuscitation

Objectives

On successfully completing this topic, you will be able to:

- understand a structured approach to neonatal resuscitation
- understand the equipment and drugs used for neonatal resuscitation.

Introduction

The resuscitation of babies at birth is different from the resuscitation of all other age groups and knowledge of the relevant physiology and pathophysiology is essential. However, the majority of newly born babies will establish normal respiration and circulation spontaneously.

Normal physiology

After the delivery of a healthy term baby the first breath usually occurs within 60–90 seconds of clamping or obstructing the umbilical cord. Clamping of the cord leads to the onset of asphyxia, which is the major stimulant to start respiration. Physical stimuli such as cold air or physical discomfort may also provoke respiratory efforts. The first breaths are especially important, as the lungs are initially full of fluid.

Labour causes the fluid-producing cells within the lung to cease secretion and begin reabsorption of that fluid. During vaginal delivery up to 35 ml of fluid is expelled from the baby by uterine contraction. In a healthy baby the first spontaneous breaths generate a negative pressure of between –40 cm H_2O and –100 cm H_2O (–3.9 and –9.8 kPa), which inflates the lungs for the first time. This pressure is 10–15 times greater than that needed for later breathing when the lungs are aerated but is necessary to overcome the viscosity of fluid filling the airways, the surface tension of the fluid-filled lungs and the elastic recoil and resistance of the chest wall, lungs and airways. These powerful chest movements cause fluid to be displaced from the airways into the lymphatics.

In a 3-kg baby, up to 100 ml of fluid are cleared from the airways following the initial breaths, a process aided by full inflation and prolonged high pressure on expiration, i.e. crying. Bypassing labour and vaginal delivery by caesarean section before the onset of labour may slow the clearance of pulmonary fluid from the lungs and reduce the initial functional reserve capacity.

The first breaths produce the baby's functional residual capacity. This is less likely to occur following caesarean delivery performed before the onset of labour. Neonatal circulatory adaptation commences with the detachment of the placenta but lung inflation and alveolar distension releases mediators, which affect the pulmonary vasculature as well increasing oxygenation.

Surfactant (which is 85% lipid) is made by type-II (granular) pneumocytes in the alveolar epithelium. Surfactant reduces alveolar surface tension and prevents alveolar collapse on expiration. Surfactant can be demonstrated from 20 weeks of gestation, but the increase is slow until a surge in production at 30–34 weeks. Surfactant is released at birth due to aeration and distension of the alveoli. The half-life of surfactant is approximately 12 hours. Production is reduced by hypothermia (less than 35°C), hypoxia and acidosis (pH less than 7.25).

Pathophysiology

Our knowledge of the pathophysiology of fetal asphyxia is based on pioneering animal work in the early 1960s. The results of these experiments, which followed the physiology of newborn animals during prolonged asphyxia and subsequent resuscitation, are summarised in Figure 7.1.

When the placental oxygen supply is interrupted the fetus initiates breathing movements. Should these fail to provide an alternative oxygen supply (as they will obviously fail to do *in utero*) the baby loses consciousness. If hypoxia continues then the respiratory centre becomes unable to continue initiating breathing and breathing stops, usually within two to three minutes (primary apnoea, Figure 7.1). Babies have a number of automatic reflex responses to such a situation, conserving energy by shutting down the circulation to non-vital organs. Bradycardia ensues but blood pressure is maintained, primarily by peripheral vasoconstriction but also by an increased stroke volume. After a latent period of apnoea (primary), which may vary in duration, primitive spinal centres no longer suppressed by the respiratory centre exert an effect by initiating primitive gasping breaths. These deep spontaneous gasps are easily distinguishable from normal respirations as they occur 6–12 times per minute and involve all accessory muscles in a maximal inspiratory effort. After a while, if hypoxia continues, even this activity ceases (terminal apnoea, Figure 7.1). The time taken for such activity to cease is longer in the newly born baby than in later life, taking up to 20 minutes.

The circulation is almost always maintained until all respiratory activity ceases. This resilience is a feature of all newborn mammals at term, largely due to the reserves of glycogen in the heart. Resuscitation is therefore relatively easy if undertaken before all respiratory activity has stopped. Once the lungs are inflated, oxygen will be carried to the heart and then to the brain. Recovery will then be rapid. Most infants who have not progressed to terminal apnoea will resuscitate themselves if their airway is patent.

Once gasping ceases, however, the circulation starts to fail and these infants are likely to need extensive resuscitation.

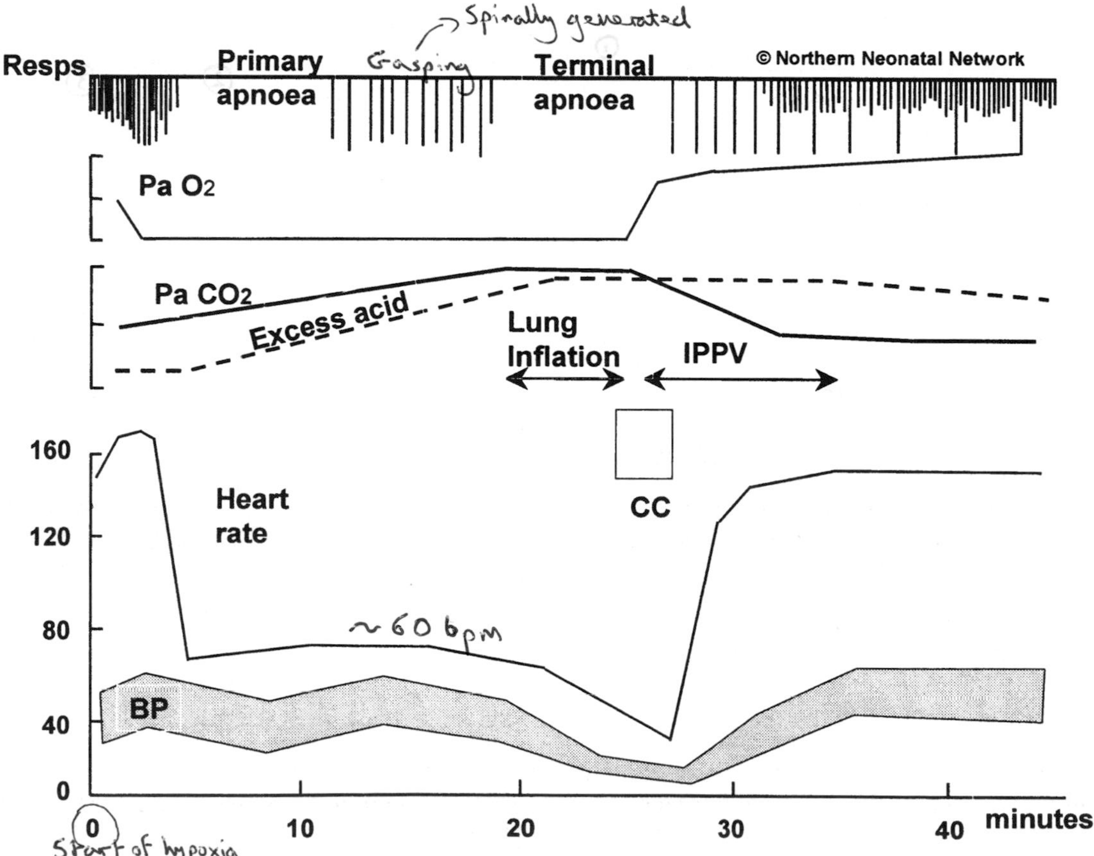

Figure 7.1 Effects of asphyxia (reproduced with permission from the Northern Neonatal Network)

Meconium

Hypoxia *in utero* in the term infant (over 37 weeks), leads to gut vessel vasoconstriction, increased peristalsis and a relaxation of the sphincters. This can result in the passage of meconium *in utero*. In addition, fetal hypoxia, as described above, if severe enough may lead to gasping and aspiration of amniotic fluid with meconium before birth.

Once the baby is delivered, meconium causes problems related to complete or partial airway obstruction. With the asphyxial insult, this combines to produce a multi-organ problem, which is fortunately relatively uncommon in the UK.

Slight colouration of liquor with meconium is not significant.

Practical aspects of neonatal resuscitation

Most babies, even those born apnoeic, will resuscitate themselves given a clear airway. The basic approach to resuscitation is Airway, Breathing and Circulation but there are a number of additions to the formula:

- Get help.
- Start the clock.
- Dry, wrap and keep baby warm.
- Assess the baby.

Call for help

- Airway
- Breathing (lung inflation and ventilation)
- Circulation

Ask for help if you expect or encounter any difficulty.

Start the clock

If available, or note the time.

Temperature control

Dry the baby off immediately and then wrap in a dry towel. Cold babies have an increased oxygen consumption and are more likely to become hypoglycaemic and acidotic, they also have an increased mortality. If this is not addressed at the beginning of resuscitation it is often forgotten. Most of the heat loss is by latent heat of evaporation – hence the need to dry the baby and then to wrap the baby in a dry towel. Babies also have a large surface area-to-weight ratio – heat can be lost very quickly.

Ideally, delivery should take place in a warm room and an overhead heater should be switched on. However, drying effectively and wrapping the baby in a warm dry towel is the most important factor in avoiding hypothermia.

A naked wet baby can still become hypothermic despite a warm room and a radiant heater, especially if there is a draught.

Assessment of the newborn

The Apgar score was proposed as a tool for evaluating a baby's condition at birth. Although the score, calculated at one and five minutes, may be of some use retrospectively, it is almost always recorded subjectively and it is not used to guide resuscitation.

Acute assessment is made by assessing:

- Colour (pink, blue, white)
- Respiration (rate and quality)
- Heart rate (fast, slow, absent)
- Tone (unconscious, apnoeic babies are floppy).

This will categorise the baby into one of the three following groups:

1. Pink, regular respirations, heart rate fast (more than 100 bpm)

These are healthy babies and they should be kept warm and given to their mothers.

2. Blue, irregular or inadequate respirations, heart rate slow (60 bpm or less)

If gentle stimulation does not induce effective breathing, the airway should be opened and cleared. If the baby responds then no further resuscitation is needed. If not, progress to lung inflation.

3. Blue or white, apnoeic, heart rate slow (less than 60 bpm) or absent

Whether an apnoeic baby is in primary or secondary apnoea (Figure 7.1) the initial management is the same.

Open the airway and then inflate the lungs.

A reassessment of any heart-rate response then directs further resuscitation. Reassess heart rate and respiration at regular intervals throughout.

White colour, apnoea and low or absent heart rate suggest terminal apnoea. However, initial management of such babies is unchanged but resuscitation may be prolonged.

Depending upon the assessment, resuscitation follows:

- Airway
- Breathing
- Circulation

with the use of drugs in selected cases.

Airway

Position the baby with the head in the neutral position. Overextension may collapse the newborn baby's pharyngeal airway just as flexion will. Beware the large, often moulded, occiput.

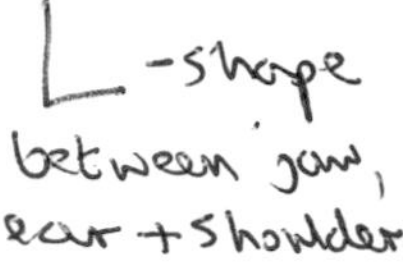

A folded towel placed under the neck and shoulders may help to maintain the airway in a neutral position and a jaw thrust may be needed to bring the tongue forward and open the airway, especially if the baby is floppy.

Gentle suction of nares and oropharynx with a soft suction catheter may stimulate respiration. Blind deep pharyngeal suction should be avoided as it may cause vagally induced bradycardia and laryngospasm.

Meconium aspiration

Meconium-stained liquor in various guises is relatively common. Happily, meconium aspiration is a rare event. Meconium aspiration usually happens *in utero* before delivery. It may be helpful to aspirate any meconium from the mouth and nose on the perineum.

If the baby is vigorous, a randomised trial has shown that no specific action (other than drying and wrapping the baby) is needed. If the baby is not vigorous, inspect the oropharynx with a laryngoscope and aspirate any particulate meconium seen using a wide bore catheter. Suction should not exceed –100 mmHg (9.8 kPa).

If intubation is possible and the baby is still unresponsive, aspirate the trachea using the tracheal tube as a suction catheter. However, if intubation cannot be achieved immediately, clear the oropharynx and start mask inflation. If, while attempting to clear the airway, the heart rate falls to less than 60 bpm then stop airway clearance and start inflating the chest.

Breathing (inflation breaths and ventilation)

The first five breaths should be inflation breaths. These should be two- to three-second sustained breaths using a continuous gas supply, a pressure-limiting device and a mask. Use a transparent, circular, soft mask big enough to cover the nose and mouth of the baby (Figure 7.2). If no such system is available then a 500-ml self-inflating bag and a blow-off valve set at 30–40 cm H_2O can be used.

The chest may not move during the first one to three breaths as fluid is displaced. Once the chest is inflated reassess the heart rate. Assess air entry by chest movement not by auscultation. In fluid-filled lungs, breath sounds may be heard without lung inflation. However, it is safe to assume that the chest has been inflated successfully if the heart rate responds.

Once the chest is inflated, ventilation is continued at a rate of 30–40 ventilations per minute.

Circulation

If the heart rate remains slow (less than 60 bpm) once the lungs are inflated, cardiac compressions must be started. The most efficient way of doing this in the neonate is to encircle the chest with both hands, so that the fingers lie behind the baby and the thumbs are apposed on the sternum just below the inter-nipple line. Compress the chest briskly, to one third of its diameter. Current advice is to perform three compressions for each inflation of the chest.

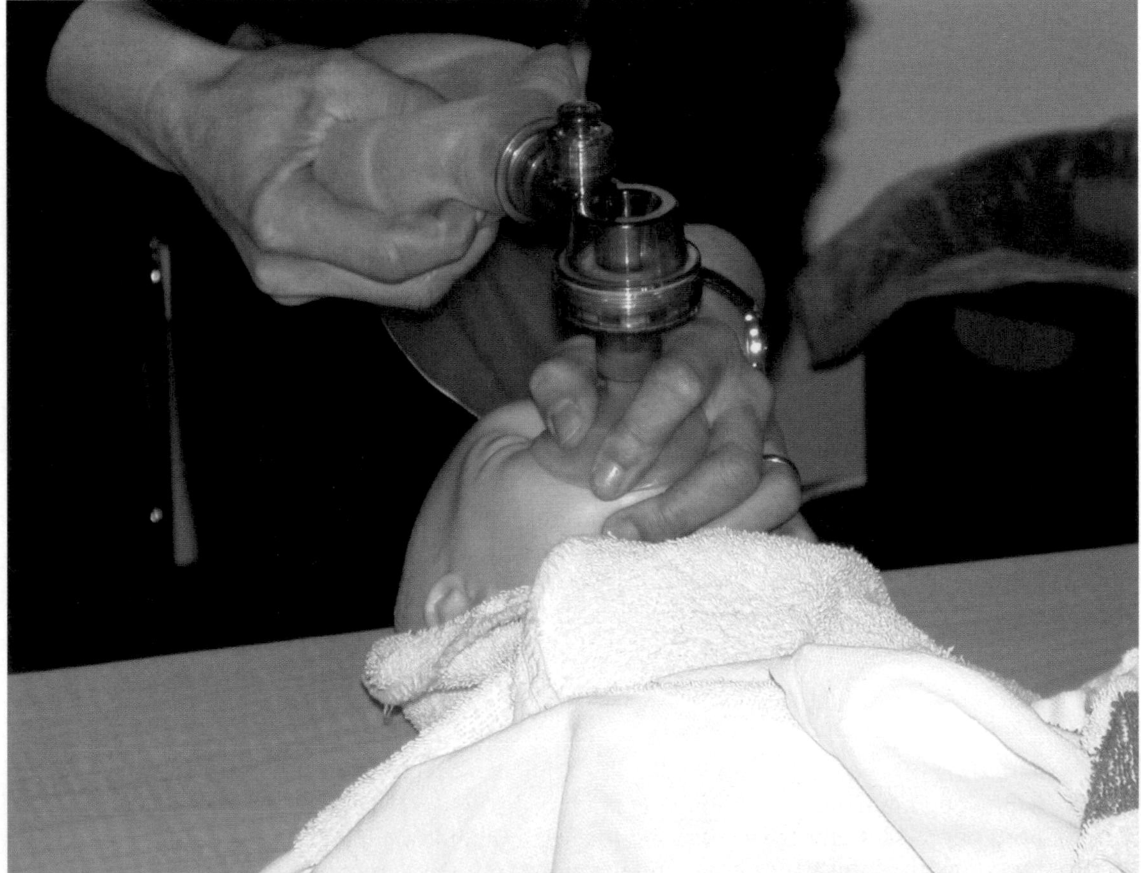

Figure 7.2 Bag value mask ventilation of neonate

The purpose of cardiac compression is to move oxygenated blood or drugs to the coronary arteries in order to initiate cardiac recovery. Thus, there is no point in cardiac compression before the lungs have been inflated. Similarly, compressions are ineffective unless interposed breaths are of good quality and inflate the chest. The emphasis must be upon good-quality breaths followed by effective compressions.

Once the heart rate is above 60 bpm and rising, cardiac compression can be discontinued.

Drugs

If, after adequate lung inflation and cardiac compression, the heart rate has not responded, drug therapy should be considered. However, the most common reason for failure of the heart rate to respond is failure to achieve lung inflation. Airway and breathing must be reassessed as adequate before proceeding to drug therapy. Venous access will be required via an umbilical venous line, as drugs should be given centrally (Figure 7.3). The outcome is poor if drugs are required for resuscitation.

Epinephrine (adrenaline)

In the presence of profound unresponsive bradycardia or circulatory standstill, 10 micrograms/kg (0.1 ml/kg 1:10 000) epinephrine may be given intravenously or endotracheally. Further doses of 10–30 micrograms/kg (0.1–0.3 ml 1:10 000) may be tried at three- to five-minute intervals if there is no response. For this drug, the endotracheal route is accepted but effectiveness is unproven in resuscitation at birth.

Bicarbonate

Any baby who is in terminal apnoea will have a significant metabolic acidosis. Acidosis depresses cardiac function and, in a highly acidotic environment epinephrine, does not bind to receptors. Bicarbonate 1 mmol/kg (2 ml/kg of 4.2% solution) is used to raise the pH and enhance the effects of oxygen and epinephrine.

Bicarbonate remains controversial and should only be used in the absence of discernible cardiac output or in profound and unresponsive bradycardia.

Dextrose

Hypoglycaemia is a potential problem for all stressed or asphyxiated babies. It is treated by using a slow bolus of 5 ml/kg of 10% dextrose intravenously and then providing a secure intravenous dextrose infusion at a rate of 100 ml/kg/day 10% dextrose. Reagent strips (such as BM Stix®) are not reliable in neonates when reading less than 5 mmol/l.

Fluid

Very occasionally, hypovolaemia may be present because of known or suspected blood loss (antepartum haemorrhage, placenta or vasa praevia, unclamped cord) or be secondary to loss of vascular tone following asphyxia. Volume expansion, initially with 10 ml/kg, may be appropriate. Normal saline can be used; alternatively, Gelofusine® (Braun) (succinylated gelatin) has been used safely. If blood loss is acute and severe, non-crossmatched O-negative blood should be given immediately. However, most newborn or neonatal resuscitations do not require fluid unless there has been known blood loss or septicaemic shock.

Naloxone

This is not a drug of resuscitation. Occasionally, a baby who has been effectively resuscitated and is pink, with a heart rate over 100 bpm, may not breathe because of the effects of maternal opiates. If respiratory depressant effects are suspected the baby should be given naloxone intramuscularly (200 micrograms in a full-term baby). Smaller doses of 10 micrograms/kg will also reverse the sedation but the effect will only last a short time (20 minutes IV or a few hours IM).

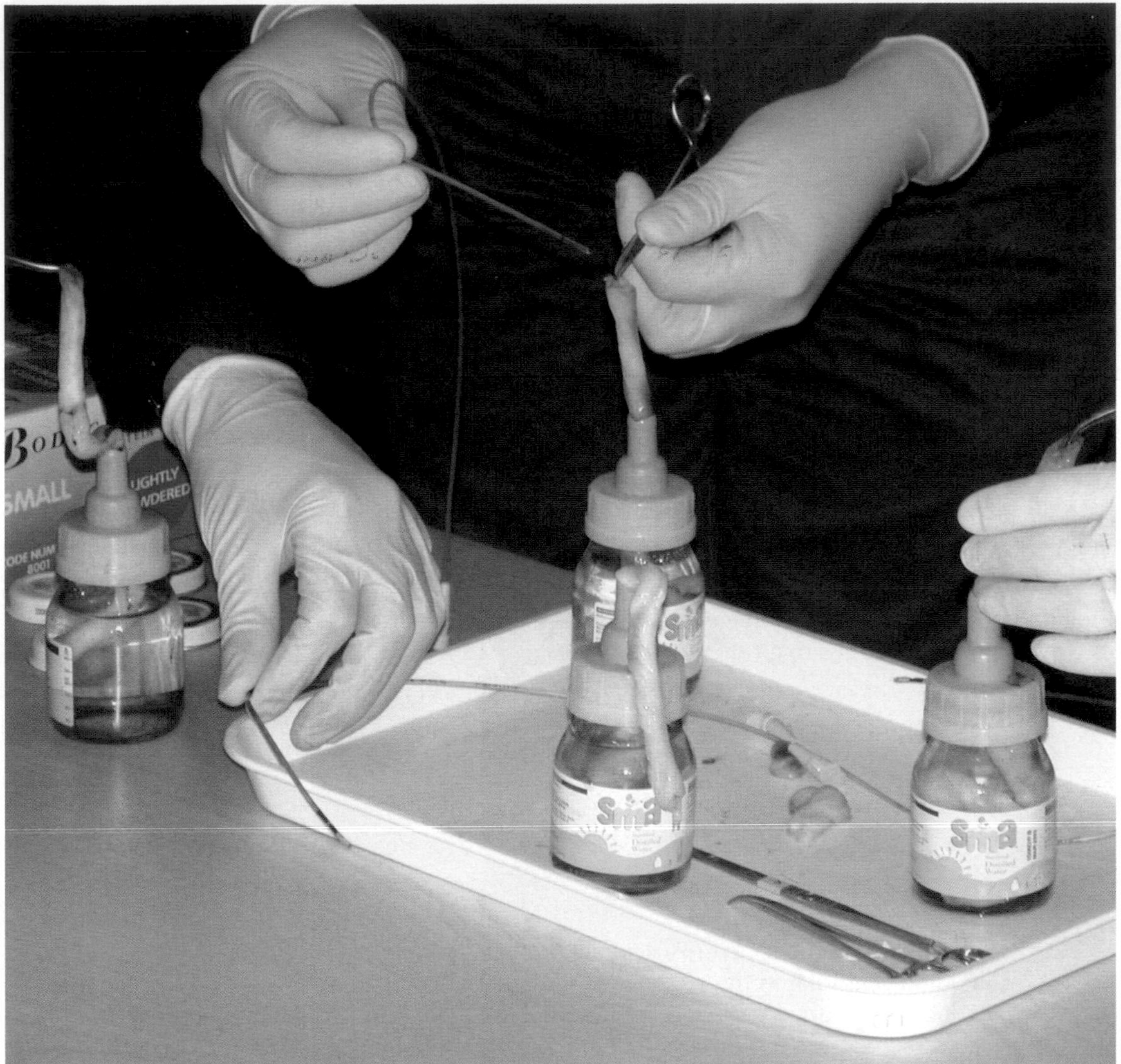

Figure 7.3 Umbilical vein catheterisation

Atropine and calcium gluconate

Atropine and calcium gluconate have no place in newborn resuscitation. Atropine may, rarely, be useful in the neonatal unit, when vagal stimulation has produced resistant bradycardia or asystole.

Response to resuscitation

Often, the first indication of success will be an increase in heart rate. Recovery of respiratory drive may be delayed. Babies in terminal apnoea will tend to gasp first as they recover before starting normal respirations. Those who were in primary apnoea are likely to start with normal breaths, which may commence at any stage of resuscitation.

Tracheal intubation

Most babies can be adequately resuscitated using a mask system. Swedish data[39] suggest that if this is applied adequately, only 1 in 500 babies actually needs intubation. However, endotracheal intubation remains the gold standard in airway management. It is especially useful in prolonged resuscitations, preterm babies and cases of meconium aspiration. It should be considered if mask ventilation has failed, although the most common reason for failure with mask inflation is poor positioning of the head with consequent failure to open the airway.

The technique of intubation is the same for infants and will be taught in the skill stations. A normal full-term newborn usually needs a 3.5-mm endotracheal tube, but 3.0-mm and 2.5-mm tubes should also be available.

Preterm babies

The more preterm a baby is, the less likely it is to establish adequate respirations. Preterm babies (less than 32 weeks) are likely to be deficient in surfactant. Effort of respiration will be increased although musculature will be less developed. One must anticipate that babies born before 32 weeks may need help to establish prompt aeration and ventilation.

Preterm babies with surfactant deficiency may need **relatively** higher inflation pressures than term babies. It is appropriate to start with a pressure of 2.0–2.5 kPa (20–25 cm H_2O) but to increase this if there is no heart rate response and chest movement is inadequate after initial breaths.

Preterm babies are more likely to get cold (higher surface area to mass ratio) and more likely to be hypoglycaemic (fewer glycogen stores).

Actions in the event of poor initial response to resuscitation

1. **Check airway and breathing.**

2. **Check for a technical fault:**
   - is oxygen connected?
   - is mask ventilation effective? Auscultate both axillae and observe movement
   - is endotracheal tube in the trachea? Auscultate both axillae and observe movement
   - is endotracheal tube in the right bronchus? Auscultate both axillae and observe movement
   - is endotracheal tube blocked? If there is doubt about the position or patency of the endotracheal tube replace it.
   - Is a longer inflation time required?

3. **Does the baby have a pneumothorax?**
   This occurs spontaneously in up to 1% of newborns but those needing action in the delivery unit are exceptionally rare. Auscultate the chest for asymmetry of breath sounds. A cold light source can be used to transilluminate the chest – a pneumothorax may show as a hyper-illuminating area.

   If a tension pneumothorax is thought to be present clinically, a 21-gauge butterfly needle should be inserted through the second intercostal space in the mid-clavicular line. Alternatively, a 22-gauge cannula may be used, connected to a three-way tap. Remember that you may well cause a pneumothorax during this procedure.

4. **Does the baby remain cyanosed despite breathing with a good heart rate?**
   There may be a congenital heart malformation, which may be duct-dependent or persistent pulmonary hypertension of the newborn.

5. **If the baby is pink with a good heart rate but not breathing effectively, it may be suffering the effects of maternal opiates.**
   In this situation, naloxone 200 micrograms IM may be given. This should outlast the opiate effect.

6. Is there severe anaemia or hypovolaemia?

In the face of large blood loss, 20 ml/kg O-negative blood or a volume expander should be given.

Discontinuation of resuscitation

Such a decision should be taken be taken by a senior member of the team, ideally a consultant. This means that help must have been called. The outcome for a baby with no cardiac output after 15 minutes of resuscitation is likely to be very poor.

Avoid 4 'H's

Hypoxia
Hypothermia
Hyperinflation
Hypoglycaemia

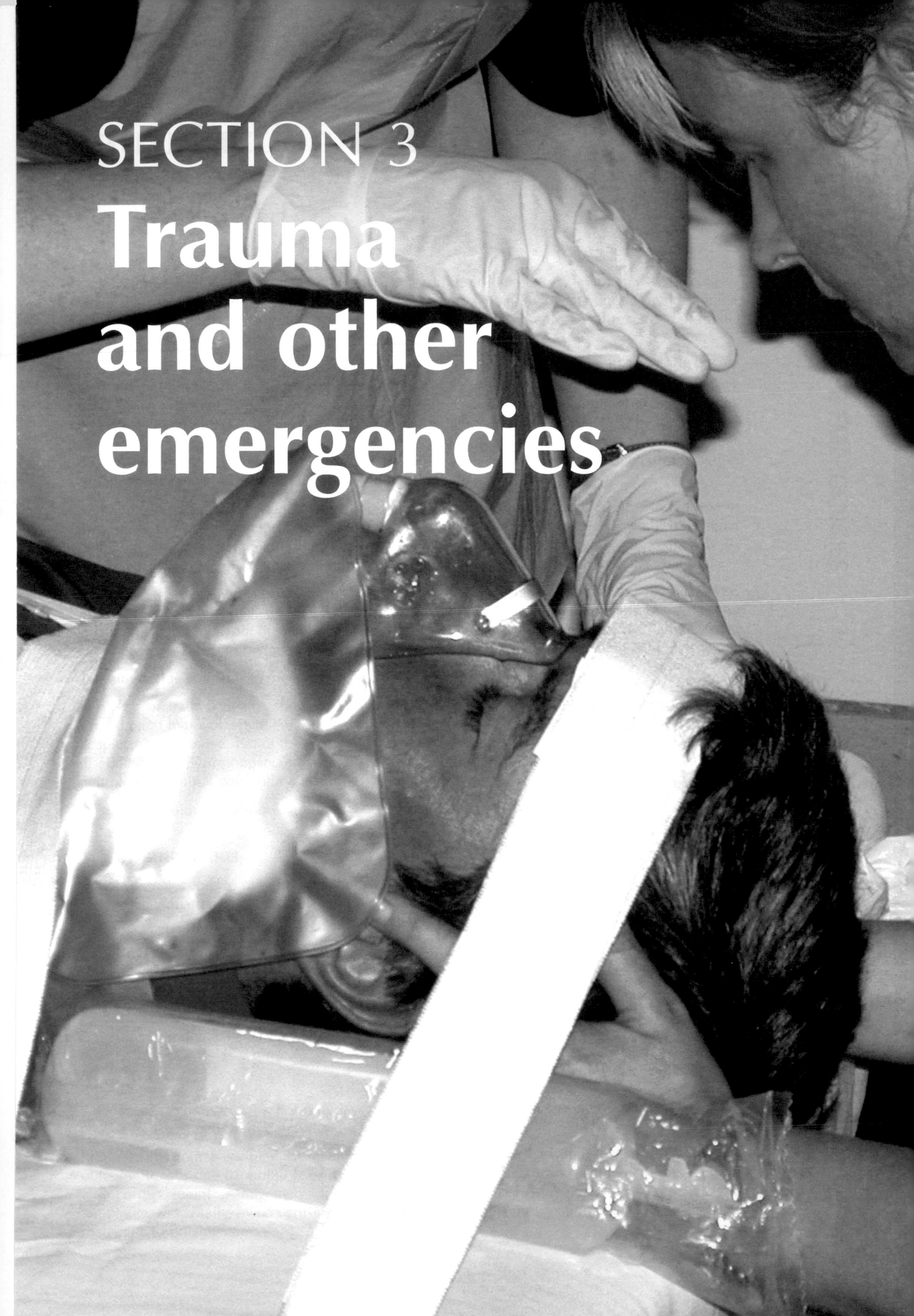

SECTION 3

Trauma and other emergencies

Consider anti-D treatment in all pregnant trauma patients, even if the trauma is minor.

Clear chronological records of assessment of injuries, treatment and reassessment findings should be made and signed, timed and dated.

Communication with the patient, with relatives and with the multidisciplinary team is essential for success.

Algorithm 8.1. Thoracic emergencies key points

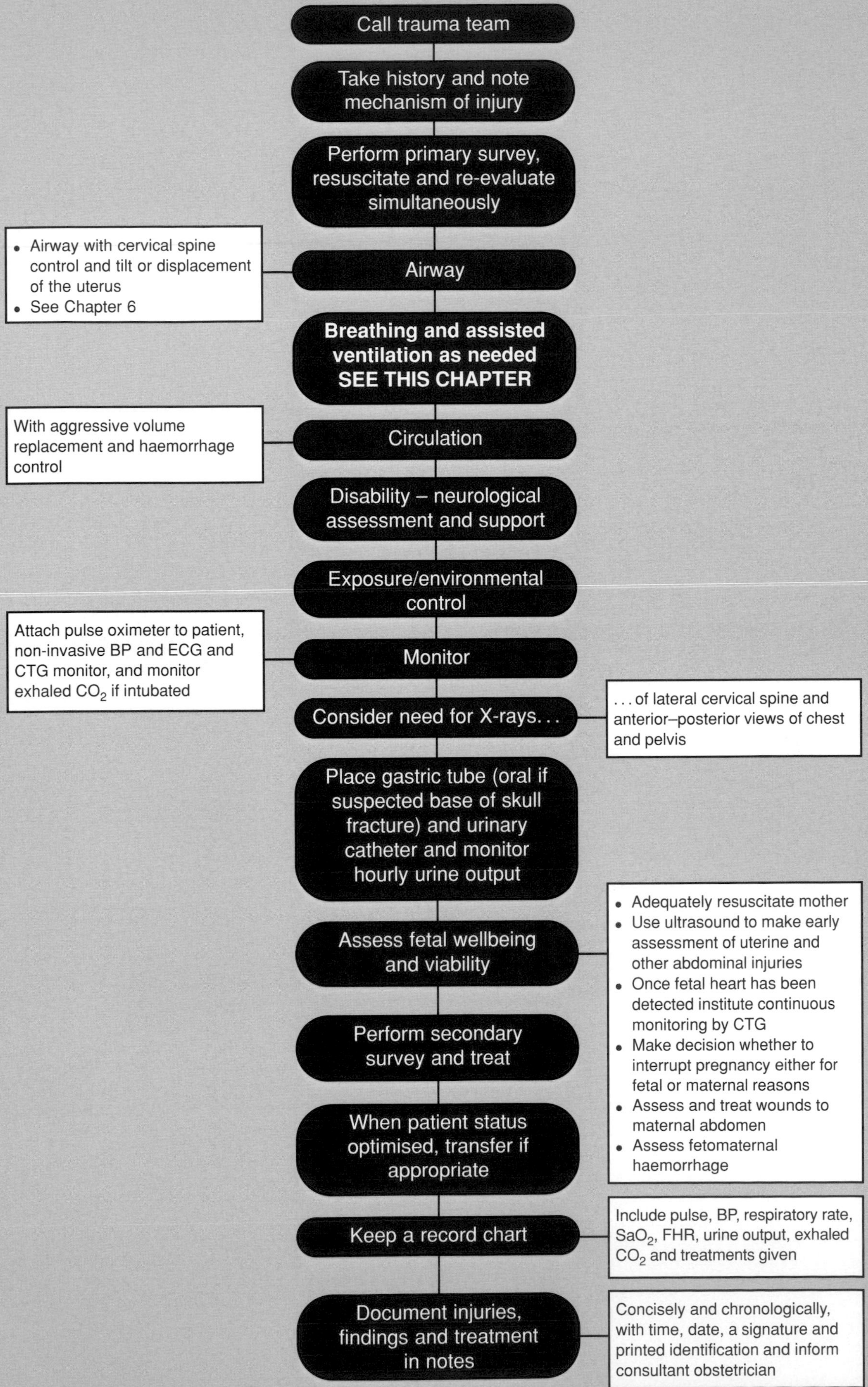

Chapter 8

Thoracic emergencies

Objectives

On successfully completing this topic, you will be able to:

- identify six life-threatening injuries
- identify six potentially life-threatening injuries
- identify the skills required to manage life-threatening injuries.

Introduction and incidence

Chest injuries are common in patients with major trauma and they are responsible for around one-quarter of the fatalities. Many of these deaths can be prevented by the prompt recognition of life-threatening conditions and the early initiation of simple methods of treatment. Very few patients will require surgery, with the majority requiring standard resuscitation and the safe evacuation of air or blood from the pleural cavity with an intercostal drain. Prompt and effective resuscitation of the mother, including the avoidance of aortocaval compression is the most effective way of ensuring good fetoplacental perfusion. Although it is an infrequent event to be presented with a pregnant patient with chest trauma, it should be pointed out that the CEMD reported five deaths from rupture of the thoracic aorta and its branches.

Types of injury

Chest injuries are usually classified as:

- penetrating
- blunt
- both.

It must be appreciated that while there may be external signs of thoracic injury, intra-abdominal organs including the gravid uterus may also have been damaged, particularly in the later stages of pregnancy. The reverse is also true, in that obvious abdominal trauma may extend into the chest. In general, penetrating injuries will require surgical exploration.

Primary survey and resuscitation

An accurate incident history is vital and should highlight potential organ-system injuries. For example, the driver of a car in collision with a tree would be at risk of a traumatic brain injury, cervical-spine trauma, traumatic aortic rupture, lung and myocardial contusion and abdominal trauma, in addition to many other bony and soft-tissue injuries.

The principles of management are:

- **primary survey and resuscitation**
  Life-threatening injuries discovered during the primary survey should be dealt with immediately.

Algorithm 9.1. Shock key points

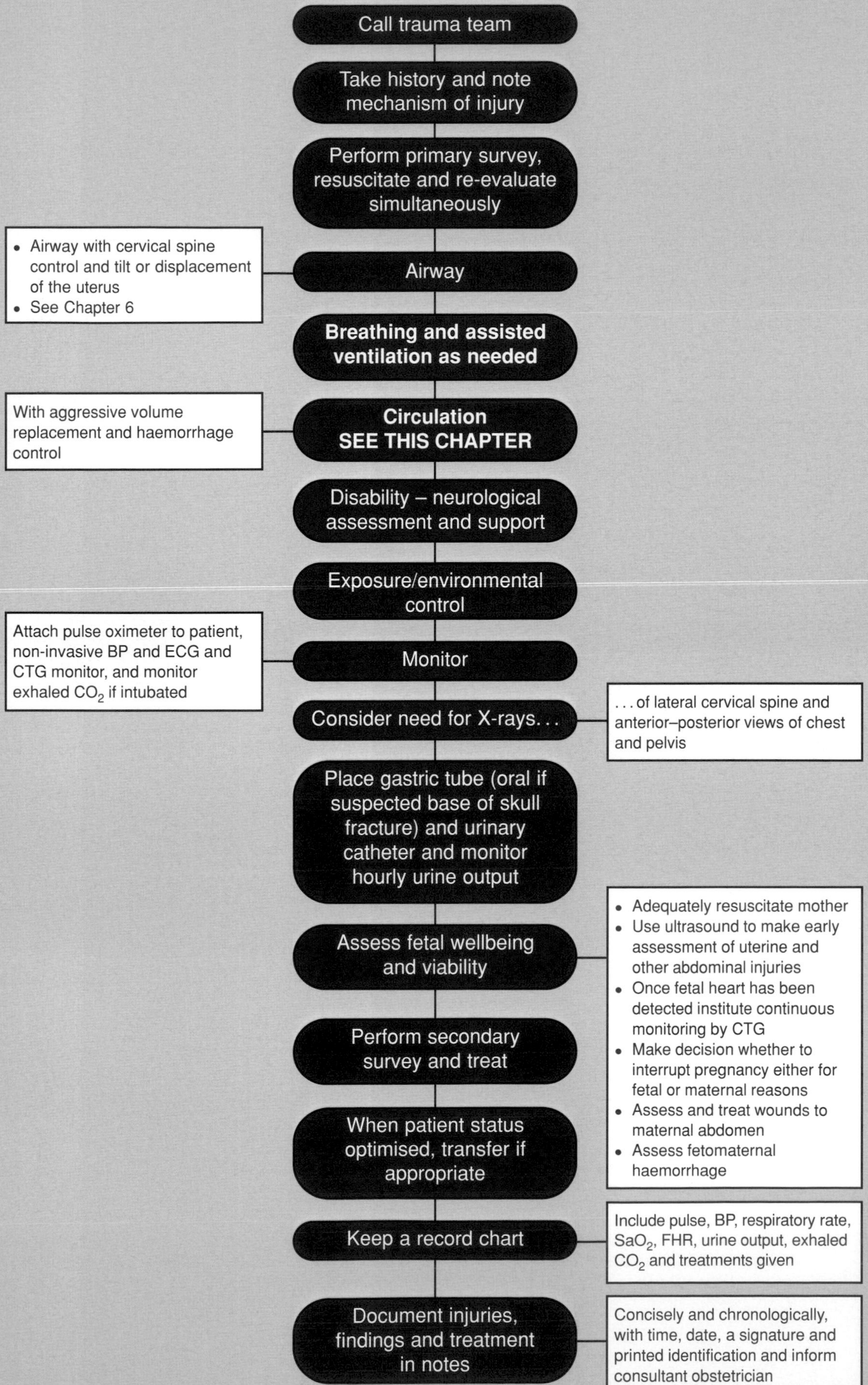

Chapter 9

Shock

Objectives

On successfully completing this topic, you will be able to:

- define shock
- relate the physiological changes to the cardiovascular system in pregnancy and how they affect the presentation of hypovolaemia
- recognise shock
- discuss the principles of treatment of hypovolaemic shock
- identify other shock syndromes and understand their management.

Introduction

Shock is inadequate tissue perfusion. Inadequate tissue perfusion means imminent cell death.

The treatment of shock is directed towards restoring cellular and organ perfusion with adequately oxygenated blood.

Physiological changes to the cardiovascular system in pregnancy

To maintain organ perfusion an adequate cardiac output is required.

Cardiac output = Stroke volume x heart rate

Stroke volume is determined by preload.

Preload denotes the venous return to the heart. In the heavily pregnant patient the uterus may lie on the vena cava and reduce the venous return to the heart.

Vena caval and aortic compression may reduce cardiac output by up to 30%. This is known as supine hypotension. To prevent this the heavily pregnant patient must always be tilted or have the uterus manually displaced to the left to reduce the pressure on the inferior vena cava.

Remember 'Hello How are you Mrs Tilt?'

Any shock is exacerbated by vena caval obstruction.

A further consideration in pregnancy is that the plasma volume and red-cell volume increase to make a total increase in circulating blood volume. The pregnant patient may lose 1200–1500 ml of blood before showing any signs of hypovolaemia (35% of her circulating blood volume). The compensatory mechanism is the shutting down of blood flow to the fetoplacental unit. Blood loss in the mother therefore may first be reflected by fetal distress. The major consideration if there is any suspicion of haemorrhage in the mother is 'Is the fetoplacental unit being perfused?' The fetal heart rate should be monitored to assess this.

In trauma, hypovolaemia is by far the most common cause of shock.

Recognition of hypovolaemia

The most common cause of hypotension in trauma is hypovolaemia but remember that hypotension is a very late sign, developing only when significant blood loss has occurred, in pregnancy particularly.

Successful outcome depends on the early recognition of shock, restoration of volume and control of haemorrhage.

Signs of hypovolaemia are:

- increase in heart rate
- cold, pale, sweaty, cyanosed skin
- alteration of mental state
- fall in urine output
- narrowed pulse pressure
- hypotension (late sign).

Mental state

If the patient is conscious and talking sensibly, he is not only breathing through an open airway, he is perfusing his cerebral cortex with sufficient oxygenated blood (50% of the normal cardiac output). Increasing hypovolaemia and subsequent cerebral hypoxia cause alterations in the level of consciousness. These alterations begin with anxiety and, if untreated, proceed through confusion and aggressiveness to eventual unresponsiveness and death.

Think of the skin, kidneys and brain as 'end organs' that monitor the adequacy of perfusion, i.e. the adequacy of circulating, oxygenated blood.

Capillary refill

This is a quantification of skin perfusion. It is performed by compressing a fingernail for five seconds. The test is normal if colour returns within two seconds of releasing compression (the time taken to say the words 'capillary refill').

Classification of circulating volume lost

Haemorrhage is the acute loss of circulating blood. In the non-pregnant adult 7% of bodyweight is circulating blood (approximately five litres in a 70 kg adult or 70 ml/kg of bodyweight). In children, circulating volume is calculated to be 8–9% of body weight (80 ml/kg of bodyweight) and in term pregnant women the circulating volume increases by about 40% (100 ml/kg of bodyweight).

This classification applies to the non-pregnant patient. It is useful in identifying the signs of hypovolaemia and relating them to level of loss.

Have a low threshold of suspicion for bleeding and fluid replacement, particularly in the pregnant patient in whom signs of hypovolaemia are only manifest when they have lost much more. Consider again: is the fetoplacental unit being perfused or has perfusion fallen due to blood loss?

Class I

Loss of less than 15% of circulating volume (up to 750 ml in a 70 kg adult). This is fully compensated by the diversion of blood from the splanchnic pool. There are no abnormal symptoms and signs other than minimal tachycardia. In otherwise healthy patients this blood loss does not require blood replacement.

Class II

Loss of 15–30% of circulating volume (750–1500 ml in a 70-kg adult) requires peripheral vasoconstriction to maintain systolic blood pressure. Symptoms are tachycardia, tachypnoea and the pulse pressure is narrowed because of raised diastolic blood pressure. Crystalloid fluid replacement will be required.

Class III

Loss of 30–40% of circulating volume (1500–2000 ml in a 70-kg adult).

There is tachycardia, tachypnoea, changes in mental status and a measurable fall in systolic blood pressure because peripheral vasoconstriction fails to compensate for the increasing loss. Note it is only at this stage of loss that there is a fall in systolic pressure. Patients with this blood loss require transfusion.

Class IV

Loss of more than 40% of circulating volume (over 2000 ml in a 70-kg adult) is immediately life threatening. Symptoms are tachycardia, fall in blood pressure, narrowing of pulse pressure, negligible urine output, altered mental status. Loss of more than 50% circulating volume results in loss of consciousness. These patients require transfusion and immediate surgical intervention.

Classification of circulating volume lost

Class	Circulating volume (%)
I	0–15
II	15–30
III	30–40
IV	> 40

Think of a tennis match!

Pitfalls in the recognition of shock

- In pregnancy, as described above.
- Infants have a resting heart rate of 160 bpm. Preschool children have a normal heart rate of 140 bpm. For children from school age to puberty the normal heart rate is 120 bpm. A tachycardia therefore is a rise in heart rate above these.
- The elderly do not always mount a tachycardia as the myocardium is less responsive to catecholamines.
- People with pacemakers have a fixed upper-heart rate.
- Athletes may have a very slow baseline heart rate.
- People on beta-blockers are relatively unable to mount a tachycardia.
- Haemoglobin level is an unreliable measure of acute blood loss. If it is low or has fallen by the early stages of shock this is suggestive of very severe loss.

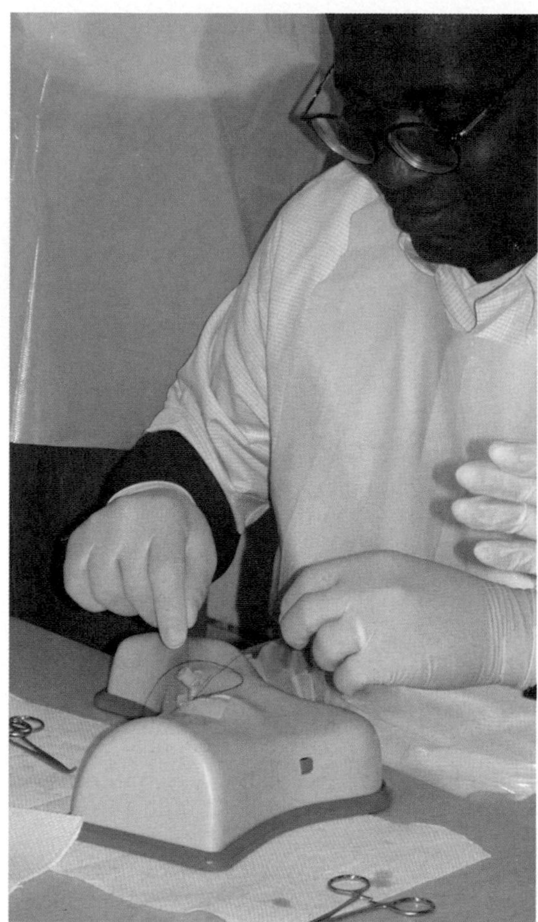

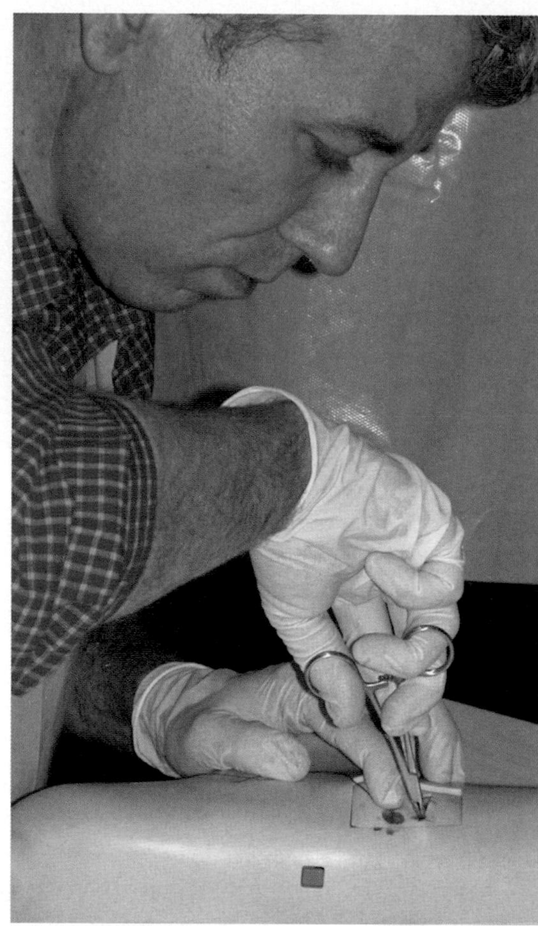

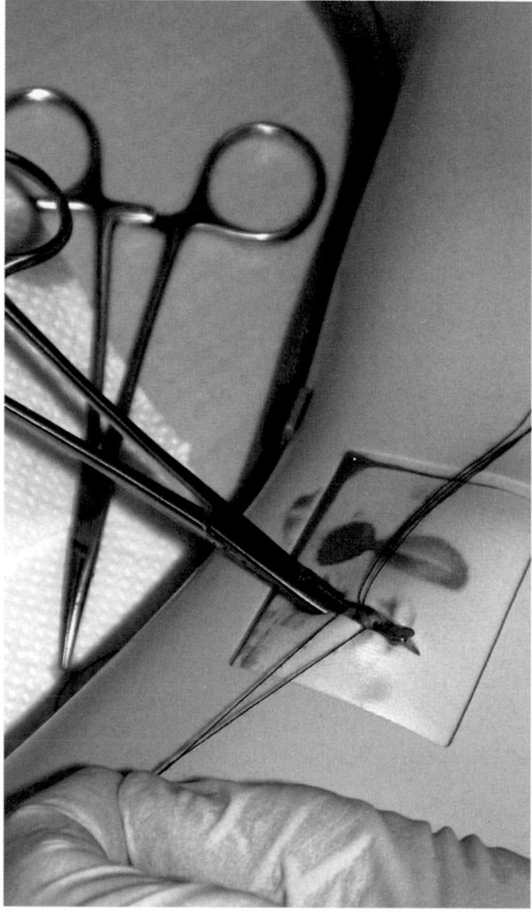

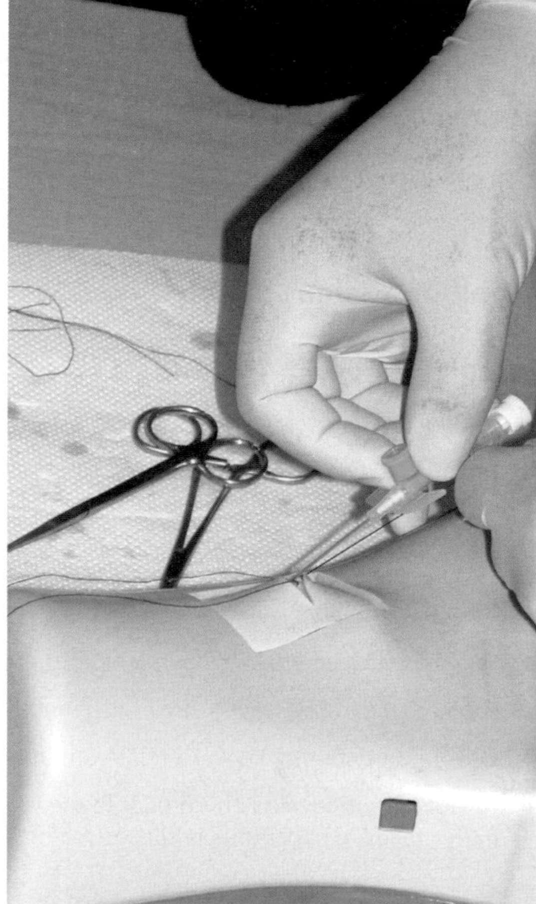

Stages in intravenous cutdown

Principles of treatment of hypovolaemic shock

Primary survey and resuscitation according to the **A**, **B**, **C** principle (see Chapter 6).

Clear the airway (protect the cervical spine when appropriate) and deliver oxygen at 10–15 litres per minute via tight-fitting facemask with reservoir bag. Correct any life-threatening breathing difficulties.

Diagnosis of hypovolaemic shock must be promptly followed by restoration of adequate circulating volume **and** stopping the bleeding. There is no place for 'hypotensive' resuscitation in the pregnant patient.

Consider haemorrhage to be of two types:

- compressible
- non-compressible.

Compressible haemorrhage is controllable by direct pressure, limb elevation, packing or by reduction and immobilisation of fractures.

In the case of pelvic fractures, although surgery may be needed, some control of bleeding may be achieved by splinting the pelvis using a pelvic splint as part of the resuscitation process (pelvic fixator).

Non-compressible haemorrhage is bleeding into a body cavity (chest, abdomen, pelvis or retroperitoneum) that can only be controlled by surgery. Call the appropriate surgeon.

Blood loss in trauma may be into five sites ('blood on the floor and four more'):

1. external ('on the floor')
2. chest
3. abdomen
4. pelvis and retroperitoneum
5. around long-bone fractures (especially the femur).

Note: The presence of significant amounts of blood in the chest will be identified during **B**reathing in the primary survey. Identification of other sites of bleeding is an essential element of **C**irculation.

You must be highly suspicious in all cases of blunt abdominal injuries.

Some idea of blood volumes lost from different injuries can be seen from the following table:

Blood volumes lost from different injuries

Injury	Blood volume lost (litres)
Closed femoral fracture	1.5
Fractured pelvis	3.0
Fractured ribs (each)	0.15
One blood-filled hemithorax	2.0
A closed tibial fracture	0.5
An open wound the size of an adult hand	0.5
A clot the size of an adult fist	0.5

Replacement of lost volume

Intravenous access is best achieved by inserting as large a cannula as possible into each ante cubital fossa. 'Short and thick does the trick'. If peripheral cannulation cannot be achieved consider:

- intravenous cutdown

- femoral vein cannulation (avoid if possible in the pregnant patient)
- central venous access, if appropriate personnel.

Always warm fluids.

Crystalloids are physiological solutions that remain only temporarily in the intravascular space. They are useful for the immediate replacement of lost volume. Initially, two litres of crystalloid (Hartmann's solution/Ringer-Lactate solution) should be infused through wide-bore cannulae.

They are therefore less effective in maintaining intravascular volume. An overload may cause pulmonary and cerebral oedema (care in pre-eclampsia/eclampsia – consider central venous monitoring). Colloids remain in the intravascular compartment and may be preferred.

Treatment regimen (non-pregnant patient)

The response to resuscitation by intravenous fluids and the need for further intravenous fluids and/or surgery can be considered under four headings:

Response	Intervention needed
Type I	Signs improve and remain improved. No further fluid challenge is required.
Type II	An initial but unsustained improvement then regression to abnormal levels of these vital signs. This means that either the fluid has been redistributed from the intravascular compartment to the extravascular compartment or blood loss continues. Give a further intravenous challenge of two units of colloid or whole blood if available. If the vital signs return to acceptable levels, the response was due to redistribution of fluid. If vital signs remain abnormal then this is a Type III response.
Type III	Continue intravenous colloid or whole blood at flow rates sufficient to sustain resuscitation. This patient needs urgent surgery within the hour.
Type IV	No response to rapid intravenous infusion of crystalloid, colloid and/or blood. This patient needs immediate surgery (to 'turn off the tap') if she is to survive.

Management problems

Cooling

Transfusion of large amounts of blood can cause hypothermia. Take measures to prevent this. Transfuse through a blood warmer and warm blood (ask staff to hold it close to their own bodies), keep patient well covered, keep ambient temperature warm, consider warming mattresses and blankets.

Continuing haemorrhage

You must consider all potential sources of blood loss. Concealed haemorrhage is life-threatening and must be in the forefront of your mind in all hypovolaemic patients who respond poorly or do not respond to treatment – response types III and IV. Urgent surgery is required. You must also consider the possibility of coagulopathy when large volumes of fluids have been infused. Remember that stored blood contains fewer clotting factors than fresh blood and fresh frozen plasma. Give FFP in conjunction with blood.

Fluid overload

Fluid overload is unlikely to occur in severely injured, previously fit young adults. Fluid replacement should be titrated against haemodynamic effects, especially when estimates of loss can be calculated from the mechanism of injury and the haemorrhage is compressible. In pre-eclampsia/eclampsia, consider early central venous pressure monitoring.

Acid-base imbalance

Metabolic acidosis may develop with severe or long-standing shock as a result of inadequate tissue perfusion and subsequent anaerobic metabolism. The way to treat is to adequately resuscitate.

Other types of shock

Hypovolaemic shock is the most common in trauma. The differential diagnosis should also include cardiogenic, neurogenic, anaphylactic and septic shock. Clues can be gained from the history, careful secondary survey, selected additional tests and the response to treatment.

Cardiogenic shock

Myocardial dysfunction may occur following cardiac tamponade, myocardial contusion, air embolus, pulmonary embolus, tension pneumothorax or myocardial infarction. Ideally, all patients with blunt thoracic injury should have constant ECG monitoring. Measuring cardiac enzymes will not alter the acute management of myocardial infarction and are poor indicators of myocardial contusion.

Neurogenic shock

Damage to some parts of the brain stem or high thoracic or cervical spinal cord produces hypotension due to interruption of the sympathetic chain, with subsequent loss of vessel tone. Sympathetic denervation also removes the cardiac response to hypotension, that is, tachycardia. The vagus is unopposed, resulting in bradycardia, which may worsen if the vagus nerve is stimulated, for example, by passing an endotracheal tube or nasogastric tube. The patient with neurogenic shock demonstrates hypotension without tachycardia. The immediate treatment of symptomatic bradycardia in neurogenic shock is atropine 0.5–1.0 mg intravenously, but isoprenaline may be required.

Septic shock

In trauma, it is most likely to occur in patients with penetrating abdominal injuries and in whom the peritoneal cavity has been contaminated by intestinal contents. It is a recognised complication of delivery. The mechanism of shock is one of vasodilatation caused by bacterial toxins. If there has been no haemorrhage (or if haemorrhage has been adequately corrected) the patient, although hypotensive, will have a tachycardia and, initially, warm pink skin and a wide pulse pressure (a full bounding pulse). The very sick septic patient will be tachycardic, cyanosed and peripherally shut down. Septic patients have a metabolic acidosis, detectable on sampling of arterial or venous blood. See Chapter 26 for the management of sepsis in pregnancy.

Anaphylactic shock

You should suspect this uncommon mechanism of shock in any patient who has recently received medication or who has been exposed to other allergens, especially when the history is not known.

It causes symptoms that can include pruritus, erythema, flushing, urticaria, angio-oedema, nausea, diarrhoea, vomiting, laryngeal oedema, bronchospasm, hypotension, cardiovascular collapse and death.

Consider as a cause of cardiac arrest.

Anaphylactic reactions usually begin within 5–10 minutes of exposure and the full reaction usually evolves within 30 minutes. In a patient with latex allergy, repeated vaginal examination with gloves containing latex and other exposure to latex can lead to anaphylaxis.

- Stop administration of drug(s)/blood product likely to have caused anaphylaxis.
- Call for help, including anaesthetist. Treat according to the ABC protocol.
- Give adrenaline/epinephrine:
  - either 0.5–1.0 mg (0.5–1.0 ml of 1:1000) intramuscularly every ten minutes until improvement in pulse and blood pressure
  - or 50–100 micrograms (0.5–1 ml of 1:10 000) intravenously titrated against blood pressure.
- If cardiovascular collapse 0.5–1.0 mg (5–10 ml of 1:10 000) may be required intravenously, in divided doses titrated against response. Give at a rate of 0.1 mg/minute and stop when a response has been obtained.
- Start intravascular volume expansion with crystalloid or synthetic colloid.
- Give secondary therapy, chlorphenamine 10–20 mg by slow IV infusion, consider ranitidine 50 mg IV and hydrocortisone 100–300 mg IV.
- Give catecholamines if blood pressure is still low.
- ADRENALINE/epinephrine 0.05–0.1 micrograms/kg/minute (approx 4–8 micrograms/minute).
  5 mg adrenaline/epinephrine in 500 ml saline gives 10 micrograms/ml.
- NORADRENALINE/norepinephrine 0.05–0.1 micrograms/kg/minute (approx 4–8 micrograms/minute).
  4 mg noradrenaline/norepinephrine in 500 ml dextrose gives 8 micrograms/ml.

Summary

- Hypovolaemia is the most likely cause of shock in most trauma patients and in the emergencies of late pregnancy.
- A high index of suspicion is essential during assessment particularly in the pregnant patient.
- Management requires replacement of lost volume and immediate control of haemorrhage either by direct compression, splintage or, where necessary, by urgent surgery.

Algorithm 10.1. Abdominal trauma and other abdominal catastrophes key points

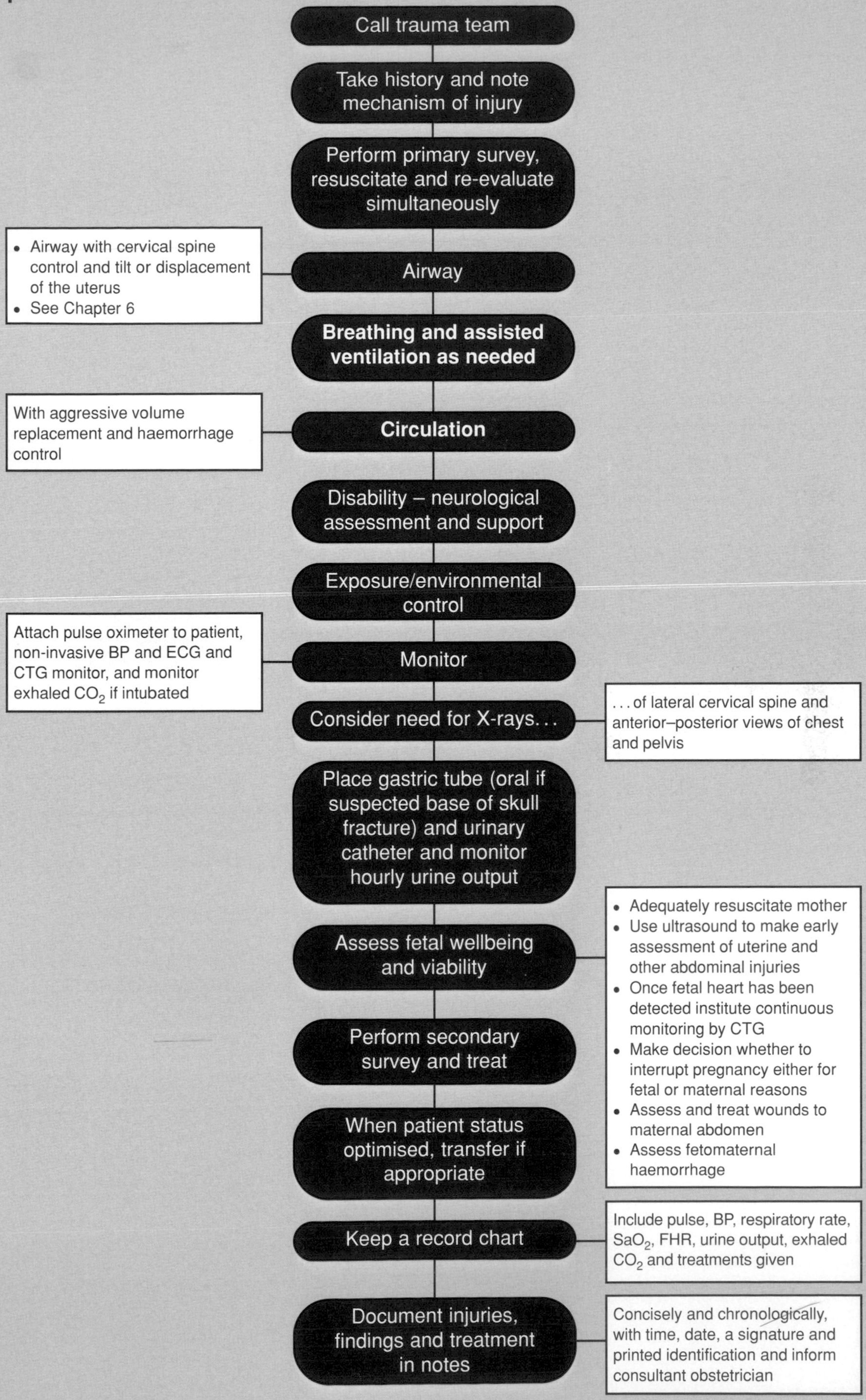

Call trauma team

Take history and note mechanism of injury

Perform primary survey, resuscitate and re-evaluate simultaneously

Airway
- Airway with cervical spine control and tilt or displacement of the uterus
- See Chapter 6

Breathing and assisted ventilation as needed

Circulation
With aggressive volume replacement and haemorrhage control

Disability – neurological assessment and support

Exposure/environmental control

Monitor
Attach pulse oximeter to patient, non-invasive BP and ECG and CTG monitor, and monitor exhaled CO_2 if intubated

Consider need for X-rays...
...of lateral cervical spine and anterior–posterior views of chest and pelvis

Place gastric tube (oral if suspected base of skull fracture) and urinary catheter and monitor hourly urine output

Assess fetal wellbeing and viability
- Adequately resuscitate mother
- Use ultrasound to make early assessment of uterine and other abdominal injuries
- Once fetal heart has been detected institute continuous monitoring by CTG
- Make decision whether to interrupt pregnancy either for fetal or maternal reasons
- Assess and treat wounds to maternal abdomen
- Assess fetomaternal haemorrhage

Perform secondary survey and treat

When patient status optimised, transfer if appropriate

Keep a record chart
Include pulse, BP, respiratory rate, SaO_2, FHR, urine output, exhaled CO_2 and treatments given

Document injuries, findings and treatment in notes
Concisely and chronologically, with time, date, a signature and printed identification and inform consultant obstetrician

Chapter 10

Abdominal trauma and other abdominal catastrophes

Objectives

On successfully completing this topic you will:

- be able to assess the patient who has sustained abdominal trauma and recognise the possibility of injury
- be able to assess the pregnant woman with abdominal pain and diagnose potentially life-threatening conditions
- be aware of the changes in anatomy and physiology that occur in pregnancy and be aware of how they may alter the response to trauma and affect presentation of acute abdominal conditions.
- be aware of the diagnostic procedures available for the investigation of abdominal trauma
- be familiar with the investigation and treatment of abdominal pain in pregnancy
- be aware of the role of ultrasound in pregnancy-related trauma, especially the role of focused abdominal sonography for trauma (FAST).
- be aware of the role of diagnostic peritoneal lavage and its indications.

Background and incidence

Abdominal injuries in pregnancy are on the increase both from accidental and non-accidental causes. Apparently fairly trivial trauma to the uterus may be responsible for potentially fatal placental abruption to the fetus. Abdominal pain in pregnancy is common, and missed or delayed diagnoses of intra-abdominal pathology are common.

Abdominal injuries are a constant source of preventable deaths associated with major trauma in the pregnant and non-pregnant patient alike. The prompt and accurate assessment of the presence of intra-abdominal injury and its likely source can be challenging, and the existence of a gravid uterus makes decision making harder. This also applies to the assessment of acute abdominal pain in pregnancy.

Obstetricians should become involved early in the trauma process when pregnancy is obvious or known, and they need to be familiar with the patterns of abdominal injury in the pregnant and non-pregnant patient and their relative overall priority. They need to be aware of the effects of pregnancy on the response to blood loss of both mother and fetus. The mother, especially in later pregnancy, tolerates blood loss well; the fetus tolerates maternal blood loss very badly.

Pregnancy may also make the assessment of the abdomen more challenging. The peritoneum is less sensitive, the omentum is less able to contain local inflammation and areas of maximum tenderness may be shifted due to organ displacement secondary to the enlarging uterus (e.g. appendicitis).

The 1997–99 CEMD report makes recommendations for the use of seat belts in pregnancy: 'Above

Ultrasound

A brief ultrasound examination of the left and right upper quadrant, the pelvis and the pericardium (focused abdominal sonography for trauma – FAST) by an experienced operator has become the initial investigation of choice in many trauma units. Good results have been achieved in pregnant trauma patients. Precise information can be obtained concerning the nature and extent of intra-abdominal bleeding and the examination is non-invasive and is easily repeatable. It may, however, fail to identify small amounts of intraperitoneal fluid, bowel or pancreatic injuries and a negative examination should be viewed with caution after a major trauma. It has the advantage that it visualises the fetal heart to obtain an accurate fetal heart rate but is not good at diagnosing an early abruption.

Computed tomography

CT scanning provides a highly sensitive and specific examination in suspected abdominal injury. The principle disadvantage is the risk associated with transfer to a remote department away from resuscitation and operative facilities. Radiation risks have been considerably reduced in recent years. CT should only be used for stable patients where further elucidation of the precise injuries are required. In the patient with a viable pregnancy, abdominal delivery followed by a trauma laparotomy is likely to be the safer option for baby and mother.

Assessment of fetal wellbeing and viability

Data on outcome after maternal abdominal trauma suggest that maternal outcomes are similar to those for non-pregnant patients but there is a high likelihood of fetal loss. It cannot be over-emphasised that the best way of achieving a good fetal outcome is by thorough evaluation and resuscitation of the mother, thereby ensuring good placental perfusion and oxygenation. Once maternal stability has been achieved and life-threatening injuries have been dealt with, delivery may be expedited if fetal wellbeing is in question. A resuscitative laparotomy may be indicated for both fetal and maternal reasons. Hypotensive resuscitation is not appropriate for the pregnant woman with a live, viable fetus. The correct treatment is to turn off the tap!

Secondary survey

A complete examination of the abdomen should be carried out regardless of whether serious injury is suspected. Even limited musculoskeletal trauma may affect the progress of the pregnancy and interrupting the pregnancy may make management easier. Regular obstetric evaluation will be required.

Solid and hollow visceral injury

Injuries to the liver and spleen are less common with the protection of the gravid uterus in late pregnancy but they still occur. If patient's cardiovascular system is stable, experienced centres may elect to treat selected patients conservatively. This is particularly the case in patients where the fetus is not viable. There should be a very low threshold for caesarean section. Hollow visceral injuries can be very difficult to detect and a high index of suspicion is required to pick them up. A careful maternal and fetal examination and ultrasound examination should reveal significant uterine injuries. Injuries to the genitourinary tract, the pancreas and retroperitoneum can be difficult to detect and specialised radiological investigations may be required.

It should be remembered that the peritoneum is less sensitive in pregnancy.

Pelvic trauma

There is very little literature concerning serious pelvic injuries in the later stages of pregnancy. However, uncontrolled haemorrhage from pelvic fractures continues to be a cause of potentially avoidable death after major trauma in the non-pregnant population and the management principles are common to both groups.

Pelvic fractures may cause fracture to the fetal head, especially if the head is engaged.

The precise mechanism of injury provides considerable information as to the type of pelvic injury sustained. An anteroposterior X-ray of the pelvis is a mandatory investigation in any major trauma. Serious injuries are usually obvious, although the pelvis may only be confirmed as the source of bleeding once abdominal, thoracic and external sources have been excluded.

Venous and arterial haemorrhage should be treated initially with manual attempts to return the pelvis to its anatomical position. Both these manoeuvres and the application of an external fixator (required to maintain anatomical reduction) may be difficult in the later stages of pregnancy. Often, delivery by caesarean section will be required to salvage the baby and achieve control of pelvic haemorrhage. It may be necessary to empty the uterus by caesarean section even if the baby is dead, in order to gain access and control haemorrhage.

A high index of suspicion of the pelvis as a potential source of life-threatening bleeding should be maintained until control by other means has been established.

Acute abdominal conditions presenting in pregnancy

Abdominal pain is common in pregnancy. Heartburn, indigestion, upper abdominal discomfort, nausea, vomiting, constipation and diarrhoea frequently occur. However, sudden onset of these symptoms accompanied by pain should ring alarm bells.

History

The acute onset of abdominal pain suggests rupturing or tearing, including ruptured ectopic, ruptured uterus, ruptured aneurysm(splenic, renal, epigastric or aortic), rupture of an abscess or perforation of an ulcer. Acute abruption also presents with severe abdominal pain and should be the presumptive diagnosis until it can be ruled out.

Pain that increases over a comparatively short time is more characteristic of acute degeneration of a fibroid, acute cholecystitis, acute pancreatitis, strangulated hernia, ureteric colic, strangulation or infarction of the bowel.

Site of the pain

Right upper-quadrant pain is fairly common in pregnancy and may be caused by a variety of conditions including, most seriously, rupture of the capsule of the liver (rarely diagnosed preoperatively) and associated with toxaemia, hepatitis, cholecystitis and pyelonephritis.

Left upper-quadrant pain is unusual but should always be taken seriously and splenic rupture and splenic artery rupture both need to be excluded. Both of these conditions occur more frequently in pregnancy.

Back pain is common in pregnancy.

Pain from pancreatitis is felt in the back and may be partially relieved by leaning forward. Pain from cholecystitis is commonly referred to the area of the lower ribs posteriorly or between the shoulder blades; hyperaesthesia may be present over the lower ribs to the right (Boas sign).

Pain from renal pathology is usually felt in the loin.

Low abdominal pain is often difficult to diagnose and is often never satisfactorily explained.

Management of the more common surgical conditions in pregnancy

Appendicitis

Appendicitis is more common in the first two trimesters but perforation is more common in the third. It has long been recognised that there is a higher morbidity for mother and baby in pregnancy and therefore a relatively high negative laparotomy is acceptable.

Laparoscopy may be helpful in early pregnancy and laparoscopic appendicectomy may be feasible. Later in pregnancy the position of the appendix shifts upwards and laterally and a muscle-splitting incision should be made over the site of maximum tenderness.

Cholecystitis

This condition should be treated in the same way in the pregnant and the non-pregnant. The trend is away from conservative management towards surgery.

Acute pancreatitis carries a 10% mortality rate in pregnancy but is fortunately uncommon.

Intestinal obstruction in pregnancy is increasing, due to the increasing incidence of surgical interventions in young women leading to adhesions.

Volvulus is increased in pregnancy.

The symptoms of intestinal obstruction, absolute constipation, vomiting and colicky abdominal pains are the same in the pregnant and the non-pregnant. Fetal assessment should be carried to determine whether the baby should be delivered at the time of laparotomy.

Fatal abdominal problems in pregnancy

The 1997–99 CEMD report listed three fatalities from intestinal obstruction, one of which is said to demonstrate the difficulty in diagnosing acute abdominal pain in pregnancy and two of which demonstrated substandard care. There were two deaths from pancreatitis, one from a splenic artery aneurysm, one from intra-abdominal bleeding, one from liver failure and one from liver rupture.

These cases point out the need to carry out a structured laparotomy when operating for malignancy and hypovolaemic shock. If a patient has hypovolaemic shock that cannot be explained by blood loss, on the floor, in the chest or due to fractures in the pelvis or long bones ('blood on the floor and four places more' – chest, abdomen, pelvis and long bones).

The laparotomy should be a structured 'trauma' laparotomy with an experienced general surgeon to hand.

It must always be remembered how well young, fit, pregnant patients compensate for blood loss.

Obstetricians should call on advice from other specialties early in cases of non-obstetric disease.

Conclusion

Acute abdominal problems in pregnancy are increasing due to increase in trauma and the increased exposure of young women to surgical procedures.

Few people have experience of dealing with major trauma in pregnancy but if the patient is pregnant the obstetrician will be involved early and their advice required.

Algorithm 11.1. The unconscious patient key points

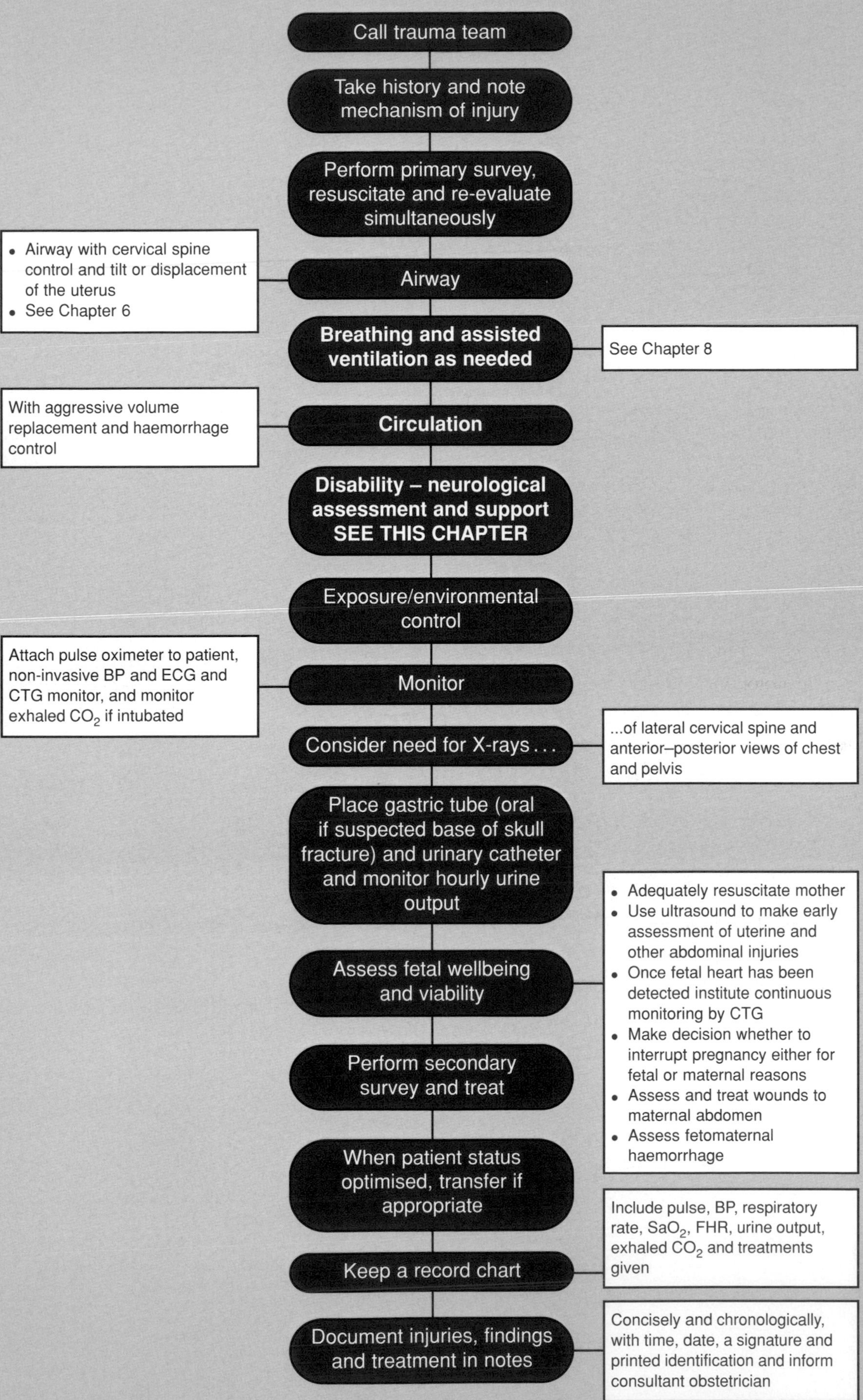

Chapter 11

The unconscious patient

Objectives

On successfully completing this topic you will be able to:

- describe the priorities in the treatment of the unconscious patient
- understand the causes of secondary brain injury and how to prevent it
- identify types of injury, particularly those that need urgent surgery, i.e. extradural and subdural haematomas.

Incidence

The 1997–99 CEMD report detailed 11 deaths due to subarachnoid haemorrhage, five due to intracerebral haemorrhage, five due to cerebral thrombosis and nine due to epilepsy. The management of the unconscious patient as a result of whatever cause should therefore be a basic skill of every obstetrician and midwife.

Primary survey and resuscitation

Primary survey and resuscitation

This follows the **A B C D E** protocol.

A – Airway

A patient with a reduced level of consciousness is more likely to have a compromised airway as the tongue falls back into the hypopharynx. Further, she is at risk of aspiration as she has obtunded laryngeal reflexes.

B – Breathing

Adequate ventilation ensures that the brain receives blood containing enough oxygen, thereby preventing further brain injury. Adequate ventilation prevents the accumulation of carbon dioxide. A rise in blood carbon dioxide levels is harmful as it causes a rise in intracranial pressure (ICP). Ventilation may be impaired by a reduced level of consciousness.

Raised intrathoracic pressure (as happens in tension pneumothorax) will compromise venous drainage from the head and raise ICP.

C – Circulation

An adequate blood pressure is required to maintain cerebral perfusion pressure. Hypotension resulting from other injuries must be swiftly recognised and managed to prevent secondary brain injury.

Never presume that the brain injury is the cause of hypotension. Scalp lacerations may bleed profusely but hypotension secondary to an isolated brain injury is uncommon and usually fatal. Always presume that hypotension is due to hypovolaemia outside the brain, not brain injury, and look for a source of blood loss elsewhere.

Cushing's response (progressive hypertension, bradycardia and slowing of respiratory rate) is an acute response to rapidly rising ICP and is a pre-morbid sign.

D – Disability

A decrease in level of consciousness is the marker of cerebral insult. Generally, the more deeply unconscious a patient becomes, the more serious is the insult. The unconscious pregnant patient may be post-eclamptic. Remember blood pressure, check for proteinuria and hyperreflexia.

A rapid assessment of conscious level is made in the primary survey using **A V P U**: is the patient **A**lert or responding to **V**oice or only responding to **P**ain or **U**nresponsive?

Causes of secondary brain injury

Primary brain injury is the neurological damage produced by the traumatic event. Secondary brain injury is the neurological damage caused by lack of oxygen delivery to the brain. Impaired oxygen delivery results from poor oxygenation of blood or reduced delivery of blood to brain tissues. There is reduced delivery of blood to the brain when the cerebral perfusion pressure in reduced. To understand this further it is necessary to understand something of the anatomy and physiology of the central nervous system.

Cerebral perfusion refers to the supply of oxygenated blood to the brain.

Cerebral perfusion pressure (CPP) depends on the blood pressure pushing blood into the brain (mean arterial pressure – MAP) and the resistance to this blood flow from the intracranial pressure (ICP).

$$\mathrm{CPP} = \mathrm{MAP} - \mathrm{ICP}$$

The skull is a rigid box containing brain, cerebrospinal fluid, blood vessels and blood and extracellular fluid.

ICP is the pressure inside the skull. Because the skull is a rigid box, an increase in the volume of anything within the box, i.e. brain, blood, cerebrospinal fluid or extracellular fluid will cause an increase in ICP.

Note:

MAP: normal value = 70–90 mmHg.

ICP: normal value = 10 mmHg.

If CPP is less than 50 mmHg, cerebral hypoxia will follow.

(There are limits beyond which the MAP itself will contribute to a rise in ICP – systolic BP > 160 mmHg).

A fall in cerebral perfusion pressure contributes to brain injury. Therefore, anything that causes a rise in ICP (such as hypoxia causing swelling of the brain, rise in carbon dioxide levels causing rise in arterial carbon dioxide levels and therefore swelling of the blood vessels) or a fall in MAP, causes secondary brain injury.

Raised ICP may also be due to obstruction of venous drainage from the head. This may be due to:

- pressure on the neck veins
- increased pressure inside the chest
- head down position.

It follows that keeping the patient well oxygenated and preventing a rise in intracranial pressure or a fall in cerebral perfusion is vital in the overall management of head injury. Consider minimising the volume (and therefore pressure effect) of any of the intracranial substances, i.e. tissue, blood, cerebrospinal fluid, extracellular fluid. Some of these are only theoretical considerations but others are practical, e.g. judicious use of fluids to minimise extracellular fluid volume, avoiding head down position to minimise blood congestion in the brain, avoid constricting devices around the neck and rises in intrathoracic pressure for the same reasons.

Assessment of fetal wellbeing and viability

When the mother is adequately resuscitated, the further wellbeing of the fetus must be considered. Timing of delivery should be considered in the patient about to undergo neurosurgical treatment, a prolonged period of intensive care or who is unlikely to recover consciousness. Delivery of the term fetus may be appropriate if a prolonged period of intensive care and nursing care is anticipated. Physiological complications that develop in the long-term intensive care patient (coagulopathy, sepsis etc.) may complicate a continuing pregnancy.

Types of head injury

Rising ICP due to brain swelling or expanding haematomas inside the head can cause a variety of neurological signs.

- **A decrease in level of consciousness is the marker of cerebral insult. Generally, the more deeply unconscious a patient becomes, the more serious is the insult.**
- Pressure on the third cranial nerve (oculomotor) will result in a dilated pupil on the same side ('ipsilateral') as the injury.
- Damage to the motor or sensory cortex (or tracts leading from them) will result in a motor or sensory DEFICIT on the opposite side to the injury.

Pressure on the brain stem, where the respiratory and cardiovascular centres lie, produces respiratory or cardiovascular abnormalities (change in heart rate and BP, change in breathing pattern and rate).

Primary brain injury may be diffuse or focal.

Diffuse primary brain injury

Blunt injury to the brain may cause diffuse brain injury, particularly when rapid head motion (acceleration or deceleration) leads to widespread damage within the brain substance. Such injuries form a spectrum extending from mild concussion to severe injury known as diffuse axonal injury.

Concussion is a brain injury accompanied by a brief loss of consciousness and, in its mildest form, may cause only temporary confusion or amnesia. With mild forms of concussion, most patients will be slightly confused and may be able to describe how the injury occurred. They are likely to complain of mild headache, dizziness or nausea. The mini-neurological examination will not show lateralising signs. With more severe concussion there is a longer period of unconsciousness, longer amnesia (for time both before and after the injury) and there may be focal signs. The duration of amnesia needs to be recorded.

Diffuse axonal injury is so severe as to cause a characteristically long coma in 44% of cases. The overall mortality rate is over 30%, rising to 50% in its most severe form. The treatment of such injury involves prolonged controlled ventilation in an intensive care unit.

Focal primary brain injury

Brain injuries that produce a contusion or haematoma in a relatively small area of the brain may be amenable to emergency surgery and the priority must be the urgent evacuation of the haematoma. These conditions must be diagnosed early, as early surgery greatly reduces the morbidity and mortality.

Contusions are caused by blunt injury producing acceleration and deceleration forces on the brain tissue, resulting in tearing of the small blood vessels inside the brain. Contusions can occur immediately beneath the area of impact, when they are known as coup injuries, or at a point distant from the area of impact in the direction of the applied force, when they area known as contrecoup injuries. If the contusion occurs near the sensory or motor areas of the brain, these patients will present with a neurological deficit. Precise diagnosis requires appropriate imaging (CT scanning). Initial treatment is supportive aimed at preventing secondary brain injury.

Haemorrhage causing haematomata within the skull may arise either from meningeal vessels or from vessels within the brain substance. It is defined anatomically; such a classification is useful as it has implications in terms of remediable surgery, urgency and prognosis.

Delay in the treatment of extradural haemorrhage beyond two hours and delay in the treatment of subdural haemorrhage beyond four hours worsens the prognosis.

Extradural haemorrhage

This is caused by a tear in a dural artery, most commonly the middle meningeal artery. This can be torn by a linear fracture crossing the temporal or parietal bone and injuring the artery lying in a groove on the deep aspect of the bone.

Isolated extradural haemorrhage is unusual, accounting for only 0.5% of all head injuries and less than 1% of injuries causing coma. The importance of early recognition of this injury lies in the fact that, when treated appropriately the prognosis is good because of the lack of underlying serious injury to brain tissue. If missed, the rapidly expanding haematoma causes ICP to rise, reducing cerebral perfusion and leading to cerebral hypoxia, coma and death.

The typical symptoms and signs of extradural haemorrhage are:

- loss of consciousness followed by a lucid interval (which may not be a complete return to full consciousness).
- secondary depression of consciousness
- dilated pupil on the side of injury
- weakness of the arm and leg on the contralateral side to the injury.

Subdural haemorrhage

This is more common than extradural haemorrhage and is found in 30% of all severe head injuries. The mortality rate is up to 60% because, in addition to the compression caused by the subdural blood clot, there is often major injury to the underlying brain tissue. The haematoma can arise from tears in the bridging veins between the cortex and the dura or from laceration of the brain substance and the cortical arteries.

The typical symptoms and signs of subdural haemorrhage are:

- levels of consciousness will vary depending on the underlying brain damage and rate of haematoma formation
- dilated pupil on the side of the injury
- weakness of the arm and leg on the contralateral side to the injury.

To differentiate subdural from extradural haemorrhage: extradural haematomas appear biconvex or lenticular in shape on CT scan.

If extradural haemorrhage is diagnosed and treated early chances of recovery are good.

Subarachnoid haemorrhage

Where haemorrhaging has occurred into the subarachnoid space, the irritant effect of the bloody cerebrospinal fluid causes headache, photophobia and neck stiffness. On its own, this is not serious but prognosis is poor if it is associated with a more severe head injury.

Intracerebral laceration

Through-and-through injuries, side-to-side injuries and injuries in the lower region of the brain stem all have a poor outcome.

All foreign bodies found protruding from the skull must be left in place; these should only be removed at a neurosurgical unit. Skull X-rays will show the angle and depth of penetration. Care must be taken during transfer to ensure that there is no further penetration.

Open brain injury in a conscious patient carries a good prognosis if surgery is not delayed. Scalp haemorrhage should be stopped, entrance and exit wounds covered with sterile dressings and the patient transferred to a neurosurgical unit.

Secondary survey

The neurological examination assesses:

- pupillary function
- lateralised limb weakness
- level of consciousness by the Glasgow Coma Scale.

The mini-neurological examination serves to determine the severity of the brain injury and the likelihood of a surgically treatable lesion When applied repeatedly, it can be used to determine objectively any neurological deterioration. It is supplemented by CT scanning.

Remember:

- ### Pupillary function

  Evaluate the pupils for their equality and response to bright light. A difference in diameter of the pupils of more than 1 mm is abnormal, but remember that a local injury to the eye may be responsible for this abnormality. Normal reaction to a bright light is brisk constriction of the pupil; a more sluggish response may indicate brain injury. A dilated pupil on the same side as the injury indicates compression of the brain on that side.

- ### Lateralised limb weakness

  Observe spontaneous limb movements for equality. If movement is negligible then you must assess the response to a painful stimulus. Any delay in onset of movement or lateralisation of movement following a painful stimulus is significant. Obvious limb weakness localised to one side suggests an intracranial injury causing brain compression on the opposite side.

- ### Level of consciousness

  Glasgow Coma Scale provides a quantitative assessment of the level of consciousness. It is the sum of scores awarded for three types of response:
  - eye opening (E)
    The scoring of eye opening is not possible if the eyes are so swollen as to be permanently shut. This fact must be documented.
  - verbal response (V)
    The scoring of verbal response is not possible if the patient cannot speak because of endotracheal intubation. This fact must be documented.
  - motor response (M).
    The best response obtained for either of the upper extremities is recorded even though worse responses may be present in other extremities.

Glasgow Coma Scale scoring

Response	Score
Eye opening	
Spontaneous, that is, open with normal blinking	4
Eye opening to speech on request	3
Eye opening only to pain stimulus	2
No eye opening despite stimulation	1
Verbal response	
Orientated, spontaneous speech	5
Confused conversation but answers questions	4
Inappropriate words, that is, garbled speech but with recognisable words	3
Incomprehensible sounds or grunts	2
No verbal response	1
Motor response	
Obeys commands and moves limbs to command	6
Localizes, for example, moves upper limb to pain stimulus on head	5
Withdraws from painful stimulus on limb	4
Abnormal flexion or decorticate posture	3
Extensor response, decerebrate posture	2
No movement to any stimulus	1

The Glasgow Coma Scale is scored differently in children.

Subsequent reassessment can be used to detect any deterioration. For example, if the Glasgow Coma Scale has decreased by two points or more, deterioration has occurred. A decrease of three points or more is a bad prognostic indicator and demands immediate treatment. Dramatic changes in the Glasgow Coma Scale are often preceded by more subtle signs indicating deterioration, notably subtle confusion or behavioural changes.

Severity of head injuries is classified as follows:

- Score 8 or less = Severe
- Score 9 to 12 = Moderate
- Score 13 to 15 = Minor

Other injuries

Scalp wounds

The scalp is arranged in layers. It is highly vascular and a laceration will often result in profuse haemorrhage. The bleeding point should be located and the haemorrhage arrested. This may include the use of haemostatic surgical clips and ligatures, particularly where the laceration is deep. Direct pressure may not be sufficient. The wound should be inspected carefully for signs of skull fracture and irrigated to remove debris and dirt.

Gentle palpation of the scalp wound wearing a sterile glove may enable you to diagnose the presence of a skull fracture. If an open or depressed fracture is detected, close the wound with sutures, apply a dressing, give antibiotics and transfer the patient to a neurosurgical unit. Do not remove any bone fragments at this stage.

Skull fractures

Although skull fractures are common, many major brain injuries will occur without the skull being fractured and many skull fractures are not associated with severe brain injury. Where the mini-neurological examination identifies the presence of a severe brain injury, time taken to search for a skull fracture should never delay definitive management. The significance of a skull fracture is that it identifies a patient with a higher probability of having or developing an intracranial haematoma. All patients with skull fractures should be admitted for observation.

Linear skull fractures

These are particularly important when the fracture crosses the line of intracranial vessels indicating an increased risk of intracranial haemorrhage.

Depressed skull fractures

All depressed skull fractures should be transferred for neurosurgical unit assessment. They may be associated with underlying brain injury and require operative elevation to reduce the risk of infection.

Open skull fractures

By definition, there is direct communication between the outside of the head and brain tissue because the dura covering the surface of the brain is torn. This can be diagnosed if brain tissue is visible on examination of the scalp wound or if cerebrospinal fluid is seen to be leaking from the wound. These fractures all require operative intervention and the risk of infection is high. Give prophylactic antibiotics.

Basal skull fractures

The base of the skull does not run horizontally backwards but diagonally. Basal skull fractures will produce signs along this diagonal line. They can be diagnosed clinically in the presence of cerebrospinal fluid leaking from the ear (otorrhoea) or the nose (rhinorrhoea). When cerebrospinal fluid is mixed with blood it may be difficult to detect.

Bruising in the mastoid region (Battle's sign) also indicates basal skull fracture but the bruising usually takes 12–36 hours to develop. Blood seen behind the tympanic membrane (haemotympanum) may also indicate a basal skull fracture.

Fractures through the cribriform plate are frequently associated with bilateral periorbital haematomas. Subconjunctival haematoma may occur from direct orbital roof fracture, in which case there is no posterior limit to the haematoma.

All these signs may take several hours to develop and may not be present in a patient seen immediately after injury. Basal skull fractures are very difficult to diagnose from plain X-ray films.

Summary

- Remember the **A B C D E** routine.
- Prevent secondary injury by: preventing hypoxia, hypercarbia and hypovolaemia.
- Establishing a working diagnosis.
- Constantly repeat the mini-neurological examination.
- Consider the best management of the fetus

Algorithm 12.1. Spine and spinal cord injuries key points

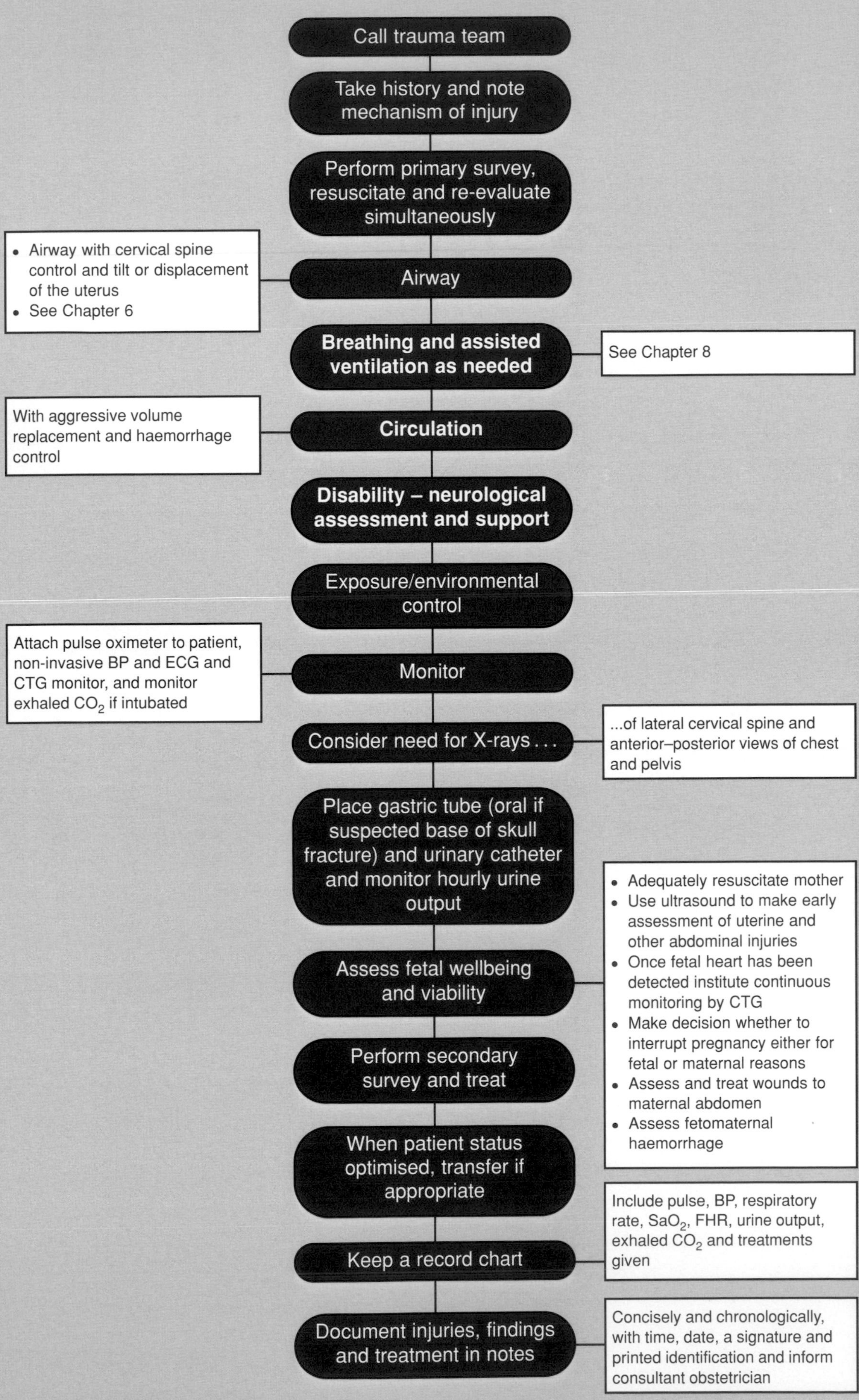

Chapter 12

Spine and spinal cord injuries

Objectives

On successfully completing this topic you will be able to:

- suspect spinal injury
- understand how to immobilise a patient
- evaluate, manage and refer a patient with spinal injury.

Introduction

In the context of this publication, spinal injuries refer to injuries to the bony spinal column, the spinal cord or both. There can be an injury to the bony spine without injury to the spinal cord, but there is significant risk of cord injury in these circumstances.

Failure to immobilise a patient with a spinal injury can cause additional neurological damage. Failure to immobilise a patient with an injury to the bony spine (without cord injury at that stage) can cause injury to the spinal cord.

A spinal injury should be suspected:

- in falls from a height
- in vehicle collisions, even at low speed
- when pedestrians have been hit by a vehicle
- where patients have been thrown
- in sports injuries, e.g. horse-riding
- in the multiply-injured patient
- in a patient with injury above the clavicle (including the unconscious patient – 15% of unconscious patients have some form of neck injury)
- in the conscious patient complaining of neck pain and sensory and/or motor symptoms.

Patients who are awake, sober, neurologically normal and have no neck pain are extremely unlikely to have a cervical spine fracture. However, neurosurgical or orthopaedic opinion should always be taken if an injury is suspected or detected.

The cervical spine is more vulnerable to injury than the thoracic or lumbar spine.

Approximately 10% of patients with a cervical spine fracture have a second associated non-contiguous fracture of the vertebral column.

Immobilisation techniques

The spine should be immobilised until spinal injury has been excluded by examination, X-ray and supplementary radiological investigations, where appropriate. Injury can only be excluded by orthopaedic or neurosurgeon or a suitably skilled A&E doctor.

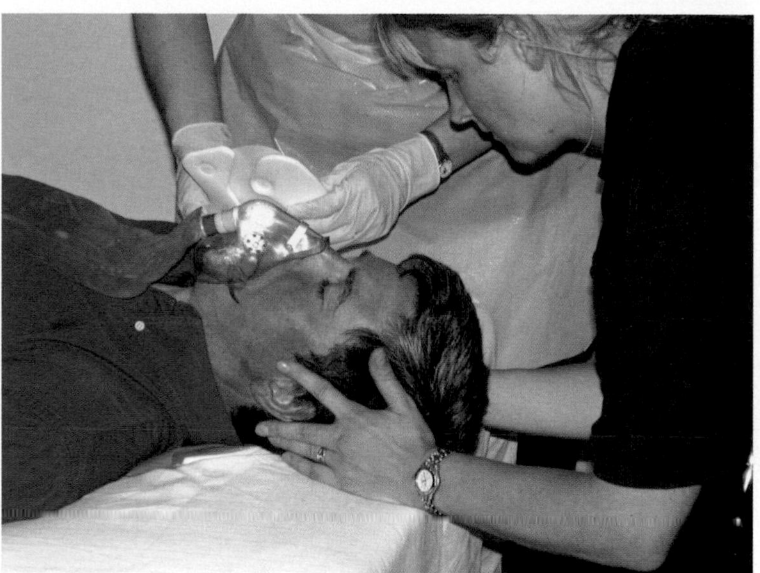

Manual immobilisation

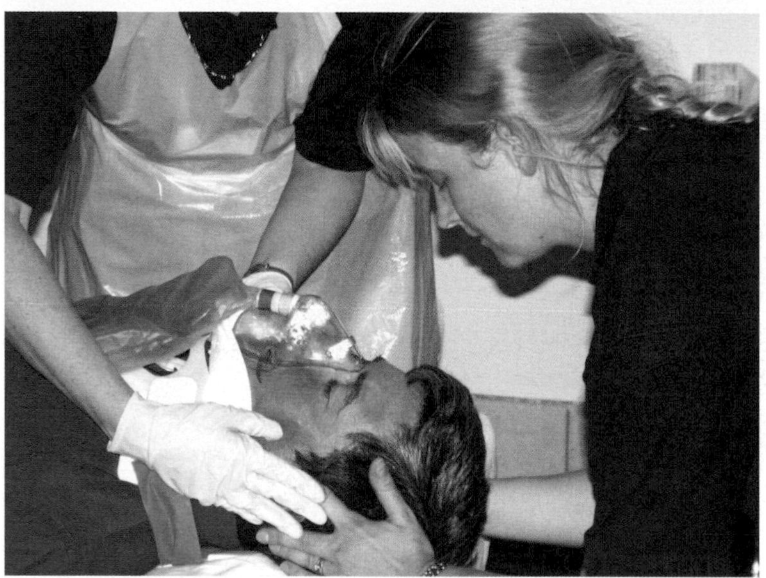

Immobilisation and collar application

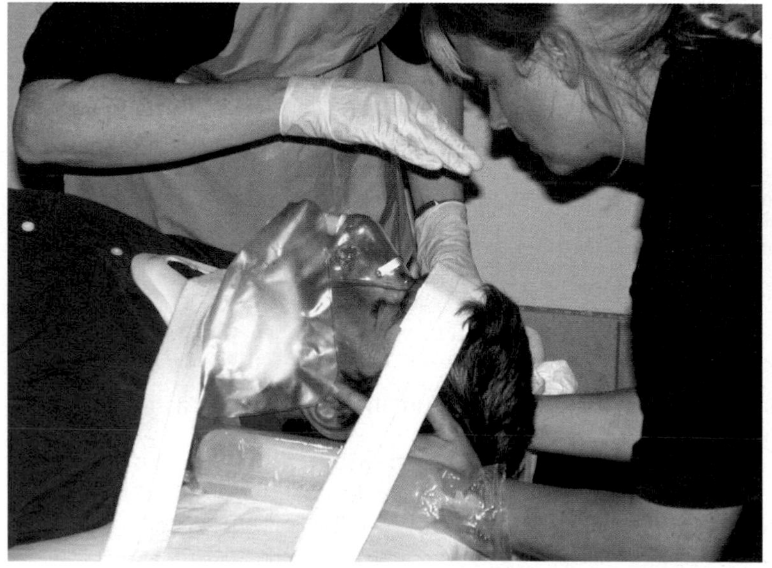

Collar, blocks (sandbags) and straps (tapes)

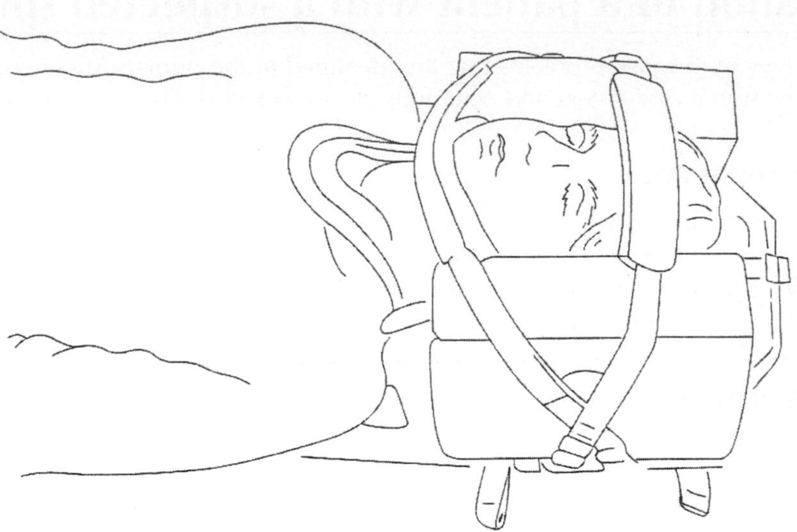

Figure 12.1 Immobilisation of the cervical spine

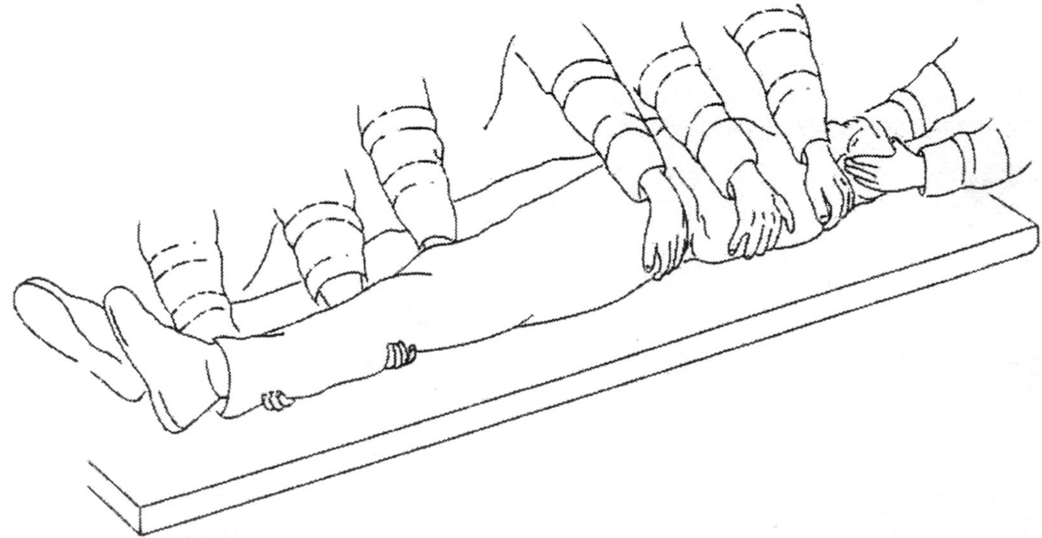

Figure 12.2 Log roll

Immobilisation should be carried out in the neutral position.

Immobilisation of the cervical spine is done by manual in-line immobilisation or by semi-rigid cervical collar, blocks on a back board and straps.

The use of a long spine board is recommended. The thoracic and lumbar spine is immobilised by a long spine board. Lying on a backboard is uncomfortable and puts the patient at risk of developing pressure ulcers. Early neurosurgical or orthopaedic opinion should be sought so that prolonged unnecessary immobilisation is avoided. To avoid supine hypotension in the heavily pregnant patient, the right hip should be elevated to four to six inches with a towel and the uterus displaced manually.

Evaluation of a patient with a suspected spinal injury

Spinal injuries may cause problems that are identified in the primary survey or the injury may be identified by spinal assessment and neurological assessment during the secondary survey.

Spinal assessment

A log-roll must be performed. This is a coordinated, skilled manoeuvre by trained personnel to turn the patient from the supine to the lateral position without causing damage to the spinal cord. Look for bruising, deformity and localised swelling of the vertebral column. Palpate for localised tenderness or gaps between spinous processes. At this point it is appropriate to carry out a rectal examination.

Neurological assessment

Of the many tracts in the spinal cord the three that can be assessed clinically are:

- **corticospinal tract** – controls muscle power on the same side of the body and is tested by voluntary movement and involuntary response to painful stimuli
- **spinothalamic tract** – transmits pain and temperature sensation from the opposite side of the body and is tested generally by pinprick
- **posterior columns** – carry position sense from the same side.

Each can be injured on one or both sides.

If there is no demonstrable sensory or motor function below a certain level bilaterally this is referred to as a complete spinal injury. If there is remaining motor or sensory function with some loss this is an incomplete injury (better prognosis). Sparing of sensation in the perianal region may be the only sign of residual function. Sacral sparing is demonstrated by presence of sensation perianally and/or voluntary contraction of the anal sphincter.

An injury does not qualify as incomplete on the basis of preserved sacral reflexes, e.g. bulbocavernosus reflex or anal wink. Priapism is due to unopposed parasympathetic drive and is suggestive of a spinal injury.

The neurological level is the most caudal segment with normal sensory and motor function on both sides.

For completeness, the key dermatomes are given here (Figure 12.3).

Each nerve root innervates more than one muscle and most muscles have innervation from more than one nerve root. Certain movements, however, are identified as representing a single nerve root.

A broad distinction can be made between lesions above and lesions below T1 (as determined by sensory and motor testing). Lesions above T1 result in quadriplegia and lesions below T1 result in paraplegia. There is a discrepancy between neurological injury level and level of bony injury because spinal nerves travel up/down the canal from the point of entry through bone to join the spinal cord. The level quoted is the neurological level.

Principles of treatment

The principles of treatment are primary survey and resuscitation, **A B C D E**, assessment of fetal wellbeing and viability, then secondary survey.

A spinal injury may present in either the primary survey or the secondary survey.

- Deal with life-threatening conditions according to the **A B C** but avoid any movement of the spinal column.
- Establish adequate immobilisation and maintain it until you are certain there is no spinal injury.
- Make an early referral to a neurosurgeon or orthopaedic surgeon if a spinal injury is suspected or detected.
- Be aware of associations of spinal injury or effects on other systems and injuries.

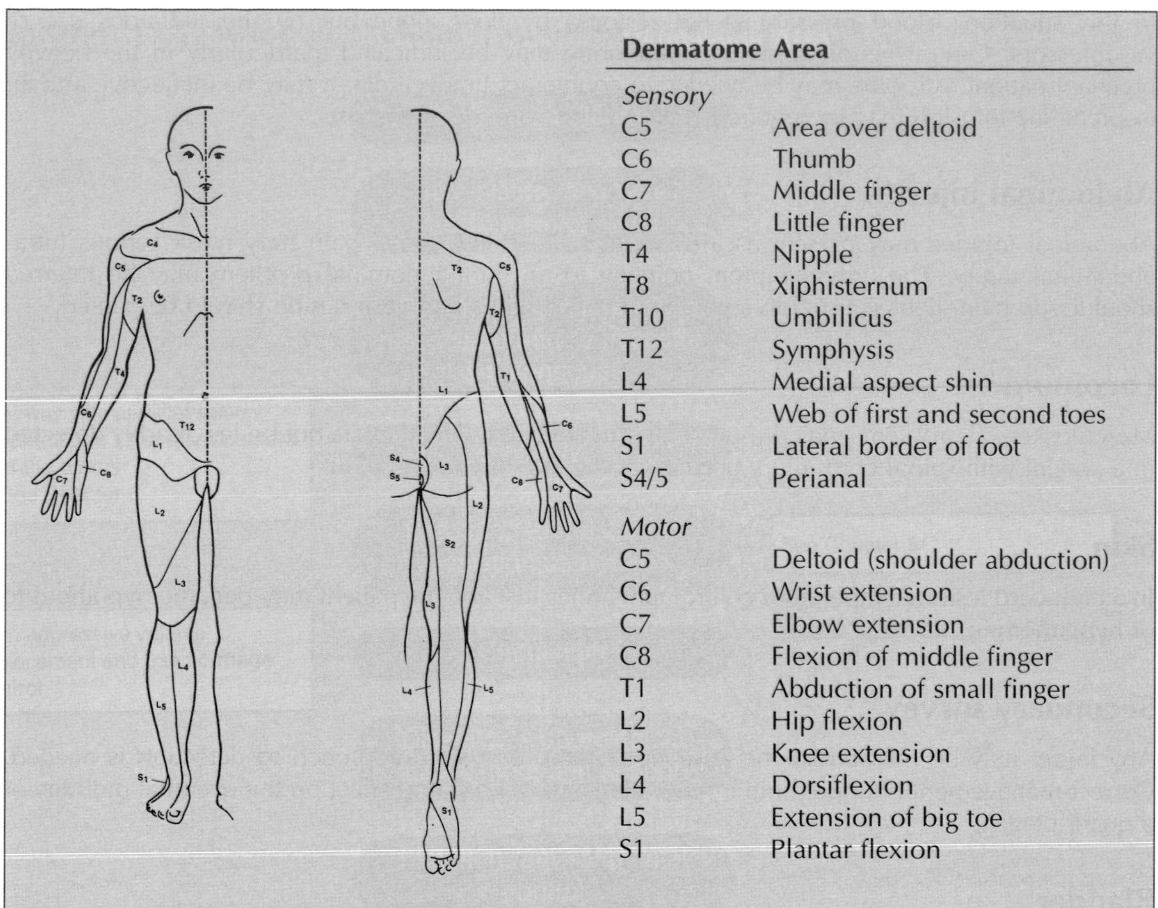

Dermatome	Area
Sensory	
C5	Area over deltoid
C6	Thumb
C7	Middle finger
C8	Little finger
T4	Nipple
T8	Xiphisternum
T10	Umbilicus
T12	Symphysis
L4	Medial aspect shin
L5	Web of first and second toes
S1	Lateral border of foot
S4/5	Perianal
Motor	
C5	Deltoid (shoulder abduction)
C6	Wrist extension
C7	Elbow extension
C8	Flexion of middle finger
T1	Abduction of small finger
L2	Hip flexion
L3	Knee extension
L4	Dorsiflexion
L5	Extension of big toe
S1	Plantar flexion

Figure 12.3 Dermatomes used for sensory and motor testing

Effect or associations identified in the primary survey

Airway obstruction

Trauma that has caused damage to the spine is likely to have caused injury above the clavicle. This may take the form of an injury to the airway or a head injury, which puts the patient at risk of airway problems.

Breathing problems

If the injury is above the fifth cervical vertebra respiration will be severely compromised. With injuries between the fourth cervical and the twelfth thoracic vertebrae there will be intercostal paralysis and, depending on the level, there may be only diaphragmatic breathing. In high thoracic injuries broncho-constriction can occur.

Complicating factors are rib fractures, flail chest, pulmonary contusion, haemopneumothorax and aspiration pneumonitis. Vigorously address these problems by providing ventilatory support, chest drainage and, if the patient can feel pain, analgesia.

Neurogenic shock

Spinal injury may cause a **C**irculation problem. Neurogenic shock results from impairment of the descending sympathetic pathways. This results in loss of sympathetic tone to the vessels and therefore vasodilatation, which causes a fall in blood pressure. Injury above the T4 level causes loss of sympathetic innervation to the heart and therefore bradycardia (failure to become tachycardic in response to hypovolaemia).

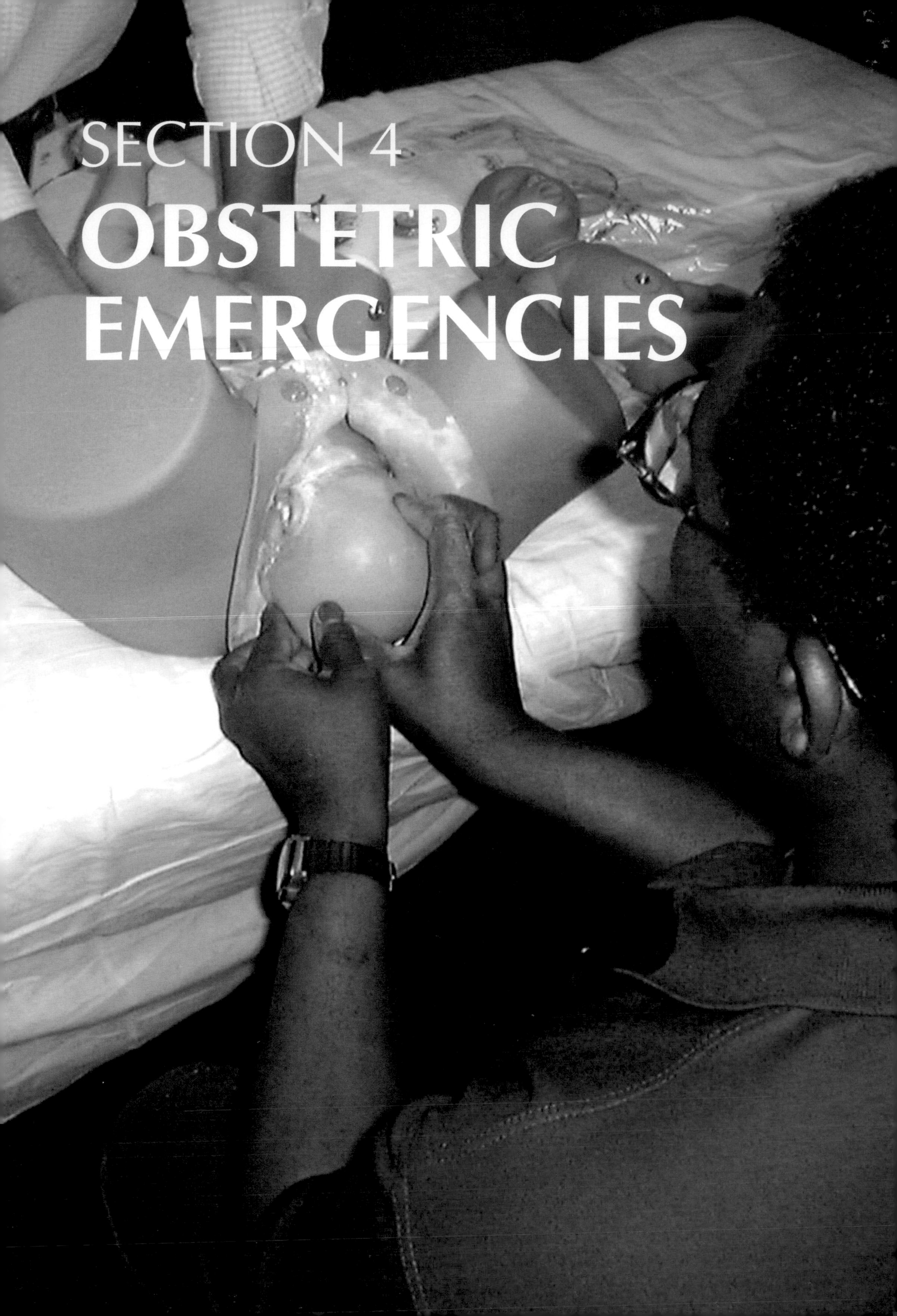

SECTION 4

OBSTETRIC EMERGENCIES

Algorithm 15.1. Pre-eclampsia/eclampsia key points

Do not leave patient alone

- Place in semi-prone position
- Call for HELP – duty obstetric and anaesthetic SpRs; senior midwife
- Inform consultants – obstetrician and anaesthetist on-call

Airway

- Assess
- Maintain patency
- Apply oxygen

Breathing

- Assess
- Protect airway
- Ventilate as required

Circulation

- Evaluate pulse and BP
- If absent, initiate CPR and call the arrest team
- Secure IV access as soon as safely possible

Control seizures

- **Loading dose $MgSO_4$:** 4 g $MgSO_4$ in 20% solution IV over 10–15 minutes. Add 8 ml of 50% $MgSO_4$ solution to 12 ml physiological saline
- **Maintenance dose $MgSO_4$:** 1 g per hour infusion Add 25 g $MgSO_4$ (50 ml) to 250 ml physiological saline 1 g $MgSO_4$ = 12 ml per hour IV
- **If seizures continue or recur:** $MgSO_4$ 2 g ≤ 70kg; 4 g ≥ 70 kg IV as per loading dose over 5–10 minutes. If this fails: diazepam 10 ml IV or thiopentone 50 mg IV paralyse and intubate
- **Monitor:** Hourly urine output, respiratory rate, O_2 saturation & patellar reflexes – every 10 minutes for first 2 hours and then every 30 minutes
  Check serum magnesium if toxicity is suspected on clinical grounds
- **Stop infusion:** Check magnesium levels and review management with consultant if:
  Urine output < 100 ml in 4 hours
  or if Patellar reflexes are absent
  or if Respiratory rate < 16/minute
  or if Oxygen saturation < 90%
- Always get suppression of reflexes before respiratory depression
- **Antidote:** 10% calcium gluconate 10 ml IV over 10 minutes

Control hypertension

- **Treat hypertension** if systolic BP > 170 mmHg or diastolic BP > 110 mmHg or MAP >125 mmHg
  Aim to reduce BP to around 130–140/90–100 mmHg
  Beware maternal hypotension and FHR abnormalities – monitor FHR with continuous CTG
- **HYDRALAZINE** 10 mg IV slowly
  Repeated doses of HYDRALAZINE 5 mg IV 20 minutes apart may be given if necessary
  Close liaison with anaesthetists: may require plasma expansion
- **LABETALOL** 50 mg IV slowly if BP still uncontrolled
  If necessary repeat after 20 minutes or start IV infusion: 200 mg in 200 ml physiological saline at 40 mg/hour, increasing dose at half-hourly intervals as required to a maximum of 160 mg/hour

If not postpartum . . . Deliver

- There is no place for the continuation of pregnancy if eclampsia occurs
- **'STABILISE' THE MOTHER BEFORE DELIVERY**
- **DELIVERY IS A TEAM EFFORT** involving obstetricians, midwives, anaesthetists and paediatricians
- Ergometrine should not be used in severe pre-eclampsia and eclampsia
- Consider prophylaxis against thromboembolism
- Maintain vigilance as the majority of eclamptic seizures occur after delivery

OBSERVATIONS

Pulse oximeter
BP
Respirations
Temperature
ECG
Test urine for protein
Hourly urine output
Fluid balance charts
FHR – monitor continuously

INVESTIGATIONS

FBC & platelets
U&Es
Urate
LFT
Coagulation screen
Group & hold serum
MSSU
24-hr urine collections for:
- total protein & creatinine clearance
- catecholamines

Chapter 15

Pre-eclampsia and eclampsia

Objectives

On successfully completing this topic you will be able to:

- treat hypertension and effect plasma volume expansion
- treat and prevent eclamptic fits
- manage/advise on fluid
- recognise and treat the complications of the condition.

Management of severe pre-eclampsia and eclampsia

- Guidelines for management must be available locally and read in full by all staff in the labour ward.
- Deviations from the guidelines must be agreed at consultant level.
- These patients should, as a minimum, be reviewed by the on-call consultant and by his/her team on a daily basis, and examined by the registrar/SHO every four hours.
- Early communication: with paediatricians, obstetric anaesthetists and intensivists, is vital.
- Fluid balance should be meticulous and no patient should be put at risk through iatrogenic fluid balance.
- Remember steroids in HELLP.

Key recommendations for pre-eclampsia and eclampsia[42]

- An obstetrician-led special team of appropriate size and composition should be set up in each unit to formulate and update pre-eclampsia and eclampsia protocols and to advise in difficult cases. They should also coordinate regular staff training.
- The need is emphasised for appropriate protocols to prevent junior staff being exposed to potentially dangerous clinical situations of which they have little experience.
- A single senior clinician should have responsibility for the overall management of each case, in particular for fluid balance. There should also be a clear system in place with regard to transfer of these patients at an appropriate stage, if necessary.
- All women should receive antenatal education so that they are aware of the symptoms associated with pre-eclampsia, its importance and the need to obtain urgent professional advice.
- There is the need for continued education of medical and midwifery staff, particularly in the community, with regard to the implications of pre-eclampsia and the need for accurate diagnosis, assessment and prompt referral when required.

Introduction and incidence

The 1997–99 report of the CEMD[4] shows a fall in the death rate from hypertensive disease of pregnancy, although it remains the second leading cause of direct death. It is suggested that the fall in the death rate may reflect the introduction of guidelines for the management of pre-eclampsia.

In an emergency situation there should be no conflict in management.

Pre-eclampsia/eclampsia remains one of the main causes of maternal mortality and morbidity in the UK.[4] However, given that eclampsia occurs in around one in 2000 deliveries,[41] most units will manage only one or two cases per year. This relative rarity increases the need for guidelines.

Definition of pre-eclampsia

Pre-eclampsia is a multisystem disorder that develops in previously normotensive women after 20 completed weeks of gestation (with no pre-existing renal disease). It is characterised by:

- hypertension (defined as blood pressure ≥ 140/90 mmHg, on two separate occasions at least four hours apart

  and

- proteinuria (**significant** proteinuria > 0.5 g in 24 hours in the absence of urinary tract infection)

both of which resolve by the sixth postpartum week.[43]

Eclampsia

Eclampsia is part of the clinical spectrum of pre-eclampsia; the seizure activity may be associated with pre-existing pre-eclampsia or it may be the first presentation of the condition. Thirty-eight percent of fits occur antenatally, 18% intrapartum and the remaining 44% postpartum, usually in the first 24–48 hours after delivery.[41]

Importance of pre-eclampsia

Pre-eclampsia is important because it constitutes a substantial risk to the pregnant woman and her unborn fetus. Hypertensive disorders of pregnancy represent the second leading cause of maternal mortality in the UK, most of these deaths being attributed to pre-eclampsia and its complications.[4]

Complications

Maternal complications	Hypertension Risk of cerebrovascular accident Renal failure Liver failure (liver rupture) Disseminated intravascular coagulation Pulmonary oedema (acute respiratory distress syndrome) Pulmonary haemorrhage Placental abruption Eclampsia (risk of aspiration pneumonia).
Fetal complications	Prematurity Intrauterine growth restriction Respiratory distress syndrome Acute fetal distress (secondary to sudden lowering of blood pressure with anti-hypertensive agents) Intrauterine death

The clinical manifestations of severe pre-eclampsia are consistent with a systemic disorder in which severe hypertension is only one aspect of the pathophysiology. Patients presenting with such multi-organ disease are often both a diagnostic and therapeutic challenge. Clinical symptoms and signs of note include:

- headache, visual disturbances, epigastric pain, vomiting
- nondependent (especially facial) or pulmonary oedema
- right upper quadrant abdominal tenderness
- optic vasospasm
- recently developed hypertension > 160/110 mmHg with proteinuria > 1 g in 24 hours
- hyperreflexia with clonus
- rapidly changing biochemical/haematological picture.

Management of severe pre-eclampsia[42]

Consider admission or, if available, review on daycare maternity ward, if:

- systolic BP ≥ 140 mmHg, or if
- diastolic BP ≥ 90 mmHg, or if
- hypertension and proteinuria ≥ +, or if
- presence of symptoms, e.g., epigastric pain, with hypertension ± proteinuria.

Inform:

- obstetric specialist registrar (SpR) and consultant
- paediatric SpR and consultant
- anaesthetic SpR and consultant.

Assess and observe/monitor:

- blood pressure
- generalised oedema
- symptoms
- optic fundi
- reflexes ± clonus
- test urine for protein
- urinary output
- fluid balance charts.
- fetal CTG and ultrasound scan on admission
- Doppler studies if available.

Investigate:

- blood:
  - FBC and platelets
  - urea and electrolytes
  - LFT
  - coagulation screen
  - group and hold serum

- urine:
  - MSSU
  - 24-hour urine collections for:
    - total protein and creatinine clearance
    - catecholamines.

Principles of management

Treat hypertension if:

- systolic BP ≥ 170 mmHg, or if
- diastolic BP ≥ 110 mmHg, or if
- mean arterial pressure ≥ 125 mmHg.

Aim to reduce BP to around 130–140/90–100 mmHg.

A rapid and precipitous fall in maternal blood pressure or maternal hypotension as a result of intravenous anti-hypertensive drugs may cause FHR abnormalities, especially in growth restricted/compromised fetuses.

Monitor FHR with continuous CTG during and after administration of intravenous drugs for 30 minutes.

Drug treatment

- **Hydralazine:** 10 mg IV slowly
  Repeat doses: 5 mg IV at 20-minute intervals may be given if necessary (the effect of a single dose can last up to six hours).

  If no lasting effect with boluses (assess over 20 minutes), consider an infusion at 2.0 mg/hour increasing by 0.5 mg/hour as required (2–20 mg/hour usually required).

  Close liaison with anaesthetists: may require plasma expansion and invasive monitoring.

- **Labetalol:** If BP still uncontrolled 50 mg IV slowly
  If necessary, repeat after 20 minutes or start IV infusion of 200 mg in 200 ml normal saline, starting at 40 mg/hour, increasing dose at half-hourly intervals as required, to a maximum of 160 mg/hour.

  If blood pressure does not respond to the above, discuss with senior renal physicians and anaesthetists.

- **Use of nifedipine antepartum**
  The decision to administer nifedipine should be made by consultant staff.

  Oral route is safer and as effective as sublingual route.

  Dose: 10 mg orally. Monitor FHR with CTG.

  Note: An interaction between nifedipine and magnesium sulphate has been reported to produce profound muscle weakness, maternal hypotension and fetal distress.[43–45]

- **Initiate steroids if gestation ≤ 34 weeks (RCOG Guideline).**[46]

- **Consider the need for anticonvulsant therapy if eclampsia imminent.**

Principles of fluid balance

BEWARE: Iatrogenic fluid overload in pre-eclampsia/eclampsia.[4]
Maintenance fluids should be given as crystalloid but additional fluid (colloid) may be necessary prior to vasodilatation to prevent maternal hypotension and fetal compromise.[47] Consideration should also be given to correcting hypovolaemia in women with oliguria.

- **Record fluid balance accurately** (including delivery and postpartum blood loss, input/output deficit)

- **Maintain crystalloid infusion** – 85 ml/hour, or urinary output in preceding hour plus 30 ml.[47]
- **Give selective colloid expansion** – prior to pharmacological vasodilatation; oliguria with low CVP
- **Give diuretics** – only for women with confirmed pulmonary oedema.
- **Apply selective monitoring of CVP**.[48]

Consider the need for in utero/neonatal transfer[47,49]

If a maternity unit does not have access to HDU/ICU, is unable to cope with maternal complications or is unable to cope with preterm babies, it may be appropriate to consider antenatal transfer of the mother. However, maternal safety must not be jeopardised and each case should be considered on its clinical merits. In some cases it is safer to deliver the mother and then consider the need for transfer of mother and/or child.

'Referral to a regional centre for advice and/or assistance should be considered in all cases of eclampsia, particularly where there are maternal complications.'[47]

Delivery

- Delivery should be a team effort involving obstetricians, midwives, anaesthetists and paediatricians.
- The need for delivery is dependent on the maternal and fetal condition.
- Either caesarean section or induction of labour may be appropriate, depending on the clinical findings.
- In eclampsia, the definitive treatment is delivery.

  *'However, **it is inappropriate to deliver an unstable mother** even if there is fetal distress. Once seizures are controlled, severe hypertension treated and hypoxia corrected, delivery can be expedited.'*[47]
- Ergometrine should not be used in cases of severe pre-eclampsia and eclampsia.
- If delivery is by caesarean section, use antibiotic prophylaxis.[50]
- Consider prophylaxis against thromboembolism (RCOG risk assessment guidelines).[51]
- An early combined obstetric and anaesthetic approach to monitoring and management provides optimal care.

Principles of care after delivery

- Maintain vigilance as the majority of eclamptic seizures occur after delivery.
- High-dependency care should be provided as clinically indicated (24 hours minimum).[47,52]
- **Consider the need for admission to ICU**.[52]
- Monitoring should be undertaken by experienced staff: a nurse/midwife should be allocated to provide one-to-one care, with input from senior medical staff.
- Maintain close attention to fluid balance.
- Reduce anti-hypertensive medication as indicated.

Follow-up

- Long-term follow-up to make sure that blood pressure resolves.
- Specific investigations:
  - anti-phospholipid antibodies
  - lupus anticoagulant
  - thrombophilia screen[53]
  - if eclampsia has occurred, consider CT scan of head.[47]

- Discuss with mother what has happened and its significance for the future.
- Inform general practitioner and community midwives.

Initial management of severe pre-eclampsia: discussion points

The aim of antenatal care is to detect patients at risk of severe pre-eclampsia and eclampsia. Greater attention should be paid to patients with specific risk factors, such as pre-existing hypertension and family history. Further evaluation can be carried out at day assessment units, if available. The majority of hypertensive patients can be managed as outpatients with no intervention except for monitoring of the patient and the fetus. However, it is estimated that 25% of hypertensive patients require admission for acute management.[54]

On admission, evaluation of the patient is performed. Management is a team approach and the relevant personnel should be informed early.

Measurement of blood pressure[55]

The usefulness of the definition of pre-eclampsia relies on accurate measurement of blood pressure. However, blood pressure is a variable and can fluctuate on a minute-to-minute basis. Equipment in hospitals can vary in readings. Routine recording in hospitals has been reported to be inaccurate because of the inconsistencies in the positioning of the patient, use of a large cuff if the patient was obese, rounding of the measurement, selection of the right or left arm and the period of pre-measurement resting.

Further, there is widespread confusion among obstetricians and midwives about which Korotkoff sound to use when measuring the diastolic blood pressure. Traditionally, the fourth sound (K4, muffling) has been recommended for use because of the perception that the fifth (K5, disappearance) may sometimes be zero in pregnancy. However, others have recommended K5 because it is nearer to the diastolic as measured by intra-arterial cannulation. The difference between the two is on average about 6–15 mmHg, so the distinction is of clinical significance. Probably the best policy at present is to record both when they are distinct and different.

Another problem includes the use of automated blood pressure monitors, some of which underestimate the blood pressure in pre-eclampsia by a mean of 8 mmHg when compared with conventional sphygmomanometry.

The above factors should be taken into account when assessing patients with pre-eclampsia/eclampsia.

Recommendation for audit

- How is blood pressure measured in your hospital? Is there a standard technique?
- When were sphygmomanometers in your hospitals assessed for accuracy? What is their intra- and inter- observer variation?
- Do staff use K4 or K5 when recording blood pressure and what measurement/s is/are recorded in the chart?

Proteinuria[56]

Apart from blood pressure measurement, analysis of the urine by dipstick for proteinuria is the most commonly performed antenatal screening test. However, urine must be obtained under sterile conditions. Dipstick estimation can be useful in the initial assessment, but the 'gold standard' is the quantitative analysis of a 24-hour urine sample.

Uric acid measurement

Uric acid rises in pre-eclampsia and is a better predictor of fetal death than blood pressure.[57] This elevation is thought to be partly due to impairment of renal tubular function and some partly due to increased production secondary to tissue damage due to ischaemia. Serial testing is advocated as a rising level indicates progression of the disease process.

Liver function tests

Disruption of liver cells leads to a release of enzymes into the circulation. The most sensitive change is seen in aspartate transaminase (AST) but there is also a rise in alanine transaminase (ALT). A rise in liver enzymes is always significant and needs to be followed closely.

Platelets

A falling platelet count in pre-eclampsia is associated with progression of the disease and a worsening outcome. Serial samples should be taken to watch for developing trends. A falling trend is of concern and can give some guidance as to the timing of delivery. If a platelet count is greater than 100 000, major coagulation problems are unlikely.[58]

In recent years, the combination of haemolysis, elevated liver enzymes and low platelet count has been described as the HELLP syndrome.[59] This is not a new phenomenon but more a new description of previously described pathological findings. If a platelet count of less than 100 000 is found, a full coagulation screen, blood film and liver function tests should be carried out as this can give information on disease progression and maternal risk.[60]

Management of hypertension

Although medical treatment for mild/moderate hypertension remains controversial, therapy for severe hypertension is well accepted.[61] The aim of treatment is to prevent cerebral haemorrhage and hypertensive encephalopathy. The 1997–99 CEMD report[4] identified intracranial haemorrhage as the main cause of maternal death in hypertensive diseases, reflecting inadequate blood pressure control. Control of the blood pressure may also allow valuable time to be gained, enabling delivery of a more mature fetus.

The most commonly used drugs are hydralazine, methyldopa, labetalol and nifedipine. At the time of going to press, the choice of the antihypertensive depends on the experience and familiarity of the attendant staff with a particular drug. Care should be taken not to reduce the blood pressure too quickly. The aim of therapy is not to normalise blood pressure but to stop the rise and to achieve a moderate fall. Blood pressure control must, if at all possible, be achieved prior to delivery but especially before intubation for general anaesthesia before caesarean section, as an acute blood pressure rise can occur.[62]

Antenatal corticosteroids to prevent respiratory distress syndrome

RCOG guidelines on the use of antenatal corticosteroid therapy, published in 1996,[46] recommended that 'every effort should be made to initiate antenatal corticosteroid therapy in women between 24 and 36 weeks of gestation in any condition requiring elective preterm delivery'. However, updated guidelines (December 1999)[63] looked at the effectiveness of antenatal steroids: 'while it is accepted that antenatal corticosteroid therapy reduces the incidence of respiratory distress syndrome (RDS), an analysis of the "number needed to treat" suggests that after 34 weeks, 94 women will need to be treated to prevent one case of RDS, while before 31 weeks one case of RDS is prevented by every five women treated'.

Antenatal corticosteroid therapy is recommended before 34 weeks.[42] Use of antenatal corticosteroid therapy between 34 and 36 weeks is a grey area and clinicians are asked to refer to the RCOG guidelines and to decide for themselves if antenatal corticosteroid therapy is indicated.

The MAGPIE trial

Even for women with severe pre-eclampsia, the risk of eclampsia is low – around 1%. Magnesium sulphate has few adverse effects.[64]

The MAGPIE trial to establish the clinical efficacy of magnesium sulphate in pre-eclampsia has now completed.[65] This trial has shown that women treated with magnesium sulphate had a 58% lower risk of seizures. Overall, 11 per 1000 fewer women had seizures when treated with magnesium sulphate

Delivery

The cure for pre-eclampsia is delivery of the fetus and placenta. However, timing of the delivery affects outcome for both mother and baby. Most maternal deaths occur postpartum. A rushed delivery in an unstable patient adds to her risk. A delay in delivery may also be associated with maternal death. Early close communication between obstetricians, midwives, anaesthetists and paediatricians is vital in management.

Fluid balance in pre-eclampsia

Most maternal deaths and significant morbidity occur after delivery.[4,66] The main cause of death in pre-eclampsia is now pulmonary oedema. The risk of pulmonary oedema is aggravated by exogenous fluid given in the belief that these women are at risk of renal failure.

Renal failure is unusual in pure pre-eclampsia and is usually associated with additional problems such as haemorrhage and sepsis.[67] If it does occur, the morbidity and mortality are low as it is usually an acute tubular necrosis that can be manage easily.[67]

Oliguria is not uncommon after delivery, occurring in about 30% of patients with severe disease. This does not require treatment, as urinary output will recover in its own time. If there is any doubt about renal function, urinary osmolality can be checked: if concentrated, renal function is satisfactory and is due to reduced renal perfusion, which will improve over time. If urine is not concentrated, renal failure is present and the renal physicians should be involved in management. There is no evidence that oliguria in the presence of concentrated urine leads to renal failure. Fluid challenges are dangerous in pre-eclampsia as much of the fluid will be lost from the vessels into the interstitial fluid, aggravating the existing tissue oedema.

Invasive monitoring is usually not necessary, and central venous pressure (CVP) lines can be misleading.[68] In pre-eclampsia, pulmonary oedema because of increased interstitial fluid, can occur in the presence of a low CVP.

It is safer to run a patient 'dry' and restrict intravenous fluids than to run the risk of pulmonary overload.

Management of imminent eclampsia or eclampsia[42]

General measures[69]

DO NOT LEAVE THE PATIENT ALONE.

CALL FOR HELP – duty obstetric and anaesthetic SpRs; senior midwife.

INFORM CONSULTANTS – obstetrician and anaesthetist on call.

Is it safe to approach the patient? Consider hazards around the patient that will affect your safety.

Prevent maternal injury during convulsion – place in semi-prone position.

Airway

- Assess.

- Maintain patency.
- Protect airway.
- Apply oxygen.

Breathing

- Assess.
- Ventilate as required.

Circulation

- Evaluate pulse and blood pressure.
- If absent, initiate CPR and call arrest team.
- Left lateral tilt.
- Secure IV access as soon as safely possible.
- Attach pulse oximeter, ECG and automatic BP monitors.
- Urinary catheter – hourly urinometer readings.
- Fluid input/output chart

Observations and investigations

- As for the management of severe pre-eclampsia.
- Consider blood gases.

Check for aspiration

Lungs should always be auscultated after the convulsion has ended.

Medication for the management of seizures

The vast majority of the initial seizures are self-limiting.[69]

MAGNESIUM SULPHATE is the anticonvulsant drug of choice.[70]

Avoid polypharmacy to treat seizures – this increases risk of respiratory arrest.

After **A B C**:

- Loading dose: 4 g IV over 10–15 minutes

  Add 8 ml 50% $MgSO_4$ solution to 12 ml of physiological saline

  = 4 g in 20 ml = 20% solution

- Maintenance Dose: 1 g per hour

  Add 25 g $MgSO_4$ (50 ml) to 250 ml physiological saline

  1 g $MgSO_4$ = 12 ml per hour IV

  1 g/hour is infused for 24 hours after last fit provided that:
  - respiratory rate > 16 bpm
  - urine output > 25 ml/hour, and
  - patellar reflexes are present

  Administer via infusion pump.

  REMEMBER TO SUBTRACT VOLUME INFUSED FROM TOTAL MAINTENANCE INFUSION VOLUME (85 ml/hour)

A higher maintenance dose may be required initially to prevent recurrent seizures – consultant must make this decision.

- If seizure continues or if seizures recur, give a second bolus of magnesium sulphate:

  2–4 g depending on weight of patient, over 5–10 minutes

  (2 g if < 70 kg and 4 g if > 70 kg)

  ONE STAT DOSE ONLY.

If seizures continue despite a further bolus of magnesium sulphate, *'options then include diazepam (10 mg) or thiopentone (50 mg IV). Intubation then becomes necessary in such women to protect the airway and ensure adequate oxygenation. Further seizures should be managed by intermittent positive pressure ventilation and muscle relaxation'*.[47]

When using magnesium sulphate:

- Monitor:
  - hourly urine output`
  - respiratory rate, oxygen saturation and patellar reflexes – every 10 minutes for first two hours and then every 30 minutes
  - serum magnesium levels if toxicity is suspected on clinical grounds.
- Request $MgSO_4$ levels if:
  - loss of patellar reflexes. Always get suppression of reflexes before respiratory depression.
  - respiratory rate < 16 breaths/minute (**CARE:** lower rate may be appropriate if on opiates)
  - urine output < 25 ml/hour for 4 hours
  - further seizures occur.

Management of imminent eclampsia or eclampsia: discussion points

Even under ideal conditions, an eclamptic fit is a dramatic and disturbing event. Doctors and midwives are severely challenged at these times by the emergency and by their own anxiety. As the vast majority of the initial seizures are self-limiting, the priority after securing maternal safety is **A**irway, **B**reathing, **C**irculation. As soon as SAFELY possible, a large secure line should be inserted and the loading dose of magnesium sulphate given.

Debate: Whether or not to give diazepam for the initial seizure

As already discussed, the majority of the initial seizures (which are uncommon events) are self-limiting and should have stopped while attendants go through **A B C**.

After the convulsion has ceased, the patient begins to breathe again and oxygenation is rarely a problem. Difficulty with oxygenation may occur in women who have had repetitive seizures or received drugs, such as diazepam, in an attempt to abolish the seizures. It is recommended that diazepam should be avoided to stop the initial seizure, especially if the patient does not have a secure intravenous line in place and someone skilled in intubation is not immediately available.

As magnesium sulphate will be given to prevent recurrent seizures, polypharmacy is extremely hazardous in women with eclampsia, as addition of diazepam or phenytoin may lead to apnoea or cardiac arrest, or both.[69]

The decision to administer diazepam should be made by the lead consultant.

Symptom correlation with the development of eclampsia

The majority of patients have one convulsion only.[70] While prodromal symptoms, particularly headache and abdominal pain, are present in most patients who fit, about 20% of patients will convulse unexpectedly, often with a normal blood pressure and no specific signs for the development of eclampsia.[70] Hyperreflexia has never been demonstrated as an accurate predictor of eclampsia. However, it is of great value as a clinical measure of magnesium toxicity.

Magnesium levels

Therapeutic 2.0–4.0 mmol/l

With increasing magnesium levels, the following may occur:

Symptoms	$MgSO_4$ level (mmol/l)
Feeling of warmth, flushing, double vision, slurred speech	3.8–5.0
Loss of tendon reflexes	> 5.0
Respiratory depression	> 6.0
Respiratory arrest	6.3–7.0
Cardiac arrest	> 12.0

Magnesium toxicity

Symptom	Treatment
Urine output < 100 ml in 4 hours	If no clinical signs of magnesium toxicity, decrease rate to 0.5 g/hour
	Review overall management with attention to fluid balance and blood loss
Absent patellar reflexes	Stop $MgSO_4$ infusion until reflexes return
Respiratory depression	Stop $MgSO_4$ infusion
	Give oxygen via facemask and place in recovery position because of impaired level of consciousness
	Monitor closely
Respiratory arrest	Stop $MgSO_4$ infusion
	Give IV Calcium gluconate
	Intubate and ventilate immediately
Cardiac arrest	Commence CPR. Stop $MgSO_4$ infusion
	Give IV Calcium gluconate
	Intubate and ventilate immediately
	If antenatal, immediate delivery
Antidote	10% Calcium gluconate 10 ml IV over 10 minutes

Prevention of recurrent seizures and magnesium toxicity

If convulsions have occurred, anticonvulsants are required. A large multicentre trial has shown that magnesium sulphate is superior to both phenytoin and diazepam.[70] The re-convulsion rates and maternal deaths were found to be significantly reduced by magnesium sulphate as compared with either phenytoin and diazepam. However, it is important to note that no treatment will completely prevent seizures. Re-convulsion rates vary between 5% and 20%.[70]

One of the main concerns that many obstetricians have is the fear of magnesium toxicity. Duley *et al.*[70] used clinical evaluation alone and showed that toxicity did not occur. Further, the adverse effects from magnesium were no worse than for diazepam and significantly less than those found with phenytoin. Using the dosage regimen, there is no need to check magnesium levels unless there is treatment failure or clinical evidence of toxicity. In most cases, therapy can be monitored safely by measurement of the patellar reflex and respiratory rate (or oxygen saturation).

HELLP syndrome[71]

HELLP is a syndrome comprising haemolysis, elevated liver enzymes and low platelets. It occurs in 4–12% of patients with severe pre-eclampsia. Hypertension is not always a clinical feature. It can occur in multiparous patients as well as primigravidae and it is associated with a high perinatal mortality rate. HELLP can present with vague symptoms of nausea, vomiting and epigastric/right upper-quadrant pain and, because of this, there is often a delay in diagnosis. A high index of suspicion is therefore required.

The management of HELLP, as for severe pre-eclampsia, is to evaluate the severity, stabilise and deliver. High-dose corticosteroids may be beneficial. The risk of recurrence of the HELLP syndrome is approximately 20%.

Contents of 'eclampsia box'[42]

Each maternity unit should have an 'emergency box' for eclampsia. This ensures that appropriate equipment is readily available.

Emergency box for eclampsia

Equipment	Quantity
Drugs	Magnesium sulphate 50%, 5 g in 10-ml ampoule x 10 ampoules Calcium gluconate 10%, 8.9 mg in 10-ml ampoule x 2 ampoules Hydralazine 20 mg in 1-ml ampoule x 2 ampoules Labetalol 200 mg in 20-ml ampoule x 1 ampoule Sodium chloride 10-ml ampoule x 10 ampoules
Intravenous fluids	250-ml bag of sodium chloride x 2 1 litre Hartmann's solution x 1 IVAC giving set x 1 IV blood giving set x 1
Venous access	20-gauge cannula (pink) x 2 18-gauge cannula (green) x 2 16-gauge cannula (grey) x 2 Tourniquet x 1 Fixation tape x 1 roll
Airway equipment	Guedel airways: sizes 4, 3 and 2 Laerdal bag, mask and valve Green oxygen tubing 2 metres Yankaeur sucker
Other equipment	50-ml syringe x 2 20-ml syringe x 2 10-ml syringe x 2 Green needles x 2 Reflex hammer x 1

Patient information

Patient information packs can be obtained from:

ACTION ON PRE-ECLAMPSIA (APEC)
31–33 College Road,
Harrow, Middlesex HA1 1EJ.
Tel: 020-8863 3271

Fax: 020-8424 0653
Help line: 020 8427 4217
Website: **www.apec.org.uk**
E-mail: **info@apec.org.uk**
Registered charity no. 1013557

Patient information: discussion points

It is recommended in *Why Mothers Die* that '*All women should receive antenatal education so that they are aware of the symptoms associated with pre-eclampsia, its importance and the need to obtain urgent professional advice*'.[4]

Audit and training

Audit

Once guidelines have been introduced, their use can be audited. It is up to each maternity unit to decide how they might audit their guidelines. With the advent of risk assessment, maternity units may consider establishing a small team consisting of a senior obstetrician, a junior obstetrician, midwife, paediatrician and anaesthetist. Each case of eclampsia would be evaluated and assessed against established guidelines. The evaluations would be presented at perinatal meetings – the remit being to educate and discuss areas where improvement could occur.

Training

The emphasis is on a 'team approach'. Communication in labour ward could be improved by:

- introduction of team scenario training on the ward – these can also help to highlight areas where improvements can occur
- discussion of RCOG Guidelines, e.g., *Management of Eclampsia* (available on the RCOG website: **www.rcog.org.uk**) –it is important that midwives and anaesthetists are involved in these discussions.

Fitness to drive after convulsions associated with eclampsia

If the classic hallmark signs of eclampsia are present and convulsions are associated with these then, once the condition is controlled and the woman is generally well, she need not refrain from driving. Since this will vary with each woman, the clinician will need to advise directly. As the convulsion is deemed to be a direct result of the eclampsia rather than an underlying liability to fits, no restrictions are placed on returning to drive.

Algorithm 16.1 Massive obstetric haemorrhage key points

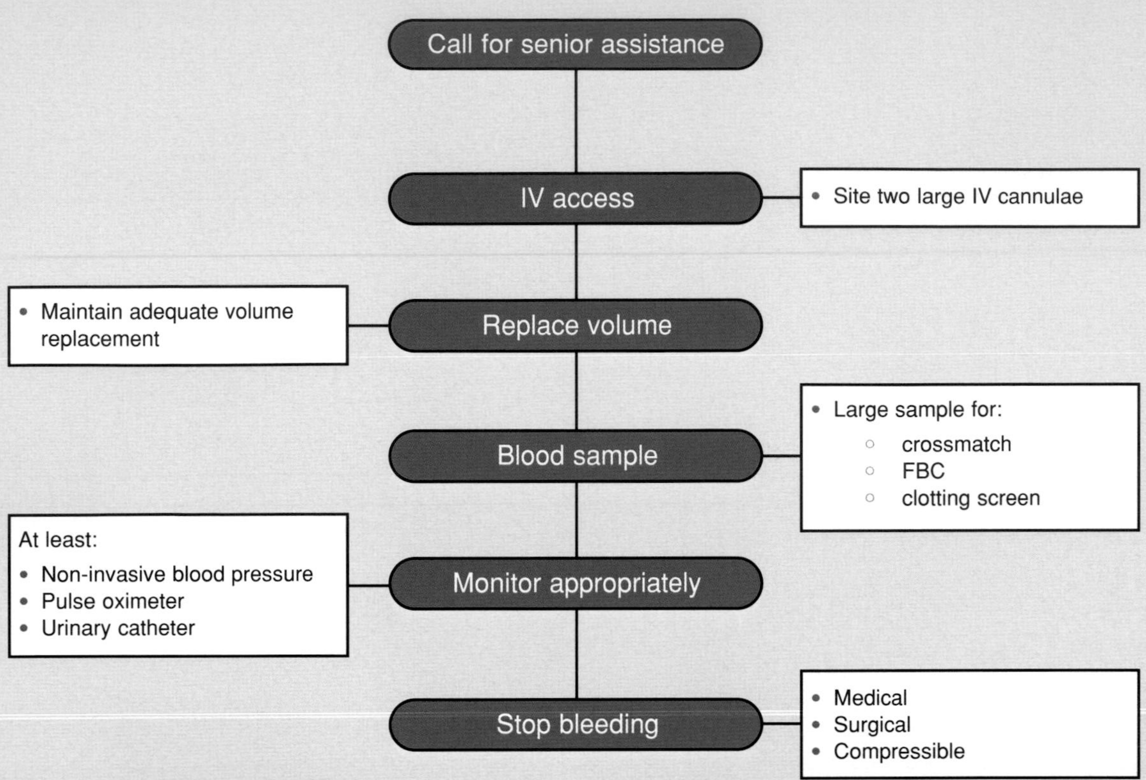

Chapter 16

Massive obstetric haemorrhage

Objectives

On successfully completing this topic you will be able to:

- manage massive obstetric haemorrhage
- understand the haematological and cardiovascular changes of pregnancy and obstetric pathologies
- recognise maternal decompensation in response to major haemorrhage
- make a plan to facilitate optimum management in your environment

Introduction

Massive haemorrhage remains a leading cause of maternal mortality despite modern improvements in obstetric practice and transfusion services. This chapter covers some aspects of particular relevance to anaesthetists. Complications of haemorrhage associated with first-trimester bleeding due to miscarriage or ectopic pregnancy have not been considered, although many general principles will apply.

Maternal mortality and incidence of massive haemorrhage

The most recent report on Confidential Enquiries into Maternal Deaths in the United Kingdom[4] details a fall in mortality rate from 5.5 per million maternities in 1994–96 to 3.3 per million maternities. Concern remains that care is not always as good as it could be, especially in cases where the problem could have been anticipated.

Mortality statistics give no data on the incidence of massive haemorrhage or on the maternal and fetal morbidity associated with haemorrhage and transfusion. Specific complications include transfusion-related reactions and infections, genital tract trauma, loss of fertility and the rare Sheehan's syndrome (hypopituitarism).

Definition and epidemiology

Massive obstetric haemorrhage has been variously defined[72] as the loss of more than 1000 ml or 1500 ml blood as either antepartum or postpartum loss. This definition is used as a marker for audit or to mobilise additional resources reserved for such emergencies. Considerable problems are recognised in the accurate measurement of blood loss and a definition based on volume alone has some shortcomings. Both visual and measured loss can be highly inaccurate and loss from placental abruption or uterine rupture may be partially or completely concealed. Underestimation of blood loss may delay active steps being taken to prepare for or prevent further bleeding.

Major causes of obstetric haemorrhage (primary or secondary)

Resulting initially in hypovolaemia:

- Uterine atony
- Placenta praevia
- Retained placenta or products of conception
- Genital tract injury including broad ligament haematoma
- Uterine rupture
- Uterine version
- Associated with ectopic pregnancy.

Associated with coagulation failure:

- Placental abruption
- Pre-eclampsia
- Septicaemia/intrauterine sepsis
- Retained dead fetus
- Amniotic fluid embolus
- Incompatible blood transfusion
- Abortion with hypertonic saline
- Existing coagulation abnormalities.[72]

Other outcomes may help in the audit of massive haemorrhage and could be used to identify problem areas requiring reorganisation or staff training. Auditing records of women requiring more than two units of blood may still underestimate mothers with a blood loss of 1000–1500 ml. A mother with an antenatal Hb of 12g/dl and a 2000-ml blood loss, replaced with colloid other than blood, might have a postnatal Hb of 8g/dl or above. This could be treated expectantly with oral iron. This mother would not appear in a review of haemorrhage based on transfusion practice, despite falling within the definition by volume of massive obstetric haemorrhage.

In a large series from California,[73] 27 of 16 462 (0.16%) women delivering in one hospital in 1988 received more than two units of blood products. Only 11 of 27 (41.0%) women had conditions that would have led to antenatal warning of massive haemorrhage, largely women with a placenta praevia. In a study from Vancouver in 1985–86,[74] 40 of 7731 (0.58%) of women delivering received more than two units of blood. Again these transfusions were described as unpredictable in 27 of 40 (67.5%) cases. Overall rates of transfusion in this series were 48 of 6049 (0.8%) for vaginal births and 52 of 1682 (3.1%) for caesarean delivery.

Summary of audit points

- Incidence of measured blood loss greater than 1000ml or 1500 ml.
- Incidence and indication for transfusion of blood products.
- Postnatal Hb fall of > 3 g/dl in women who have not been transfused. This may identify women with unrecognised significant loss at the time of delivery.[75]
- Critical incident reporting. A report of difficulties encountered in obtaining staff, equipment or blood products filed by the personnel involved in each critical event for discussion with staff in all disciplines.
- Morbidity represented by circulatory collapse, organ failure, transfer to the intensive care unit, genital tract trauma and loss of fertility.

Guidelines for the management of massive haemorrhage

Many units will have developed local guidelines to be followed in the event of massive haemorrhage, as recommended in the CEMD reports. Each will have its own problems, depending on staff availability and the geography of the hospital. They will include details of senior staff to be contacted in obstetrics, anaesthetics and haematology.[76] A management protocol should be agreed by the clinical and laboratory staff and will a provide a focus for regular audit.

Practical management

Organisation

The pivotal factor in the management of a massive obstetric haemorrhage is the restoration of the circulating blood volume. Failure to maintain adequate tissue perfusion leads to loss of vital organ function and care becomes increasingly more complex. Experienced staff – obstetricians, anaesthetists and midwives – should be called.

The blood bank technician should be alerted to the situation, as should the consultant obstetrician and haematologist. One member of the resuscitation team should be assigned to record the patient's vital signs, urinary output, type and quantity of fluid replacement, drugs given and the timing of the events.

Restoration of circulating blood volume

1. Position the mother in the left lateral position, where possible, to minimise the effects of aortocaval compression. Lateral tilt with a wedge is also used but may not be adequate. This is vital when obstetric procedures are in progress, when manual displacement of the uterus by an assistant may be necessary. If an epidural is in use, compensatory lower-limb vasoconstriction will be limited, so the effects of positioning may be more marked. Head-down tilt can be used as a short-term measure to improve venous return but this may compromise respiration.
2. Administer a high concentration of oxygen (10–15 litres per minute) to the mother, regardless of her oxygen saturation. If the baby is undelivered, increasing the maternofetal oxygen gradient may help oxygen transfer, so supranormal values of maternal PO_2 may be valuable.
3. Assess the airway and respiratory effort. Intubation may be indicated to protect the airway, if the mother has a depressed conscious level due to hypotension, or to maximise oxygenation using 100% oxygen.
4. Establish two 14-gauge intravenous lines and take 20 ml blood for diagnostic tests.[77] Lower limb or femoral access should be avoided.

Diagnostic blood tests

Diagnostic test	Blood required
Full blood count/platelet count	2.5 ml in EDTA
Crossmatch	10–15 ml in plain bottle
Coagulation screen (thrombin time and fibrinogen assay)	4.5 ml in citrate
FDP/D-dimers	2.0 ml in EACA antifibrinolytic agent)

5. Initial volume replacement should consist of up to two litres physiological saline or Hartmann's solution, followed by plasma expanders until blood is available. Large volumes of crystalloid may be undesirable in view of the relatively low oncotic pressure in pregnancy.
6. If the haemorrhage is life threatening, transfuse uncrossmatched O rhesus-negative blood otherwise transfuse ABO and rhesus D-compatible blood as soon as feasible.

7. At an appropriate moment, move the mother to a place where there is adequate space, lighting and equipment to continue resuscitation and treatment.

Component blood therapy

Blood

Fresh whole blood is not used in adult practice in the UK because release from the blood bank less than 24 hours after collection does not allow completion of a full infection screen.[77] After 48 hours storage, viable platelet numbers and the function of important clotting factors (factors V and VIII) are already reduced. Stored whole blood is rarely available, so concentrated red cells comprise the mainstay of treatment for volume replacement and the restoration of the oxygen-carrying capacity of blood. Each pack contains approximately 220 ml red cells and 80 ml saline-adenine-glucose-mannitol (SAG-M) solution, giving it a shelf life of 35 days. The haematocrit varies from 55% to 70% so a plasma substitute needs to be given in appropriate amounts to provide the additional volume required. Frequent checks of the haematocrit are helpful to guide massive transfusions, particularly when adequate measurement of loss is impossible.

Full crossmatching of blood may take up to an hour. In an emergency group-specific blood should be used. The patient's blood group and presence of abnormal antibodies are usually established during pregnancy, which facilitate the provision of blood when needed. The use of group-specific blood following antibody screening carries a risk of less than 0.1% of a haemolytic transfusion reaction, which rises to 1.0% if group-specific blood is used without antibody screening.[77] In most circumstances, issuing of group- and rhesus-compatible blood should be possible within five minutes. O Rh-negative blood should be available on the labour ward for dire emergencies but this carries a small risk of sensitisation to 'c' antigen with possible problems for future pregnancies. It should rarely be needed.

In order to reduce the transmission of the CJD virus, the blood is further leucodepleted. At present, there is no specific test to check the blood for this virus.

Alternatives to homologous blood transfusion

Interest in reducing homologous transfusion[78] has increased in recent years and some alternatives have been tried in obstetric practice.

- Autologous blood transfusion by antenatal donation
  This appears to be a safe technique in pregnancy, although its use is likely to be restricted to women who are at high risk of needing a blood transfusion, e.g. placenta praevia, or for whom blood is not readily available due to maternal antibodies to blood antigens. Unfortunately, many obstetric transfusions are unexpected, which limits the use of this technique.[79,80]

- Cell salvage procedures
  A number of techniques exist to recover blood for reinfusion from clean operative sites. Aspirated blood is anticoagulated, filtered, washed and the red cells resuspended in saline before reinfusion. Their use is thought to be safe in obstetric practice.[81]

Warmers, filters and high-pressure infusers

All large-volume infusions should be warmed, but it is mandatory to avoid infusing cold fluid directly into the heart through a CVP line. Desirable properties of a warmer include speed and ease of operation, rapid warm-up time, ability to warm adequately at high infusion rates and safety to avoid overheating.

More recent developments have moved away from the use of traditional water baths to dry warmers, which avoid the potential electrical hazards of water baths and are more easily portable. The patient should also be kept warm, as hypothermia will exacerbate poor peripheral perfusion, acidosis and coagulation abnormalities. Any benefits from the use of blood filters may be outweighed by the deleterious effect on the speed of transfusion.

High-pressure infusion devices are essential. Hand inflated pressure bags are effective but labour intensive. More sophisticated high-pressure infusers use pressure from gas cylinders to provide very high flows. Hazards of any high-pressure infusion include fluid overload and air embolism.

Defective blood coagulation

In a previously healthy woman, a clotting-factor deficiency is unlikely to occur until around 80% of the original blood volume has been replaced. Large infusions of replacement fluids, e.g. plasma substitutes, and red cells suspended in additive solutions will dilute further the coagulation factors and platelets, causing a dilutional coagulopathy. This, in combination with hypotension-mediated endothelial injury, may trigger disseminated intravascular coagulation (DIC) and the downward spiral into coagulation failure.[82]

Clotting factors and platelets

Fresh frozen plasma (FFP) is separated from whole blood within six hours of donation and stored for up to one year at –20°C to –30°C. FFP provides all the clotting factors required and should be infused at 12–15 ml/kg approximating to an initial 4–5 unit transfusion. Ideally, four units of FFP should be given for each six units of rapidly transfused blood to maintain the coagulation factors and fibrinogen above a critical level. Guidance should be sought from the results of clotting tests if these can be obtained quickly. Cryoprecipitate contains more fibrinogen than FFP but lacks antithrombin III (coagulation inhibitor), which is depleted in obstetric-related coagulopathies. Cryoprecipitate may be useful if the patient develops profound hypofibrinogenaemia.

Platelet packs have a limited shelf life of five days and should be transfused through a platelet filter. They are rarely indicated above a platelet count of 50×10^9/l but may be required to raise the level to $80–100 \times 10^9$/l if surgical intervention is planned.

Recently, methylene blue-treated FFP has become available. Methylene blue helps to inactivate the CJD virus. The FFP so treated is 10–15 times more expensive than its untreated form. At the moment, therefore, it is only available for children in the UK.

Evaluation of response

Healthy women can maintain a normal or even high blood pressure while large volumes of blood are lost intra-abdominally. Most, but not all, women will demonstrate a tachycardia if bleeding significantly but paradoxical bradycardia[83] has also been observed. Essential monitoring should include pulse, blood pressure (direct or indirect), respiration rate, oxygen saturation and fluid balance. Regular checks of the haematocrit, clotting studies and blood gases will help guide resuscitation.

A central venous pressure (CVP) line has been strongly recommended to avoid undertransfusion or fluid overload.[84] Insertion should not delay initial resuscitation but if peripheral access is inadequate this route may be used for volume replacement, providing a short large-bore catheter is inserted. If DIC is suspected or established, CVP insertion is more hazardous. The antecubital fossa should be considered for both CVP and pulmonary artery catheters, as this site is more easily compressed.[80] If these veins have already been used for smaller-gauge cannulae, exchange sets enable the upgrading of a smaller cannula to one with a larger bore using a Seldinger technique.

Pulmonary capillary wedge pressure and cardiac output measurements via a pulmonary artery catheter should be used appropriately.

Indications for insertion of a pulmonary artery catheter in the management of haemorrhage

- Hypotension unresponsive to fluid therapy
- Oliguria despite adequate CVP
- Coexisting relevant disease e.g. cardiac failure
- Co-existing severe sepsis
- Co-existing severe pre-eclampsia
- Management of pulmonary oedema

Remedy the cause of bleeding.

Detailed algorithms to assist obstetricians in decision making for common problems can be found in other texts.[85] Anaesthetists need to be aware of the drugs that may be used and the surgical options to arrest haemorrhage.

Interventions for the management of haemorrhage

- Empty uterus:
  - deliver fetus if undelivered.
  - remove placenta or retained products of conception.
- Oxytocics/ergometrine/prostaglandin.
- Massage and bimanual compression of the uterus following delivery.
- Repair of genital tract injury, e.g. vaginal/cervical lacerations.
- Uterine packing or Rusch balloon.
- Compression of the aorta (temporary control).
- Internal iliac artery/uterine artery ligation.
  This may be ineffective because of rapid opening of collateral channels. This intervention is more likely to be attempted in women of low parity in order to maintain fertility and proceeds to hysterectomy in 50% of cases.
- Hysterectomy.
- Arterial embolisation.
  There are a small number of reports of this technique in obstetric practice.[86] Access is usually obtained via the femoral artery, from where the bleeding point is identified by contrast injection. The feeder artery is catheterised and embolised with absorbable gelatin sponge (Gelfoam®, Upjohn), usually resorbed in ten days. This procedure seems to be a useful addition to the management of obstetric haemorrhage in centres with suitably trained staff. Appropriately sited catheters have been positioned preoperatively in women at very high risk, e.g. placenta accreta.

Drugs

Oxytocin

Drugs used as prophylaxis to maintain a well-contracted uterus include oxytocin (Syntocinon®, Alliance) 5 units IM or IV and oxytocin 5 units ergometrine 0.5 mg (Syntometrine®, Alliance). The recommended dose after caesarean section (*BNF*) is 5 units by slow IV injection immediately after delivery. Oxytocin has a shorter duration of action and is used as an infusion to maintain a contracted uterus (40 units in 500 ml 0.9% saline over four hours). Adverse effects include hypotension due to vasodilatation when given as a rapid intravenous bolus and fluid retention. The intramuscular use of ergometrine (0.5 mg IM) is relatively contraindicated in pre-eclampsia due to its hypertensive action.

A Cochrane systematic review has been carried out on umbilical vein injection for the management of retained placenta. This review has suggested that the umbilical vein injection of saline solution with oxytocin appears to be effective in the management of retained placenta. The reviewers suggested that, as the numbers of included trials are small, further research is required in the area.

Prostaglandins

Although injectable prostaglandins appear to be effective in preventing postpartum haemorrhage, concerns about safety and use limit their suitability for routine prophylactic management of the third stage. However, injectable prostaglandins should continue to be used for treatment of postpartum haemorrhage when other measures fail.

Prostaglandins from the E and F groups stimulate myometrial contraction and have been used for refractory haemorrhage due to uterine atony. Prostaglandins E_2 (PGE_2), prostaglandin F_2 (PGF_2) and its analogue 15-methylprostaglandin F_2 have been used either intramuscularly, intravenously, injected directly into the myometrium or as an intramyometrial infusion. There are reports of prostaglandin pessaries being placed in the uterine or vaginal cavities. PGE_2 and PGF_2 have differing effects on the cardiovascular system. The magnitude of these effects will depend on the dose given and the mode of administration, remembering that an intramyometrial injection could be rapidly absorbed into the circulation.

Use of PGE_2 results primarily in vasodilatation with a fall in systemic and pulmonary vascular resistance and resulting fall in blood pressure. Cardiac output can be maintained by an increase in heart rate and stroke volume. Both severe hypotension following intramyometrial injection and paradoxical severe hypertension following intravenous injection have been reported after the use of this drug.

Intrauterine infusions of PGE_2 (7.5 micrograms/minute) via a Foley catheter have been used successfully without significant reported adverse effects.

Intravenous infusions (10 micrograms/minute) have also been used. It is available as dinoprostone (Prostin E2®, Pharmacia) at two strengths: 1 mg/ml and 10 mg/ml, and should be diluted to a solution of 1.5 micrograms/ml.

Carboprost (Hemabate®, Pharmacia) is a potent synthetic analogue of PGF_2 (15-methyl PGF_2) for deep intramuscular injection and licensed for use in postpartum haemorrhage. Suggested dose is 250 micrograms repeated if required. The interval should not be less than 15 minutes, with a total recommended dose of 2 mg. It has been used successfully following failure of conventional treatment. It is not licensed for intramyometrial use.[87] Failure of carboprost to control haemorrhage has been associated with the presence both chorioamnionitis and coagulation abnormalities. Serious adverse effects include bronchospasm, pulmonary oedema and hypertension.

Misoprostol is cheap, stable and seems to be effective.

An increase in intrapulmonary shunting with an accompanying fall in PO_2 has been described following the use of both PGF_2 and carboprost. Oxygen saturation monitoring should be used for women receiving this drug. It should be used cautiously in women with pre-eclampsia or cardiac problems.

Other

Aprotinin and/or tranexamic acid may be options.

Obstetric interventions

Massive obstetric haemorrhage usually occurs intrapartum or within the first hour after delivery. The most common cause is uterine atony with or without retained placental tissue. Other causes include damage to the genital tract or coagulation disorders.

If a uterus fails to respond to a rubbed-up contraction, oxytocic agents should be used and an intramuscular injection of carboprost administered. When a uterus fails to respond it may be due to retained tissue and once resuscitation is effective the uterine cavity needs to be explored. During any exploration the vagina and cervix need to be examined to exclude lacerations.

Uterine packing has been reported with a successful outcome in the management of haemorrhage from an atonic uterus where conservative measures have failed.[88] More recently, the use of a hydrostatic balloon has been advocated as an alterative method for controlling haemorrhage.[25] The inflated Rusch balloon can conform to the contour of the uterine cavity and provides an effective tamponade.

Life-threatening haemorrhage can also be treated by arterial embolisation.[89]

If the haemorrhage continues then a variety of surgical techniques can be employed before a hysterectomy is performed. Bilateral uterine artery ligation has proved helpful in 95%[90] of cases. A stepwise uterine devascularisation has also been described:

1. unilateral uterine artery ligation at the upper part of the lower segment
2. bilateral uterine artery ligation at the upper part of the lower segment
3. lower uterine vessel ligation after mobilisation of the bladder and ureter
4. unilateral ovarian vessel ligation
5. bilateral ovarian vessel ligation.

Steps 1 and 2 have been reported as being effective in over 80% of cases.

Bilateral internal iliac artery ligation has been reported as being successful in half the cases associated with an atonic uterus and placenta accreta.[91] Recognised complications of this procedure include ligation of the external iliac artery, trauma to the iliac veins, ureteric injury and retroperitoneal haematoma.

There have been five successful cases reported of the use of a brace (B-Lynch) suture, which compresses the uterus avoiding compromise of the major vessel (see Figure 16.1).[92]

If the haemorrhage cannot be adequately stemmed then a hysterectomy is warranted but a delay in performing the surgery is likely to lead to a poorer outcome.

Anaesthetic management for obstetric haemorrhage

The general approach should be the same regardless of the aetiology of the haemorrhage. The anaesthetist needs to be able to assess the patient quickly, initiate or continue to resuscitate to restore the intravascular volume and provide safe anaesthesia.

Important points in the assessment will include:

- previous medical, obstetric and anaesthetic history
- a working diagnosis
- current vital signs and laboratory results
- an examination of the cardiovascular and respiratory systems
- an assessment of the upper airway as regards ease of intubation for rapid sequence induction of anaesthesia.

Prophylaxis against acid aspiration is recommended for all patients.

Regional or general anaesthesia

The presence of cardiovascular instability is a relative contraindication to regional blockade. The accompanying sympathetic blockade has the potential to worsen hypotension due to haemorrhage. There are no controlled data comparing techniques in the context of haemorrhage for either maternal or fetal outcomes. Choice for each case will depend on discussion with both the mother and surgeon involved.

If cardiovascular stability has been achieved and there is no evidence of coagulation failure, regional anaesthesia can be used.[93] This may be particularly appropriate for elective cases or where a working epidural has been in place during labour. Continuous epidural block is preferred to a single-injection spinal technique, to allow better control of blood pressure and for prolonged surgery. Adequate quantities of blood, equipment, intravenous lines and monitoring must be available to cope with further bleeding. The height of the block needs to be well maintained to allow intra-abdominal handling of viscera without discomfort.

When bleeding is torrential and cardiovascular stability cannot be achieved, rapid sequence induction of general anaesthesia is more appropriate. Induction agents with minimal peripheral vasodilator action, such as ketamine 1–2 mg/kg (Ketalar®, Parke-Davis) or etomidate 100–300 micrograms/kg (Hypnomidate®, Janssen-Cilag) should be considered and in extreme circumstances adrenaline and atropine should be ready in case of cardiovascular collapse on induction. Ventilation with high concentrations of oxygen may be needed until bleeding is controlled.

Volatile agents have been associated with increased blood loss due to their relaxant effects on uterine muscle.[94,95] Anaesthesia should be maintained with intravenous agents if uterine atony is a problem. If uterine relaxation is specifically required e.g. evacuation of retained placenta or uterine inversion, volatile agents and beta-adrenergic drugs have been used. More recently, nitroglycerin has been successfully used both intravenously and as a sublingual spray, with the major advantage of rapid onset and short duration of action.[96]

Placenta praevia

A woman with a placenta praevia has a considerable risk of haemorrhage at some time during pregnancy or delivery. Anaesthetic considerations for caesarean section include the position of the placenta and the likelihood of placenta accreta (see below). A posteriorly positioned placenta should not require surgical access to the uterus through the placental bed and therefore blood loss is usually reduced. Regional anaesthesia may be used.

In all cases, preparations for massive haemorrhage should be made, including immediate availability of crossmatched blood. Similar preparation should be made for women taken to theatre for vaginal examination to evaluate a possible low-lying placenta. The presence of the placental bed in the lower uterine segment results in less effective uterine contraction, so these women are also at increased risk of postpartum haemorrhage.

Placental abruption

The incidence of antepartum haemorrhage is 3%: 1% from placenta praevia, 1% from abruption and 1% from other causes.

Signs of abruption are sudden onset of severe abdominal pain and tenderness, shock and a hard, woody uterus. However, with a posterior abruption (i.e. with a posterior placenta), the abdomen may be soft. Fetal heart sounds may be muffled or absent: abdominal ultrasound is often necessary to establish the presence or absence of a fetal heart.

If there is a fetal death in association with abruption then the abruption is major and represents significant maternal blood loss. The blood loss may be without any vaginal loss (concealed) and may be compensated for in the maternal circulation by the shutting down of the blood supply to the fetoplacental unit. It is therefore frequently underestimated. As a rule of thumb, an abruption resulting in fetal death requires maternal transfusion (estimate the blood loss, double it and double it again and that would be the amount of blood which would need to be transfused).

Initial management is:

- **A B C**
- send blood samples for tests including Kleihauer
- deliver the fetus
- treat coagulopathy.

If significant haemorrhage has occurred and the fetus is viable, consider immediate delivery by caesarean section if necessary. Consider induction but if the fetus is viable the method of delivery is almost always caesarean section unless the cervix has dilated rapidly and the fetal heart trace is very good. There can be a problem in that, with the contractions of labour, the abruption is likely to worsen with increasing separation from the uterine wall: a fetal scalp clip is essential.

If the fetus is dead, a vaginal delivery is usually possible. Despite the woman not being in established labour at the time of the abruption, following rupture of the membranes labour tends to progress apace.

Monitor for hypovolaemia during labour and consider caesarean section if the woman does not labour fairly quickly.

Early delivery protects against the severity of DIC. DIC is due in part to the massive release of thromboplastins from the damaged uterus.

Small abruptions are often difficult to diagnose, as ultrasound is not diagnostic in the early stages. Small abruptions develop into large abruptions!

A major abruption results in the delivery of a large retroplacental clot.

An abruption results from the separation of the placenta from the uterine wall and blood being driven into the myometrium with resulting damage and release of thromboplastins and bleeding into the myometrial layers (Couvelaire uterus). This damage interferes with uterine contractility, causing atony and it therefore predisposes to postpartum haemorrhage. Alongside this, there may also be a coagulopathy. Abruption and intrauterine death are both causes of DIC, further predisposing to postpartum haemorrhage.

Expect massive postpartum haemorrhage. The underestimation of blood loss antepartum makes the effect of further bleeding less well tolerated and significant cardiovascular compromise can occur, together with further exacerbation of DIC secondary to more blood loss and blood transfusion.

- Consider CVP monitoring, involve senior staff and arrange for high-dependency care postoperatively.
- There is a possibility of caesarean hysterectomy. Senior staff should be involved.

Important points to remember:

- Haemorrhage is concealed and therefore can be grossly underestimated.
- The mother protects her own circulation from the effects of hypovolaemia by shutting down the supply to the fetoplacental unit, so signs of blood loss are nor reflected in maternal signs.
- Fetal death is a sign of a major abruption.
- Delay in delivery makes DIC more likely.
- Expect postpartum haemorrhage because the uterus is atonic and there may be DIC.
- The effect of postpartum haemorrhage is greater in the patient who is already hypovolaemic because the APH has been underestimated.

Placenta accreta/increta and percreta

These conditions of abnormal placental adherence or invasion of the myometrium are often associated with massive haemorrhage. There is an increasing incidence of placenta praevia/accreta in association with previous caesarean section,[97] a trend that will presumably continue with the rising caesarean section rate. In some cases an antenatal diagnosis of placenta praevia/accreta may have been made. Caesarean hysterectomy may be required and blood loss can be massive. The presence of the fetus can raise dilemmas, where an option beneficial to the fetus may increase risk for the mother. Finally, the isolation of many obstetric theatres and the frequent lack of facilities for major monitoring and rapid transfusion, as found in most cardiac or major trauma theatres, require careful planning to allow optimal care during these occasional but life-threatening emergencies.[98]

There have been a few case reports on the management of morbidly adherent placenta using methotrexate. Limited experience has suggested that methotrexate is particularly useful in the treatment of placenta percreta with bladder invasion due to the rapid resolution of the vascular invasion of the bladder.

Bleeding associated with caesarean section

Certain deliveries are more likely to result in damage to the uterus. Some presentations lead to difficulties extracting the baby. Abdominal deliveries carried out at full dilatation, especially after a failed instrumental delivery, are particularly likely to cause damage to the uterus or vagina.

The uterine incision may extend into the broad ligament, tearing the uterine artery and leading to brisk bleeding. It will usually be helpful to exteriorise the uterus so that the posterior aspect of the uterus and broad ligament can be examined. The anaesthetist should be consulted if the surgery is being carried out under regional block. The proximity of the ureter must be borne in mind and an effort made to sweep the bladder down and with it the ureter. This will enable better access to the uterine vessels. Realistically, if bleeding is heavy it may be very difficult to identify the ureter and the first priority is to control haemorrhage: better a live patient with a damaged ureter than a dead patient with an intact urinary tract. Expert urological help should, of course, always be requested if damage is suspected.

Tears down into the vagina may be difficult to control and it may be useful to have a second surgeon operating from the vaginal end.

Troublesome haemorrhage from the angle of the uterine incision may be controlled by the insertion of an O'Leary suture to control the uterine artery. Efforts should be made to identify the ureter.

Bleeding at caesarean section, when the uterus is relaxing, may be controlled by the B-Lynch brace suture (Figure 16.1). This only is appropriate if bleeding is due to atony.

Bleeding from a relaxing uterus can also be controlled with a balloon catheter, e.g. the Rusch urological catheter. The uterus is closed and the catheter is inserted into the uterus and inflated with up to 500 ml of fluid.

Identification and ligation of the internal iliacs will result in a 77% reduction in pulse pressure distal to the ligation. The ligation is done in continuity and the vessel is not divided.

Techniques for difficult deliveries

Suspect that difficulties may arise, for example, in cases of caesarean section at full dilatation. Examine the patient yourself vaginally and try to disimpact the head. At caesarean section, slowly pass the hand deep into the lower segment and slowly lift the head out. It is important to make sure that your hand is far enough down so that the head does not become laterally hyperflexed during extraction. A useful technique to avoid this is to stand on the patient's right and, instead of using the right hand to lift the fetal head out of the pelvis, pass the left hand behind the baby's head, allowing the head to be lifted out through the uterine incision with less risk of lateral flexion and extension of the uterine incision.

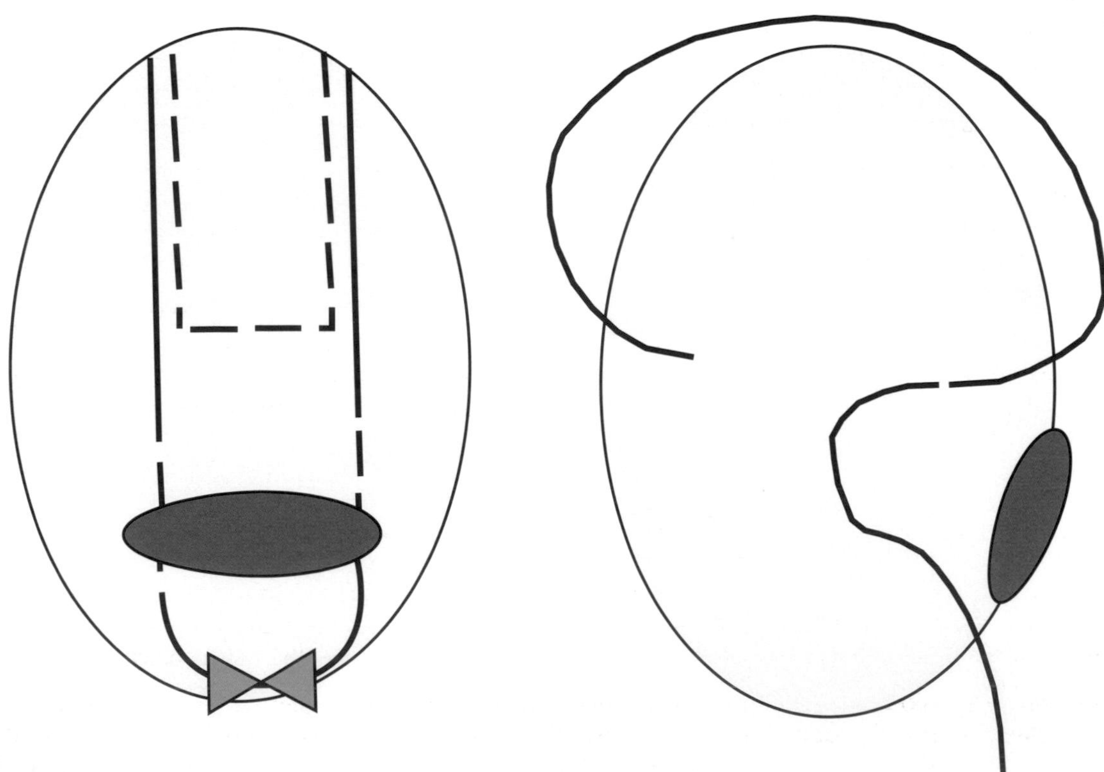

Figure 16.1 B-Lynch brace suture

For shoulder presentation with a prolapsed arm, consider Patwardhan's procedure, which involves delivering the breech first. In most cases this can be carried out through a transverse incision in the uterus, although the incision can be easily extended by converting it to a 'J' shape. The hand is passed upwards until a leg is reached and either the leg or the breech is delivered and the rest of the delivery is as for a caesarean breech delivery. This technique can also be used if the head is deeply engaged and disimpaction is unsuccessful.

The trapping of the head of a breech at caesarean section, especially a premature breech, is particularly stressful for the obstetrician. Ask the anaesthetist to administer a uterine relaxant. Ensure that both abdominal and uterine incisions are adequate. Attempt to pass your hand alongside the baby's head and apply Wrigley's forceps.

Consider converting the incision to a 'J' incision by extending upwards from the angle of the incision. This heals much better than a 'T' incision and may be less likely to rupture in a further pregnancy or labour.

A premature infant in the transverse or breech position with absent liquor may best be managed with a vertical incision in the uterus.

Placenta praevia/accreta

A traditional lower segment caesarean section can be carried out in the majority of cases of placenta praevia, even if anterior. The placenta does not need to be cut through but can usually be swept off the uterine wall and the baby delivered.

Troublesome bleeding can be controlled by a hydrostatic balloon as described above.

The hydrostatic balloon can also be used in cases of placenta accreta where there is pressure to conserve the uterus.

Summary

There are few controlled trials of treatment options in this field due to the relative rarity of cases, the urgent nature of the condition and the difficulty in obtaining ethical approval and consent for trials during pregnancy. Some information may be gained from assessing recent advances in related fields such as haemorrhage due to trauma,[99] although the major cardiovascular and haematological changes of pregnancy, and the particular pathologies unique to pregnancy such as pre-eclampsia, contribute additional challenges and require additional understanding.

Algorithm 17.1 Management of shoulder dystocia key points

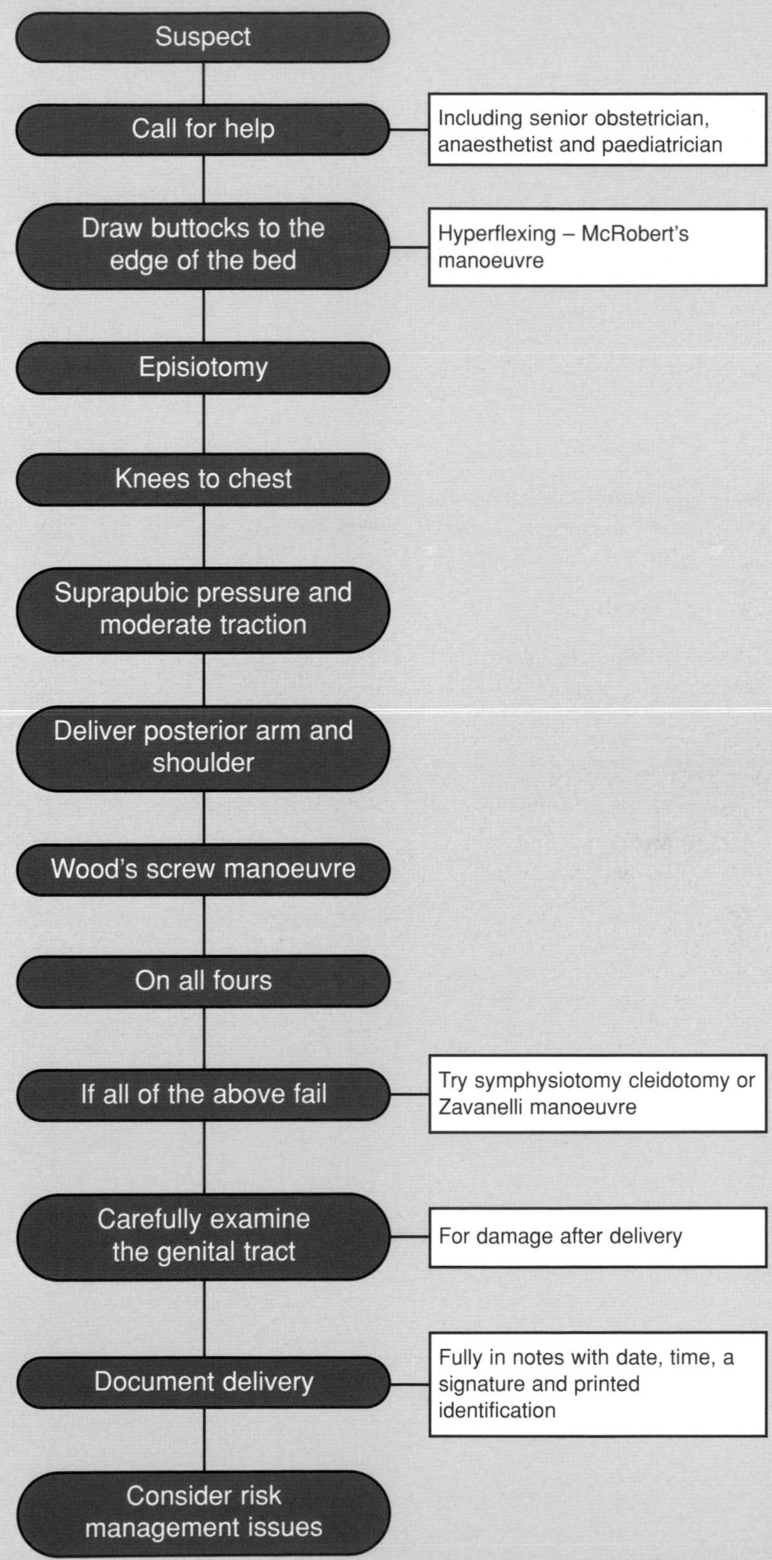

Chapter 17

Management of shoulder dystocia

Objectives

On successfully completing this topic you will:

- know how to predict shoulder dystocia
- know what should be done when risk factors for shoulder dystocia are identified
- have a plan of action.

Introduction

Shoulder dystocia remains one of the most dreaded obstetric complications and one that is often unanticipated. It is one of the primary causes of perinatal mortality and morbidity, maternal morbidity, and a costly source of litigation.

This chapter is an abbreviated update of a previous review of the subject.[100] A review of the current publications about shoulder dystocia revealed a selection in reference. We aimed to conduct, as far as possible, a complete review of the literature. In order to do this, we carried out Medline and EMBASE online searches for all publications in the last seven years (up to August 2002). Older references were sought through previous reviews and chapters on the subject.

Definition and incidence

The term shoulder dystocia has been used to describe a range of difficulties encountered with delivering the shoulders after delivering the head. Discrepancies in the definition, the degree of difficulty and the variation in manoeuvres used have resulted in differences in the reported incidence of this obstetric emergency.

Many attempts have been made to standardise the definition. Most recently, Spong *et al.*(1995)[101] proposed defining shoulder dystocia as prolonged head-to-body delivery time (more than 60 seconds) or the need for ancillary obstetric manoeuvres. The latter part of the definition agreed with Resnik's (1980)[102] definition of shoulder dystocia as 'a condition requiring special manoeuvres to deliver the shoulders following an unsuccessful attempt to apply downward traction'.

Benedetti (1989)[103] gave a more descriptive definition to the condition, but with no reference to the degree of the difficulty. He defined shoulder dystocia as 'arrest of spontaneous delivery due to impaction of the anterior shoulder against the symphysis pubis'. Gibb (1995)[104] defined three degrees of shoulder dystocia varying from 'slight difficulty' with the shoulders associated with a normal mechanism of rotation, through to severe, bilateral dystocia with both shoulders stuck above the brim.

Standardising the definition will not only make it easier to report the incidence but also will make it possible to compare the effectiveness of the different manoeuvres. We propose here to keep the definition of Resnik.

The reported incidence of shoulder dystocia varies between 0.15% and 2% of all vaginal deliveries. Sandmire and O'Halloin (1988)[105] stated that there was no evidence of increased incidence and, indeed, better treatment of diabetes mellitus should result in a reduced incidence.

Fetal mortality and morbidity

Shoulder dystocia is still a significant cause of term fetal mortality. In the Confidential Enquiry into Stillbirths and deaths in Infancy (CESDI) annual report for 1993,[106] shoulder dystocia was responsible for 8% of all intrapartum fetal deaths. Although, on the whole, fetal mortality from shoulder dystocia has improved over the last 30 years,[107] there is no room for complacency. Indeed, the Fifth CESDI annual report (1998)[108] published the discussions of an expert focus group that looked critically at 56 cases of death associated with shoulder dystocia. Forty-seven percent of these babies had died, despite delivery within five minutes. In 37 cases (66%), the level of substandard care offered by professionals was graded at 'level 3' (i.e. a different management would have likely resulted in an improved outcome). Although 65% of cases were delivered by midwives, approximately one-third were delivered by medical staff, emphasizing the need for ALL professionals involved in delivery to be aware of appropriate drills. Although the CESDI reports have produced interesting and pertinent findings, the data are difficult to quantify because of the lack of adequate denominator data.

Fetal morbidity

- Cerebral hypoxia
- Cerebral palsy
- Fracture clavicle and/or humerus
- Brachial plexus injuries

Following delivery of the head, the umbilical cord pH falls by 0.04 units per minute[109] As a result, delay in completing the delivery may result in asphyxia and, if the interval between head and trunk delivery is prolonged, permanent neurological deficit may occur. Delivery should occur within five minutes and permanent injury is progressively more likely with delays above ten minutes. Boyd *et al.*[110] found abnormal CNS signs and convulsions in 2 of 70 babies who suffered shoulder dystocia (2.9%). In another study, shoulder dystocia was responsible for 7.5% of all term infants who suffered neonatal seizures in the first 72 hours of their lives.[111] Due to the poor association between the parameters used to define birth asphyxia (i.e. pH, Apgar score, etc.) it is difficult to ascertain the incidence of permanent CNS deficit resulting from shoulder dystocia.

Brachial plexus injuries are common in shoulder dystocia.[112,113] Erb's palsy is the most common presentation. Baskett[114] reported that in a ten-year series (1980–89) there were 44 cases of Erb's palsy, 33 of which were associated with shoulder dystocia. Erb's palsy presents as internal rotation and adduction of the shoulders and extension and pronation of the elbow.

The incidence of brachial plexus injuries varies significantly between different papers but it has been decreasing. Rubin *et al.*[115] reported an incidence of 100% in 1964, while Gordon *et al.*[116] reported an incidence of 48% in 1973 and, more recently, Baskett and Allen (1995)[117] reported an incidence of 13% in 1995. Most babies with Erb's palsy improve quickly and it usually resolves within six months. Nocon *et al.*,[118] after reviewing 28 brachial plexus injuries from a cohort of 12 523 deliveries, found that all but one injury had resolved by six months.

Interestingly, Jennett *et al.*[119] found that intrauterine maladaptation may play a role in brachial plexus impairment and they stated that brachial plexus impairment should not be taken as *prima facie* evidence of birth-process injury. The mechanism of damage may not always be clear, as brachial plexus injury has also been reported at caesarean section, in the opposite arm to the trapped shoulder, and also without any recorded dystocia.[120–122] Sandmire *et al.*[123] found that only 50% of cases of Erb's palsy were associated with shoulder dystocia. The relative risk of developing Erb's palsy was 4.7 times higher after a precipitate second stage. The authors implied that the prevention of many cases of Erb's palsy was outside the attendant's control. Gerhman *et al.*[124] showed that the use of more invasive means of treating shoulder dystocia (i.e. removing the posterior arm) were not associated with an increased risk of brachial plexus injury compared with more benign 'external' manoeuvres (e.g. suprapubic pressure): 21/158 versus 27/127. Wolf *et al.*[125] found 62 cases of brachial plexus injury in 13 366 deliveries (an incidence of 0.46%); 22 recovered completely within one month, while a further23 had delayed but complete recovery. Of 17 with residual paresis, 11 underwent surgery but only three had severe paresis. The most significant marker to predict the likelihood of 'non-recovery' was a birthweight of over 4000g (odds ratio = 51).

Musculoskeletal injuries in the form of fractured clavicle or humerus can also happen. Nocon *et al.*[118] found 14 fractured clavicles in 185 cases of shoulder dystocia. These fractures usually heal quickly and have a good prognosis.

Maternal morbidity

Postpartum haemorrhage is common following shoulder dystocia. Benedetti *et al.*[126] reported a blood loss of more than 1000 ml in 68% of their cases. Vaginal and perineal lacerations are also common following delivery of shoulder dystocia. Moller-Bek and Laurberg[127] found a strong association between shoulder dystocia and fourth-degree (anal sphincter and anal mucosa injury) perineal tears. Uterine rupture may also happen, especially if undue abdominal force is used.

Risk factors

The issues that lend themselves for discussion are:

- How specific and sensitive our methods to predict macrosomia?
- What is the right course of action if macrosomia is predicted?

Risk factors for shoulder dystocia

Antepartum	Intrapartum
Fetal macrosomia	Prolonged first stage
Maternal obesity	Prolonged second stage
Diabetes	Oxytocin augmentation of labour
Prolonged pregnancy	Assisted delivery
Advanced maternal age	
Male gender	
Excessive weight gain	
Previous shoulder dystocia	
Previous big baby	

It seems that most of the antenatal risk factors are so common that they lack sensitivity and specificity. Moreover, the majority of cases of shoulder dystocia occur without any risk factors.[117] A retrospective analysis of 12 532 deliveries,[118] concluded that of most of the 'traditional' risk factors for shoulder dystocia have no predictive value. Therefore, although it is clear that there is a strong correlation between fetal weight and shoulder dystocia, all professionals need to be prepared for unexpected shoulder dystocia at all deliveries.

Intrapartum risk factors

Secondary arrest and slow progress in the first stage have been associated with increased incidence of shoulder dystocia.[128,129] McFarland *et al.*[130] reviewed 276 cases of shoulder dystocia and compared them with 600 deliveries in the same period. They concluded that labour abnormalities were comparable in the shoulder dystocia and in the control groups, both in the active phase and in the second stage, and, as a result, these labour abnormalities may not serve as clinical predictors for subsequent development of shoulder dystocia. Acker *et al.*[131] found that, in the birthweight group of 4000–4999 g, no specific labour abnormality was clearly predictive of shoulder dystocia. However, in the birthweight group of 5000 g or more, labour arrest heralded a shoulder dystocia in 55% of cases. Langer *et al.*[132] found that the duration of labour and other labour abnormalities may increase the risk of shoulder dystocia but they did not show how this can predict shoulder dystocia.

Shoulder dystocia is more frequently encountered in assisted vaginal deliveries. Boekhuizen[133] analysed 256 vacuum extractions and 300 forceps deliveries. They found an incidence of 4.6% of shoulder dystocia compared with 0.17% of all cephalic vaginal deliveries. Keller *et al.*[134] found that the use of forceps was clearly associated with increased risk of shoulder dystocia. This emphasises the importance of particularly careful abdominal and vaginal assessment before performing assisted deliveries for clinically macrosomic babies.

How does shoulder dystocia happen?

In the slighter degrees the cause may be failure of the shoulders to rotate into the anteroposterior diameter as they traverse the pelvic cavity. The posterior shoulder usually enters the pelvic cavity while the anterior shoulder remains hooked behind the symphysis pubis.

In the more severe forms of shoulder dystocia both shoulders do not cross the pelvic brim.[104]

Strategies suggested for prevention and management of shoulder dystocia

- Identifying risk factors
- Training and teaching
- Prevention – caesarean section for macrosomic babies
- Early induction of labour to prevent macrosomia
- Risk assessment – documentation of risk factors, events and their timings
- Early detection – turtle sign
- Plan of action.

These individual items will now be reviewed in light of the available evidence.

Identifying risk factors

Identify the risk of shoulder dystocia antenatally and recommend clearly in the mother's notes that an experienced obstetrician should be available for second stage.

Training and teaching

In the CESDI annual report for 1993[106] it is stated that:

'There should be regular rehearsals of emergency procedures, and training sessions in the management of rare or troublesome complications for obstetricians and midwives involved in care. Such complications include obstructed delivery ... and shoulder dystocia'.

In one questionnaire survey that involved 120 midwives assessing their training, 80% felt they did not have any theoretical training in shoulder dystocia and more than 95% felt they did not have any practical training, more than 98% expressed a need for more theoretical and simulated training to manage shoulder dystocia.[100] More than 60% of midwives involved in this survey said they would use fundal pressure and apply strong traction to the fetal neck, two actions known to increase the incidence of brachial plexus injury and fracture clavicle.[135]

Prevention

Prevention by performing caesarean section for macrosomic infants

Langer *et al.*[132] reviewed a total of 75 979 vaginal deliveries in the period from 1970–85. These patients were stratified into diabetic and non-diabetic groups. The incidence of macrosomia, defined as birthweight of 4000 g or above, was 7.6% in the non-diabetic group and 20.6% in the diabetic group. Patients were further subdivided by weight categories at 250-g intervals. Eight percent of shoulder dystocia occurred in the diabetic group when birthweight was 4250 g or above; 20% of shoulder dystocia occurred in babies weighing 4500 g or above in the non-diabetic group. The authors concluded that a trial for vaginal delivery for non-diabetic fetuses weighing 4000 g or more is recommended. They recommended an elective caesarean section for diabetics with estimated fetal weight of 4250 g and non-diabetics with estimated fetal weight of 4500 g or above. Clearly, the difficulty in complying with the latter recommendation is that it is so difficult to obtain an accurate estimate of fetal weight as indicated above. Baskett *et al.*[117] concluded, after a large review, that 'to prevent neonatal morbidity, we have to perform 54 additional caesarean sections on the basis of estimated fetal weight or 4500 g or more, to prevent one case of brachial palsy'.

Diani *et al.*[136] found that expectant management of 482 infants with suspected birthweight of 4000 g and above was safe unless there was a reason for caesarean section. In their review, 396 of 482 infants with a birthweight of 4000 g or above achieved normal delivery with no single case of birth trauma. Increased caesarean section for macrosomia from 8% in the sixties to 21% in the eighties did not improve perinatal outcome.[110]

In the CESDI annual report for 1993,[106] there were 29 fetal deaths due to shoulder dystocia and ten of these babies (35%) weighed less than 4 kg. O'Leary *et al.*[137] concluded that most cases of shoulder dystocia occur in babies of average weight.

Most cases of shoulder dystocia can be overcome without trauma to mother or baby if proper precautions are taken and abdominal delivery is not 100% safe for the baby. Naef *et al.*[138] reported that 50% of cases of shoulder dystocia occurred in normally grown fetuses and 98% of macrosomic fetuses who were delivered vaginally did not have shoulder dystocia.

Spellacy *et al.*[139] reported an incidence of 2.6% of birth trauma to babies 4500 g delivered by caesarean section. Jakobovits[140] reported that brachial plexus injury may occur before delivery.

Even if we agree with performing a very large number of caesarean sections to reduce the incidence of shoulder dystocia by 50–60%, we have first to find a way of accurately estimating fetal weight at term. As was shown earlier, the sensitivity and specificity of tests for diagnosing macrosomia is not satisfactory. We conclude that a policy of elective caesarean section for all clinically big babies will not be effective in reducing the incidence of shoulder dystocia and subsequent brachial plexus injuries.

Prevention by induction of labour for suspected macrosomia

Induction of labour has been considered as an option for managing mothers with suspected macrosomic babies, to try reduce the incidence of shoulder dystocia and subsequent birth trauma. Friescen *et al.*[141] reviewed 186 mothers with suspected macrosomic fetuses at term. Labour was induced in 46 cases, 23.9% of them needed caesarean section while, with spontaneous onset of labour in 140 cases, the caesarean section rate was 14%. This difference was statistically significant, regardless of parity or gestational age. The frequencies of shoulder dystocia, one-minute Apgar score of less than seven and abnormal umbilical blood gas were not different. The authors concluded that spontaneous labour is associated with a lower chance of caesarean section than induced labour, when the birthweight is 4000 g and above.

Weeks *et al.*[142] reached a similar conclusion after reviewing 504 patients who delivered infants weighing 4200 g or above. Caesarean section was performed in 52% of predicted macrosomic group due to high induction of labour rate (42.5%) compared with 30% in the non-predicted group. Combs *et al.*[143] showed a caesarean section rate of 57% in mothers induced for suspected macrosomia for failed induction, compared with 31% in those allowed a spontaneous onset of labour. The high rate of induction of labour and caesarean section did not reduce the incidence of shoulder dystocia. They concluded that mothers with macrosomic fetuses can safely be managed expectantly unless there is a medical reason for induction of labour.

The situation in women with diabetes is different for reasons mentioned earlier. Acker *et al.*[131] recommends caesarean section for babies with an estimated fetal weight of 4000 g or above. Langer *et al.*[132] recommend caesarean section for an estimated fetal weight of 4250 g and above. Kjos *et al.*[144] recommend induction of labour for diabetics at 38 weeks, especially if the diabetic control has not been ideal, to avoid shoulder dystocia and birth trauma.

Risk assessment

Although we have reached the conclusion that most cases of shoulder dystocia are unpredictable, we recommend documenting in the notes the risk factors, especially if they are multiple. We recommend the presence of an experienced clinician during the second stage. We recommend documenting events and manoeuvres in the notes and keeping accurate times in the notes.

Early detection

- Head bobbing' – i.e. the head coming down towards the introitus with pushing, but retracting well back between contractions.
- 'Turtle sign' at delivery – i.e. the delivered head becomes tightly pulled back against the perineum.

A plan of action

As shoulder dystocia is infrequently predictable, every clinician should be armed with a plan of action, i.e. a sequence of manoeuvres.[107,120,145,146] All manoeuvres result from one (or a combination of) the following three mechanisms:

1. increase in the available pelvic diameters
2. narrowing of the transverse (bisacromial) diameter of the shoulders by adduction and/or
3. movement of the bisacromial diameter into a more favourable angle relative to the anteroposterior pelvic diameter (e.g. into the oblique).

PLAN OF ACTION

1. Call for help.
2. Draw buttocks to the edge of the bed.
3. Episiotomy.
4. McRoberts' manoeuvre with or without moderate traction.
5. Suprapubic pressure with moderate traction.
6. Deliver posterior arm and shoulder.
7. Internal rotational manoeuvres (including Woods' screw manoeuvre).
8. Change of position ('all-fours' or 'Gaskin' manoeuvre).
9. If all the above fail, try symphysiotomy, cleidotomy or Zavanelli manoeuvre.

Call for help

This includes calling the most experienced obstetrician available, a paediatrician and an anaesthetist, and other nursing and ancillary staff as available.

Episiotomy

This is recommended to allow more room for manoeuvres such as delivering the posterior arm or internal rotation of the shoulders. Although it has been suggested that episiotomy does not affect the outcome of shoulder dystocia,[118] there is strong evidence to suggest that the incidence of vaginal lacerations with shoulder dystocia is high and performing an episiotomy to reduce the chance of having severe lacerations is recommended.

The main reason for recommending an episiotomy is to allow the operator more space to use the hollow of the sacrum to perform the different internal manoeuvres.

McRoberts' manoeuvre (with or without moderate traction)

Both thighs are sharply flexed, abducted and rotated outwards. The legs should not be placed in lithotomy poles as this would limit the amount of flexion obtained. This position serves to straighten the sacrum relative to the lumbar vertebrae and causes cephalic rotation of the pelvis to occur which helps free the impacted shoulder.[147,149] Gonik *et al.*[149] tested McRoberts' position with laboratory maternal pelvic and fetal models. Their findings showed that this manoeuvre reduced the amount of traction needed and the likelihood of subsequent brachial plexus injuries or fractured clavicle. For this reason patients should be put in McRoberts' position before applying appropriate traction on the fetal neck.

Allen *et al.*[150] also used models to measure objectively the degree of clinician-applied load in routine and difficult shoulder dystocia deliveries. The average combined force for a normal delivery was 84 N, with a 473 N-cm neck-bending moment. For a shoulder dystocia delivery the equivalent average forces were 163 N and 700 N-cm. Clavicular fracture can occur at peak force magnitudes around 100 N. Lurie *et al.*[146] reviewed 76 cases of shoulder dystocia and found that McRoberts' manoeuvre was sufficient to achieve delivery of the impacted shoulder in 67 cases (88%). McRoberts' manoeuvre is associated with the least neonatal trauma.[117]

Suprapubic pressure (with moderate traction)

Suprapubic pressure is applied to adduct and internally rotate the anterior shoulder and thus reduce the bisacromial diameter and push the anterior shoulder underneath the symphysis pubis.[146] A 'cardiac massage' grip is used, with pressure applied to the posterior aspect of the shoulder with the heel of the hand. It is important to know where the fetal back lies so that pressure is applied in the right direction. At this stage only moderate traction is applied. Strong traction as well as fundal pressure should be avoided. If continuous pressure is not successful, a 'rocking' movement may be tried. This is also known as the 'Rubin I' manoeuvre. Baskett *et al.*[117] stated that increased traction on the head was associated with the greatest degree of neonatal trauma.

Gross *et al.*[135] warned against fundal pressure. Strong pushing may have similar effects and we recommend that maternal efforts should be discouraged until shoulder displacement is achieved, as these could increase the impaction of the shoulders and increase the neurological and orthopaedic complications.

Deliver posterior arm and shoulder

The hand of the operator should be passed up to the fetal axilla and the shoulder hooked down (Figure 17.1). There is always more room in the hollow of the sacrum. Traction on the posterior axilla usually enables the operator to bring the posterior arm within reach.

The posterior arm can then be delivered or, if the cubital fossa is within reach, backward pressure on it will result in disengagement of the arm, which will then be brought down. This is achieved by getting hold of the hand and sweeping it across the chest and fetal face.[146] This process is similar to the Pinard method for bringing down a leg in breech presentation.

This procedure is usually successful.

Internal rotatory manoeuvres

These various manoeuvres are often confused with each other and are often incorrectly described in the literature.

Rubin II

The operator inserts the fingers of one hand vaginally, positioning the fingertips **behind** the anterior shoulder. The shoulder is pushed towards the fetal chest (adducting the shoulders and rotating the bisacromial diameter into the oblique). If unsuccessful, this can then be combined with the Woods' screw manoeuvre.

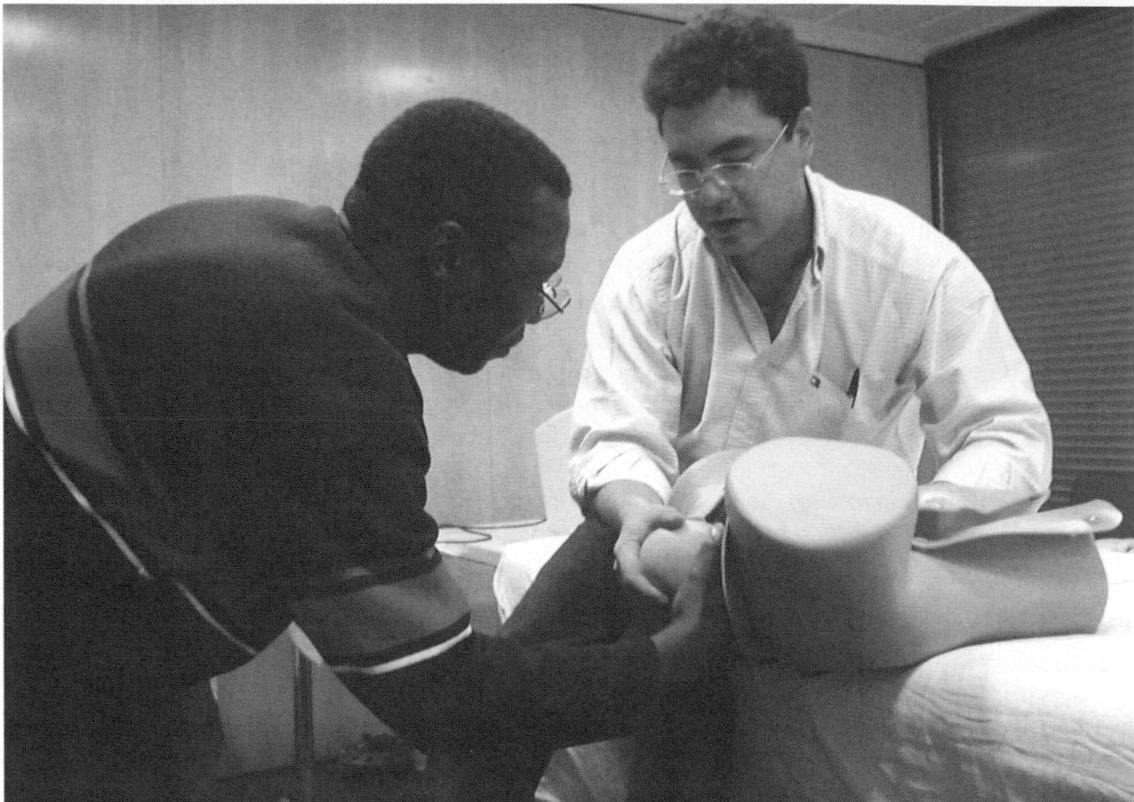

Figure 17.1 Delivering the posterior arm and shoulder

Woods' screw

This was described by Woods in 1943.[151] The fingers of the opposite hand are inserted vaginally to approach the posterior shoulder from the **front** of the fetus, aiming to rotate the shoulder towards the symphysis pubis. The Rubin II and Woods' screw can be combined to rotate the shoulders through 180 degrees (like a thread on a screw). It is important not to twist the fetal head or neck.[146,147,152]

Reverse Woods' screw

If the above fail, the fingers of the hand used for the Rubin II manoeuvre are placed on the **posterior shoulder from behind** and an attempt is made to rotate in the **opposite** direction to the original Woods' screw. If successful, the shoulders will rotate 180 degrees in the opposite direction and deliver. These manoeuvres are all eloquently described by Gobbo and Baxley.[153]

Change of position

All-fours position ('Gaskin' manoeuvre)

The maternal weight lies evenly on the four limbs and this increases the anteroposterior diameter of the inlet and facilitates other manoeuvres.[154] The posterior shoulder (with respect to the maternal pelvis) may be delivered first in this position. Midwives will often use this manoeuvre early in the management of shoulder dystocia.

In a series of 82 cases of shoulder dystocia among 4452 deliveries (incidence 1.8%) all babies were delivered successfully with this manoeuvre in a mean time of 2.3 minutes (range 1–6 minutes).[155,156] There were no cases of mortality and no cases of brachial plexus injury. One baby suffered a fractured humerus.

Obstetricians should consider the merits of this alternative approach.

Other measures

Zavanelli manoeuvre

This has been named after the physician who first performed the manoeuvre in 1978. It describes reversal of the delivery process by rotating, flexing and reinserting the head into the vagina, followed by caesarean section, i.e. after failure of all manoeuvres to overcome shoulder dystocia, restitution and neck extension are reversed and the head recoils into the vagina. O'Leary and Gunn[137] described the need for a tocolytic. They used 0.25 mg subcutaneous terbutaline. They depressed the posterior vaginal wall and used firm and constant pressure on the head. Those who have had the experience of applying this technique reported very good outcomes.

O'Leary *et al.*[157] reported 59 women whose babies underwent cephalic replacement. All but six were successfully replaced and delivered by caesarean section without excessive maternal or fetal morbidity.

Descriptions in the literature report an almost automatic ease in performance of Zavanelli manoeuvre and a complication-free procedure. However, Graham *et al.*[158] reported how difficult the process can be. O'Leary[157] reported three cases of hysterectomy due to uterine rupture during the procedure. Spellacy[159] reported three cases of severe perinatal hypoxia that ultimately resulted in brain damage and/or death. O'Leary,[157] in spite of being an advocate of the procedure, recommends that it should be used as a last resort.

Symphysiotomy[160]

This requires inserting a urethral catheter to move the urethra to one side. Two assistants support the legs after taking them out of the stirrups. An incomplete midline cut in the symphyseal joint is made. This, in addition to an episiotomy, will increase the space available and facilitate the delivery of the shoulders. The danger of performing this uncommon procedure in an emergency situation by an operator who has never performed it before must carry a considerable risk. Reid and Osuagwu[161] described the successful use of the technique in two difficult cases of shoulder dystocia. They emphasised the importance of supporting the woman's legs when the incision is made, in order to prevent sudden abduction.

Intentional fracture of the clavicle

This is really a manoeuvre of last resort.

Approaches advocated by other authors

Several authors have advocated the use of similar systematic approaches to the hands-on management of shoulder dystocia.[107,120,153,162,163] They vary in the order in which manoeuvres may be recommended, but the more important principle of having an order, a logical and calm approach, is advocated by all. Two examples are given below, both of which use mnemonics as an aide-memoire.

The Advanced Life Support in Obstetrics (ALSO) approach[153] uses the mnemonic 'HELPERR' (the order of manoeuvres is not mandatory).

HELPERR

H – Help (call for plenty)

E – Evaluate for episiotomy

L – Legs (McRoberts')

P – Pressure (suprapubic)

E – Enter (rotational manoeuvres)

R – Remove the posterior arm

R – Roll (Gaskin manoeuvre)

Magowan[164] also uses a mnemonic approach: 'PALE SISTER'.

PALE SISTER

P – Prepare – have a plan

A – Assistance

L – Legs (McRoberts')

E – Episiotomy

S – Suprapubic pressure

I – Internal rotation (Woods')

S – Screw (reverse Woods')

T – Try recovering posterior arm

E – Extreme measures

R – Repair, record and relax

Guidelines may differ at the point where internal manoeuvres are required. Should one 'enter and rotate (the shoulders)' first or 'enter and remove (the posterior arm)' first? Roberts[107] clearly states that there is no scientific evidence on which to base this choice. Therefore, it should be left to the attending professional to use the manoeuvre with which they are MOST FAMILIAR AND MOST COMFORTABLE. In a survey of obstetricians, Johanson and Wykes[164] found that 56% would attempt delivery of the posterior arm first and 36% the internal rotatory manoeuvres first.

For the purposes of the MOET course, where the majority of attendees are obstetricians, the course manual suggests removal of the posterior arm first. However, it is recommended that candidates should be familiar with the rotatory movements as well.

Medico-legal aspects

Leigh and James[165] discussed the medico-legal aspects of shoulder dystocia in a commentary in the *British Journal of Obstetrics and Gynaecology*. They pointed to 'an epidemic of cases involving shoulder dystocia where negligence is alleged'. Courts have found in favour of the professionals involved when the allegations have been that shoulder dystocia 'should have been predicted' and caesarean section offered in order to avoid the complication. It was accepted that the majority of cases are unpredictable and that professionals could not be expected to predict this catastrophe antenatally. However, in many cases, there were no departmental guidelines available for the management of shoulder dystocia once it had occurred. Inappropriate manoeuvres such as excessive lateral traction and fundal pressure would not be acceptable and indeed would be difficult to defend in present-day practice.

Units should continually review and revise their management guidelines with reference to changing, evidence-based practice. It is accepted that it is not possible to produce Grade A (randomised controlled trial) evidence in this field.

Conclusion

Although shoulder dystocia is usually an unpredictable obstetric emergency, having guide lines and a plan of action plus being vigilant to the possibility of shoulder dystocia should minimise the fetal and maternal trauma.

It is important that every institution has a guideline, with which ALL staff are familiar and comfortable. The setting up of mock 'fire-drills' has been recommended by CESDI and many of the authors referenced in this chapter. Confidence with this rare emergency can be enhanced with the use of fire drills and by completing structured skills-training courses such as the one you are attending.[166,167]

Algorithm 18.1 Prolapsed umbilical cord key points

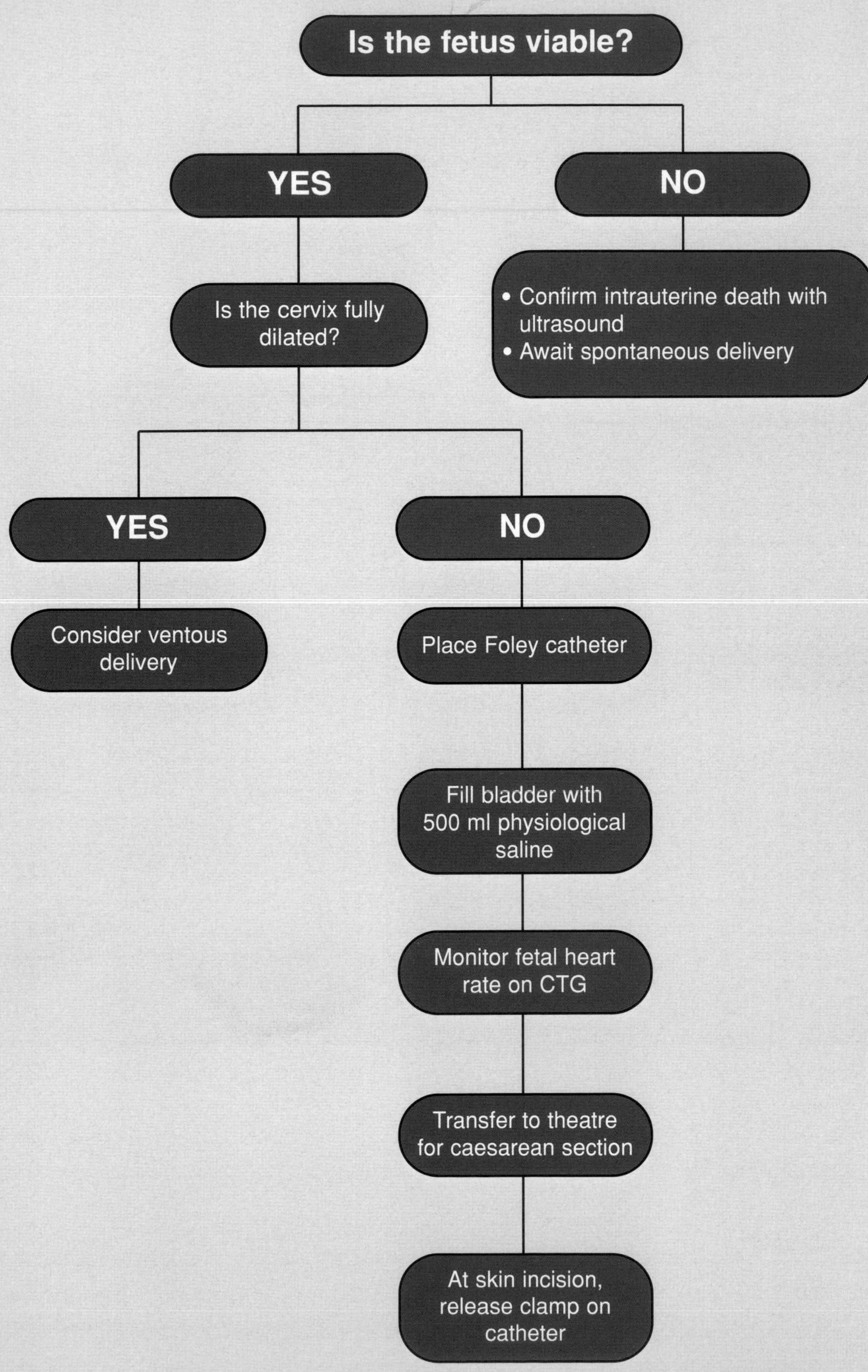

Chapter 18

Prolapsed umbilical cord

Objectives

On successfully completing this topic you will be able to:

- manage prolapse of the umbilical cord to improve perinatal outcome
- safely and efficiently manage umbilical cord prolapse to minimise maternal risk.

Definition

In this condition a loop of umbilical cord is below the presenting part and the membranes are ruptured.

Incidence

Umbilical cord prolapse occurs in approximately 0.2% of all births.[168,169]

A high percentage of mothers are multiparous. The incidence of prolapsed cord was 0.6% of all births in 1932 and the reduction in frequency of the complication probably reflects changes in obstetric practice, with increased use of elective and intrapartum caesarean section for a non-cephalic or an unengaged presenting part and a more active approach to intrapartum management of the very preterm fetus.[170]

Risk

In cord prolapse the fetal perinatal mortality has been as high as 25–50% from asphyxia due to:

- mechanical compression of the cord between the presenting part and bony pelvis, and
- spasm of the cord vessels when exposed to cold or manipulations.

However, the perinatal mortality rate associated with umbilical cord prolapse has fallen over the past 50 years. Rates reported as high as 375 per 1000 between 1924 and 1948,[171] have fallen to between 36 and 162 per 1000 within the past few decades.[169,172–174] The cause of death for infants born after umbilical cord prolapse now seems to be related more to the complications of prematurity and low birthweight than to intrapartum asphyxia *per se*.[169,174]

It is considered that part of the fall in perinatal mortality is due to the more rapid and frequent use of caesarean section once prolapsed cord has been diagnosed. However, given the association between umbilical cord prolapse and preterm birth, improvements in neonatal intensive care are probably more important.[170,175]

Aetiology/risk factors

The presenting part does not remain in the lower uterine segment due to:

- Fetal causes
  - Malpresentations; e.g. complete or footling breech, transverse and oblique lie
  - Prematurity
  - Polyhydramnios
  - Multiple pregnancy
  - Anencephaly
- Maternal causes
  - Contracted pelvis
  - Pelvic tumours

Other predisposing factors

- Low-grade placenta praevia
- Long cord
- Sudden rupture of membranes in polyhydramnios

Risk factors

In one series, obstetric interventions (such as amniotomy, scalp electrode application, intrauterine pressure catheter insertion, attempted external cephalic version, expectant management of premature rupture of membranes) preceded 47% cases of umbilical cord prolapse.[176]

Diagnosis

Vaginal examination

If the cord is prolapsed it is necessary to detect whether it is pulsating, i.e. live fetus or dead.

Ultrasound

This is done in order to confirm a fetal heart if the facility is rapidly available.

In addition, it can occasionally diagnose cord presentation. Colour flow Doppler sonography can diagnose cord presentation which is likely to be the harbinger of cord prolapse and in turn its potential complications may be avoided.[177] This is only recommended of there is reason to suspect cord presentation and if clinically indicated.

Obstetric management of umbilical cord prolapse

This has largely been unchanged since the 1950s. The approach, if the baby is alive and of a viable gestation, continues to be elevation of the presenting part and rapid delivery, usually by caesarean section.[169,170,174,178]

The evidence suggests that the interval between diagnosis and delivery is significantly related to stillbirth and neonatal death, although Prabulos and Philipson[179] suggest that the time from diagnosis to delivery may not be the only critical determinant of neonatal outcome, particularly with frank cord prolapse. Tchabo[180] reported that approximately 25% of umbilical cord prolapses occur outside the hospital. Indeed, in the Oxford study,[169] the only baby that died was the first of twins, where the cord prolapse occurred at home; the woman was transferred to hospital and subsequent delivery took 100 minutes. This suggests that umbilical cord prolapse occurring at home carries a worse prognosis. Dare[181] reported an incidence of cord prolapse of 76.7% in unbooked patients, with a perinatal mortality rate of 86.4%.

In a study by Critchlow *et al.*,[169] in 709 cases of cord prolapse, there were only three who presented with an intrauterine death. Although the risk factors already discussed are important, the majority of babies in this study were of normal birthweight and at term with cephalic presentation.

Early diagnosis is important and, in this, continuous electronic fetal monitoring may be of assistance as fetal heart rate changes frequently recur.[169,173]

A management plan is shown in Algorithm 18.1.

Traditionally, management of umbilical cord prolapse has included knee–chest or Trendelenburg positioning and manual elevation of the presenting part of the fetus above the pelvic inlet, to relieve cord compression. Provided that delivery is not imminent and the fetus is viable, this traditional management occurs while preparations for emergency caesarean section are made.[182]

At this time, an absence of audible fetal heart tones and a non-pulsatile cord maybe noted. Increasing the intravenous fluid rate, administering oxygen by facemask and discontinuing the oxytocin infusion are indicated. If the umbilical cord protrudes through the introitus, it may need to be moistened with sterile gauze soaked in warm, physiological saline. Driscoll *et al.*[183] demonstrated the importance of prompt ultrasound assessment in a patient presenting with the absence of cord pulsation and inaudible fetal heart tones. They found that fetal heart movements could be visualised, even in the absence of cord pulsation and inaudible heart tones.

Various attempts to accomplish a safe vaginal delivery after the diagnosis of umbilical cord prolapse have been reported. Barrett[184] manually replaced the prolapsed cord in the uterine cavity in six cases where the patient was remote from delivery. Of these, five had a successful 'funic reduction', followed by a normal vaginal delivery. This potentially beneficial management needs further evaluation in larger studies.

An advance in the management of umbilical cord prolapse has been the development of bladder filling. Bladder filling was first proposed by Vago in 1970[185] as a method of relieving pressure on the umbilical cord. Bladder filling raises the presenting part of the fetus off the compressed cord for an extended period of time, thereby eliminating the need for an examiner's fingers to displace the presenting part.[185,186] A number-16 Foley catheter with a 5-ml balloon is placed into the urinary bladder. The bladder is filled via the catheter with physiological saline by a standard infusion set. The quantity to be instilled has varied from 400–750 ml in the different reports.[182,186,187] The quantity of saline needed is determined by the appearance of the distended bladder above the pubis, with 500 ml usually being sufficient.[185] The balloon is then inflated, the catheter is clamped and the drainage tubing and urine bag are attached and secured.

Bladder filling has an additional advantage in that the full bladder may decrease or inhibit uterine contractions. In a series by Chetty and Moodley[187] there were no cases of perinatal mortality. All the babies had Apgar scores of six or more and the mean elapsed time from diagnosis to delivery was 69 minutes. Eight patients in their study delivered after an elapsed time of 80 minutes or more. Caspi *et al.*[186] and Katz *et al.*[182] found no perinatal deaths when bladder filling was used to manage umbilical cord prolapse.

Given that there is no evidence of fetal distress, it may be reasonable to proceed with a regional block. The bladder is emptied by unclamping the catheter before opening the peritoneal cavity for caesarean delivery. Some authors have suggested the continuous usage of beta-sympathomimetic drugs to inhibit uterine contractions such as terbutaline sulfate.[182,188]

Umbilical cord prolapse at full dilatation with a live viable fetus is one of only two situations where the vacuum extractor may be used with an unengaged head. This is discussed in the section on instrumental vaginal delivery.

Summary

Obstetricians assume a dual role in the provision of health care for both mother and fetus during labour. Umbilical cord prolapse continues to be associated with poor perinatal outcome in some cases despite emergency delivery in a modern high-risk obstetric unit. It is important that staff are fully aware of the procedures to be followed, which will ensure that they are carried out as efficiently and successfully as possible.

Algorithm 20.1 Retained placenta key points

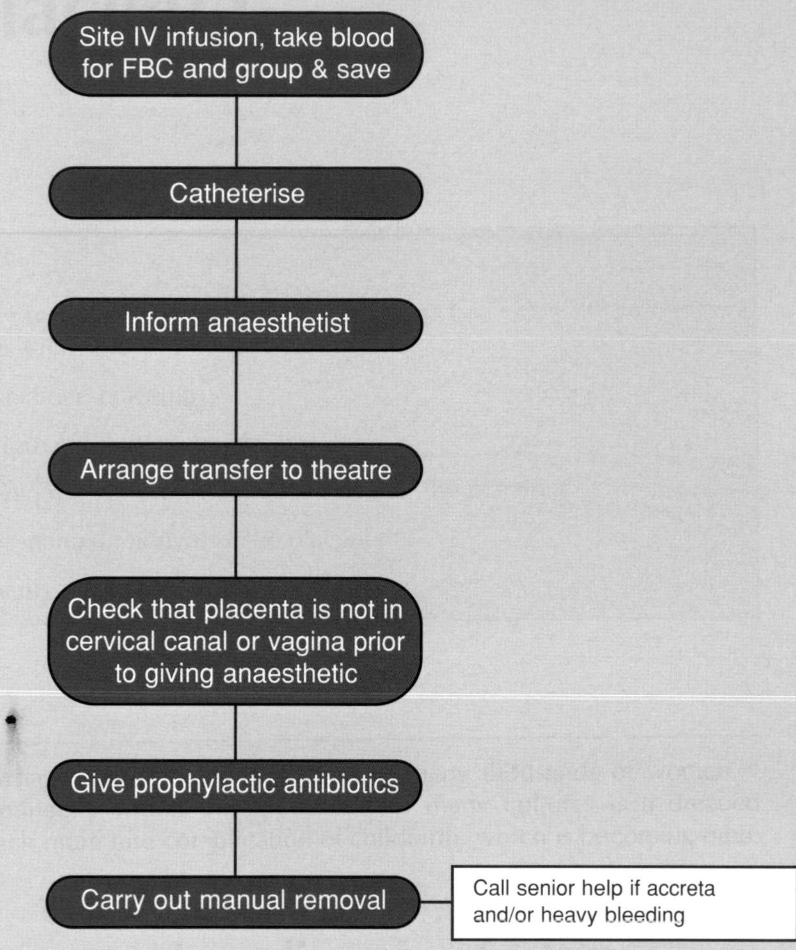

The most extreme form of placental retention is placenta accreta, where the placenta is morbidly adherent to the uterus. Miller *et al.*[210] reviewed hospital records of all cases of histologically confirmed accreta and found 62 (1/2510) among 155 670 deliveries.

Factors predisposing to retained placenta and placenta accreta

In a systematic review, which included the Hinchingbrooke trial, manual removal of the placenta was found to be more likely with active management of labour than with expectant management (2.1% cf. 1.5%)[211] and was more likely with the longer-lasting uterotonic agent ergometrine 500 micrograms and oxytocin 5 units/ml (Syntometrine®, Alliance) than with oxytocin (Syntocinon®, Alliance) alone (2.5% versus 1.6%).[212] Oxytocin induces strong rhythmic uterine contractions, principally in the upper part of the uterus, whereas ergometrine, which has no physiologically produced counterpart, produces spasm of smooth muscle throughout the body and in the uterus affects primarily the lower segment and cervix.[213] Syntometrine was developed for intramuscular use and begins to have an effect after about two minutes as the oxytocin starts to work; the ergometrine acts about four to five minutes later, causing the uterus and cervix to clamp down.[204] These findings support the link between uterine constriction and placental retention (or entrapment).

A number of authors have undertaken multivariate risk factor analyses for 'retained placenta'.[210,214–206)] Among the common risk factors for retained placenta are:

- previous retained placenta
- multiparity
- induced and preterm labour
- small placenta
- history of previous instrumentation of the uterus (caesarean section, sharp or suction curettage)
- placenta praevia
- leiomyomas.[210,214,215]

Soltan and Khashoggi found a significant association with placental weight of less than 601 g.[216]

The timing of placental delivery appears to relate closely to the gestation. Life-table analyses predicted that 90% of placentas would spontaneously deliver by 180 minutes at 20 weeks of gestation, by 21 minutes at 30 weeks and by 14 minutes at 40 weeks.[203] Romero *et al.*[208] noting the increased incidence of retained placenta in preterm pregnancies, speculated that the relatively larger size of a preterm placenta may require more uterine work and time.

There is a highly significant association between raised serum alphafetoprotein (AFP) and placenta accreta.[217] Aberrant maternal–trophoblastic interaction in the placental bed is thought to be a key to the understanding of the pathogenesis of morbid placental adherence.[218]

Placenta accreta is becoming more common and over the last 40 years the incidence has increased ten-fold. This phenomenon is due to the fact that lower segment caesarean section appears to increase the risk of subsequent placenta praevia and there is a well-documented association between placenta praevia and previous caesarean section with placenta accreta.

In a large cohort study from Taiwan,[219] risk factors for placenta accreta were:

- placenta praevia (OR 54.2; 95% CI 17.8–165.5)
- abnormally elevated second-trimester AFP (> 2.5 MoM) (OR 8.3; 95% CI 1.8–39.3)
- raised β-hCG (OR 3.9; 95% CI 1.5-09.9)
- being 35 years and older (OR 3.2; 95% CI 1.1-09.4).

In another series, placenta accreta occurred in 55/590 (9.3%) of women with placenta praevia and in 7/155 080 (1/22 154) without placenta praevia.[210]

Among women with placenta praevia, the risk of accreta ranged from 2% in women less than 35 years of age with no previous caesarean deliveries to almost 39% in women with two or more previous caesarean deliveries and an anterior central placenta praevia.[210]

Management of retained placenta

In one survey of home deliveries, 68% of emergencies related to retained placenta.[220] Vincent[223] described a number of traditional beliefs and practices related to delivering the placenta. There is an awareness of the risks of retained placenta and its link to haemorrhage is widely recognised. As a consequence, delivery of the placenta is considered of prime importance and many techniques have been devised for facilitating this. The majority of manoeuvres, described across cultures, relate to pulling on the placenta, squeezing the uterus and increasing intra-abdominal pressure by inducing vomiting. Inducing vomiting has been described in widely differing cultures across different continents.[221]

Current conventional management of retained placenta involves a general or regional anaesthetic and manual removal. This therefore requires transfer to an operating theatre and a high level of expertise. In some situations, transfer to theatre might take many hours or even days. Sawhney and Gopalan found considerable delay in referral and nearly a third of women were admitted in shock.[220]

The management of the postpartum patient with retained placenta therefore requires adequate resuscitation with fluids, oxygen and appropriate monitoring of blood pressure, oxygen saturation and urine output. Blood should be crossmatched.

Anaesthetic management should ensure the provision of cervico-uterine relaxation and analgesia at the same time as minimising risks of anaesthesia in general and postpartum haemorrhage in particular. Inhalation anaesthetic agents have been used for years to produce uterine relaxation but this effect requires high drug levels. Thus, endotracheal intubation is required, followed by another two to four minutes to achieve the depth of anaesthesia necessary for endometrial relaxation. There is concern that this form of anaesthesia will delay recovery of uterine contractility and also delay awakening from anaesthesia. There are thus complexities to the use of general anaesthesia.

As a consequence there has been an interest in using regional anaesthesia. However, one study[222] suggested that there was a greater incidence of long-term backache in patients who had extradural anaesthesia specifically for manual removal of placenta, compared with patients who had a general anaesthetic for the same procedure (this was not a randomised trial).

In addition to possible anaesthetic complications, manual removal of placenta itself carries further risks of haemorrhage and trauma. A significant association between manual removal of the placenta and postpartum endometritis has also been shown.[223] It is also possible that separation of mother and baby immediately after birth will affect bonding and breastfeeding.

Consequently, there has been considerable interest in finding a non-invasive treatment of retained placenta. In one trial, 37 women with retained placenta were randomised to have intra-umbilical vein injection of prostaglandin F_2, oxytocin or physiological saline or to immediate manual removal of the placenta. Spontaneous separation of the placenta occurred in all ten women after injection of prostaglandin and in six of ten that received oxytocin.[224] In the UK, Gazvani *et al.*[225] found a similar clinically important benefit from giving intra-umbilical oxytocin, compared with saline.

Carroli and Berger[209] have reviewed those studies that have examined the use of intra-umbilical oxytocic agents. In their review, injection of saline solution with oxytocin after 15 minutes of placental retention was associated with a significant reduction in the need for manual removal of placenta (117/234,50%, versus 129/220, 59%). Pipingas *et al.*[226] suggested that the most likely explanation for the observed beneficial effects of volume infused oxytocin would be a direct action on the myometrium underlying the unseparated placenta.

Given the strong association between retained placenta and uterine hypercontractility, it would appear to be logical to examine tocolytic possibilities. Amyl nitrate has been used for many years to relax the uterus but this requires breaking the ampoule in a breathing bag and administering via an anaesthetic system. Moreover, amyl nitrate is flammable and potentially explosive in oxygen and has adverse effects of headache, flushing and hypotension. No controlled studies have been done.

Glyceryl trinitrate (GTN) has come to the attention of obstetricians as a potent tocolytic agent. GTN is a nitric oxide donor and nitric oxide is a potent endogenous smooth-muscle relaxant in vasculature, gut, genitourinary tract and the uterus. This may be useful for aiding fetal delivery; for example, it has been used successfully for urgent tocolysis in cases of difficulties with delivery at caesarean section[227,228] and GTN has also been used intravenously to provide tocolysis for intrapartum external cephalic version (ECV).[229]

GTN has also been tried for the third-stage complications. It has been used in the management of inverted uterus.[230] Intravenous GTN has also been used successfully, in doses ranging from 50–250 micrograms for placental extraction, with minimal adverse effects.[231–233] The onset of action is within one minute and uterine contractility is restored by five minutes. However, it requires dilution, a time-consuming process with the possibility of error. Sublingual GTN has a rapid onset of action and has been used in the acute cardiac setting in place of the IV formulations. Sublingual GTN is an easy way of administering the drug and has been used in a pilot study in three patients requiring vaginal delivery of retained placenta, at an initial dose of 800 micrograms.[234] Rapid uterine relaxation was obtained with no observed adverse effects. Laslett and Baker[235] have shown that sublingual GTN has a quicker effect if administered by spray than by tablet.

A placebo-controlled trial of sublingual GTN spray for ECV has been completed. The agent was well tolerated with no significant adverse effects noted.[236]

Audit

- All women with retained placenta should have a senior doctor present.
- Time from delivery to delivery of placenta should be less than 90 minutes.
- Postnatal Hb should be checked prior to discharge.
- Prophylactic antibiotics should be given.
- A large blood sample should be taken.
- Peripheral line x 1 should be inserted.
- If the patient was ever shocked: BP, pulse and urine output monitoring should be undertaken.

Future research

A placebo-controlled trial of GTN, with reduction in need for manual removal of placenta as the main endpoint, would be of value.

Algorithm 21.1 Face presentation key points

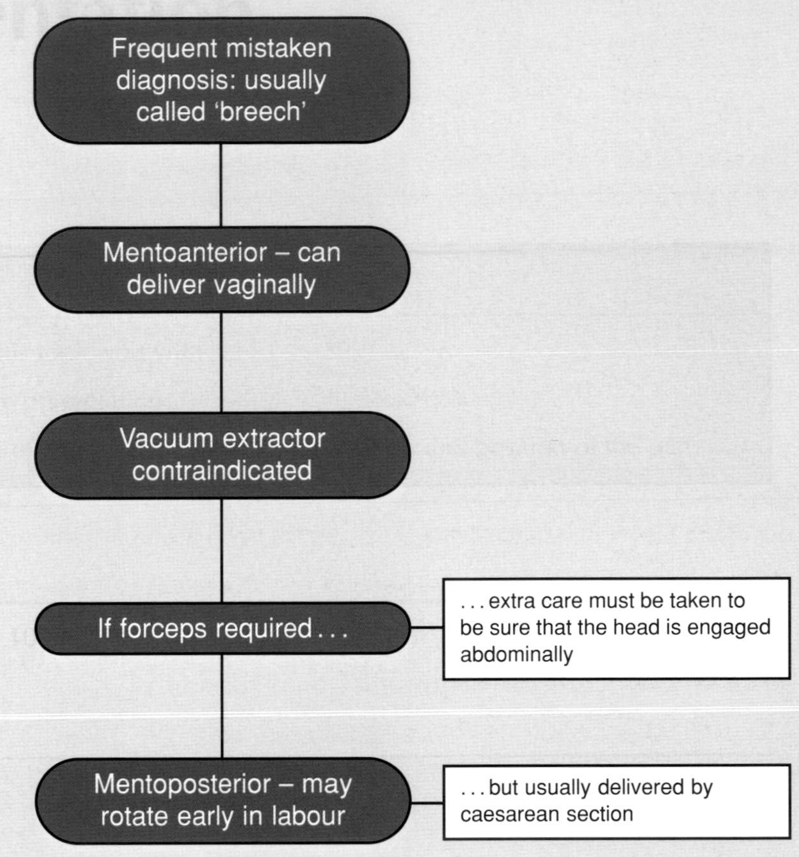

Algorithm 22.1 Ruptured uterus key points

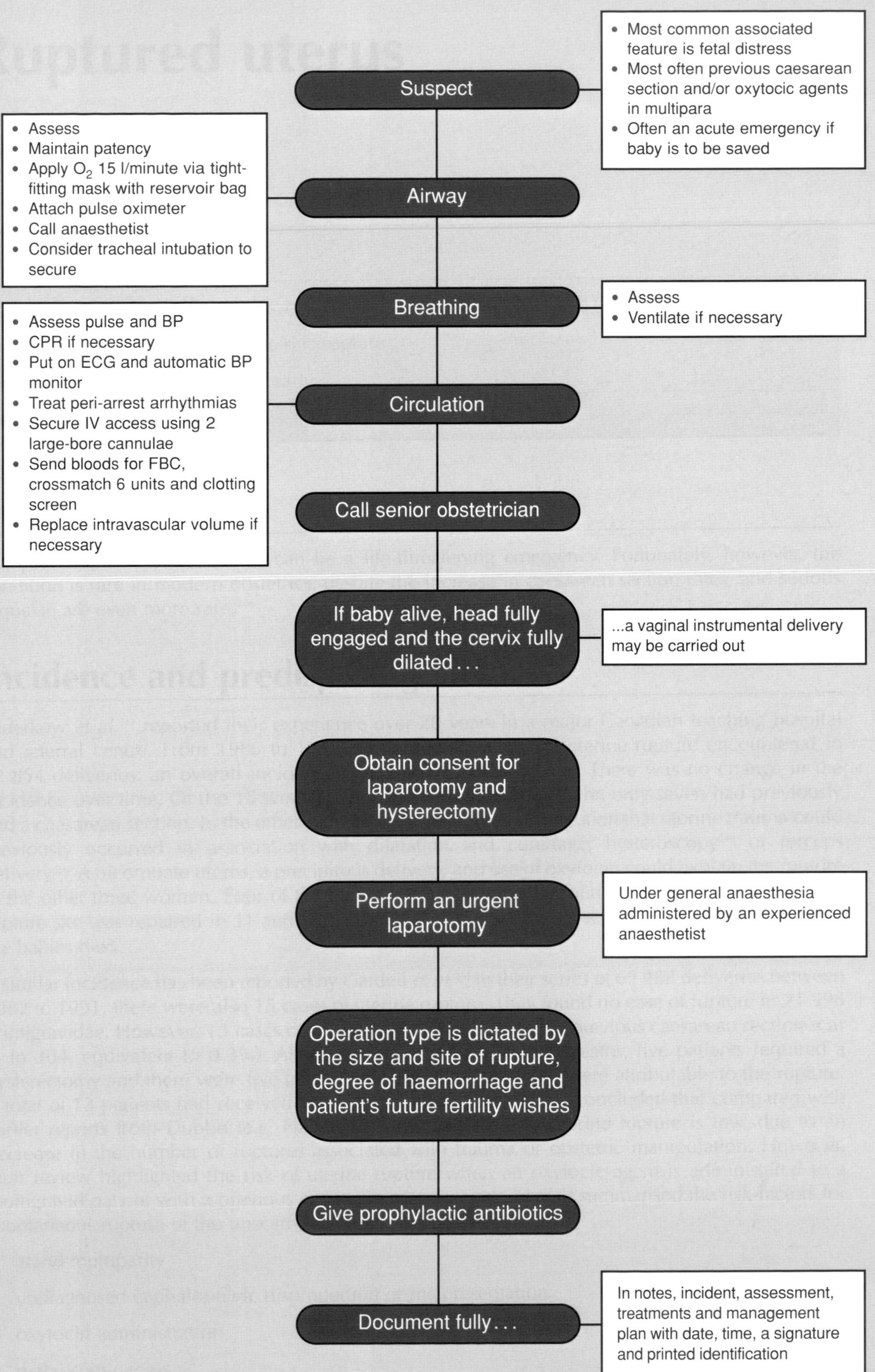

- The operator is six times more likely to cut the baby when the presenting part is breech – beware! Gently elevate the breech while cutting through the lower segment. Use your finger to make the final entry.[289]

Trial of vaginal breech

- The mother should be counselled again, and she should confirm her informed choice of vaginal delivery.
- Advise theatre and the on-call anaesthetist.
- Although epidural anaesthesia is frequently recommended, this is not essential and may be associated with more prolonged labours and an increase in caesarean section. Pethidine, where required, and a prepared anaesthetist for the second stage are a reasonable alternative. An epidural may be of benefit with the preterm breech, to prevent pushing through an incompletely dilated cervix.
- Fetal monitoring should be continuous.
- Amniotomy may be used to accelerate labour, to check for the presence of meconium in the amniotic fluid or to allow for the use of internal fetal heart rate or intrauterine pressure monitoring. If spontaneous rupture of membranes occurs, perform a vaginal examination to check for cord prolapse.
- Fetal blood sampling can be undertaken from the buttock and should be on the same basis as would be indicated with cephalic presentations.
- Oxytocin can be used for delay but, as expected, with caution. Progress should be documented in the partogram and should be as expected for a cephalic presentation.
- An obstetrician with **adequate** experience in delivering breech babies vaginally should undertake or supervise the management of the second stage.
- The basic principles in delivering a breech are those of not interfering.
- Active pushing should not be encouraged until the breech has descended to the pelvic floor. Some practitioners believe that the upright position is physiologically and anatomically advantageous at this stage.
- An episiotomy may be needed. If so, do not perform it too soon. Wait until the anus is visible over the fourchette before carrying out an episiotomy (undertaking this too soon can result in both a caesarean wound and an episiotomy). Protect the fetal bottom from being cut with your left hand.
- The breech will usually rotate spontaneously to lie with the sacrum anteriorly (rarely it will try to turn posteriorly – this must be prevented).
- Extended legs are delivered by flexion at the knee joint and extension at the hips.
- Conventionally, a loop of cord is brought down; very rarely (likely apocryphal) a short cord will prevent descent of the body. It will need division and quick delivery. The breech is supported by the accoucheur.
- As the mother pushes, the anterior shoulder scapula tip will become visible. This is a signal to run a finger over the shoulder and down to the elbow to deliver the arm. The other shoulder will rotate anteriorly (spontaneously) to allow similar delivery of the other arm.
- The baby lies supported as the head engages. Delivery of the head is straightforward with Mauriceau–Smellie–Veit manoeuvre in some cases. However, another doctor or midwife must always be scrubbed to assist, as there may be delay at this point. If there is delay at this point, the assistant holds the body upwards and arms out of the way and the forceps are applied.
- If the head does not come at this point, put a weighted speculum into the vagina (this may allow the baby to breath). Consider symphysiotomy.

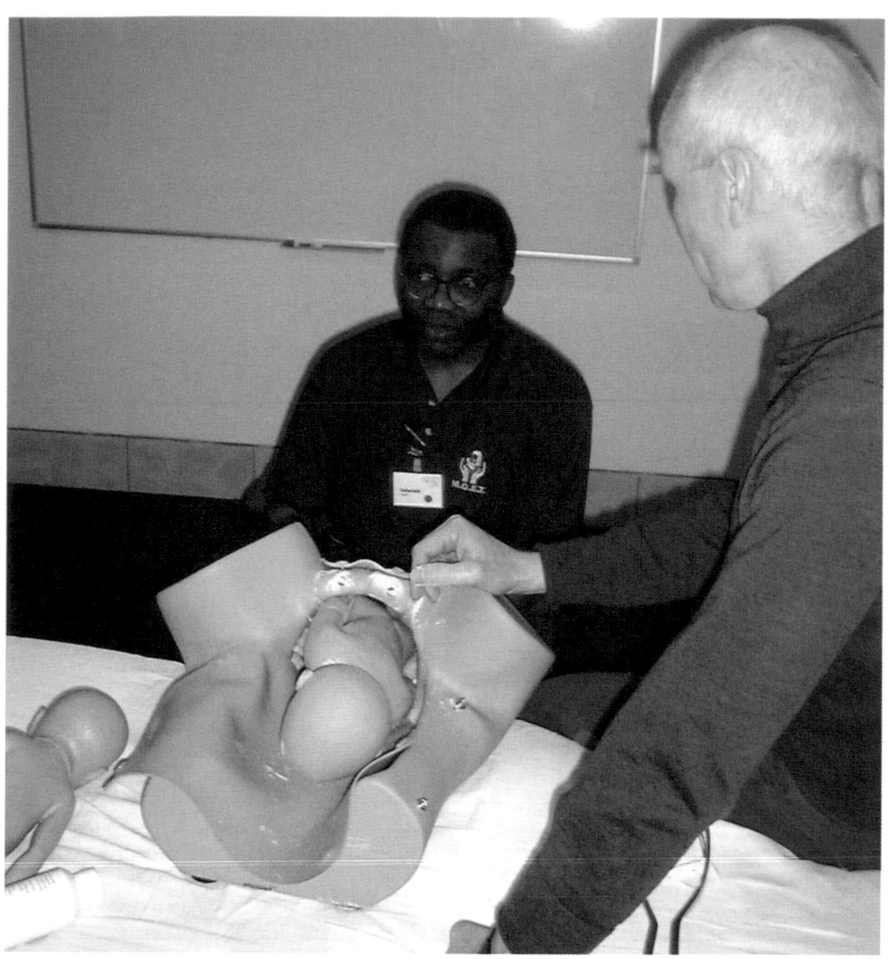

Breech delivery

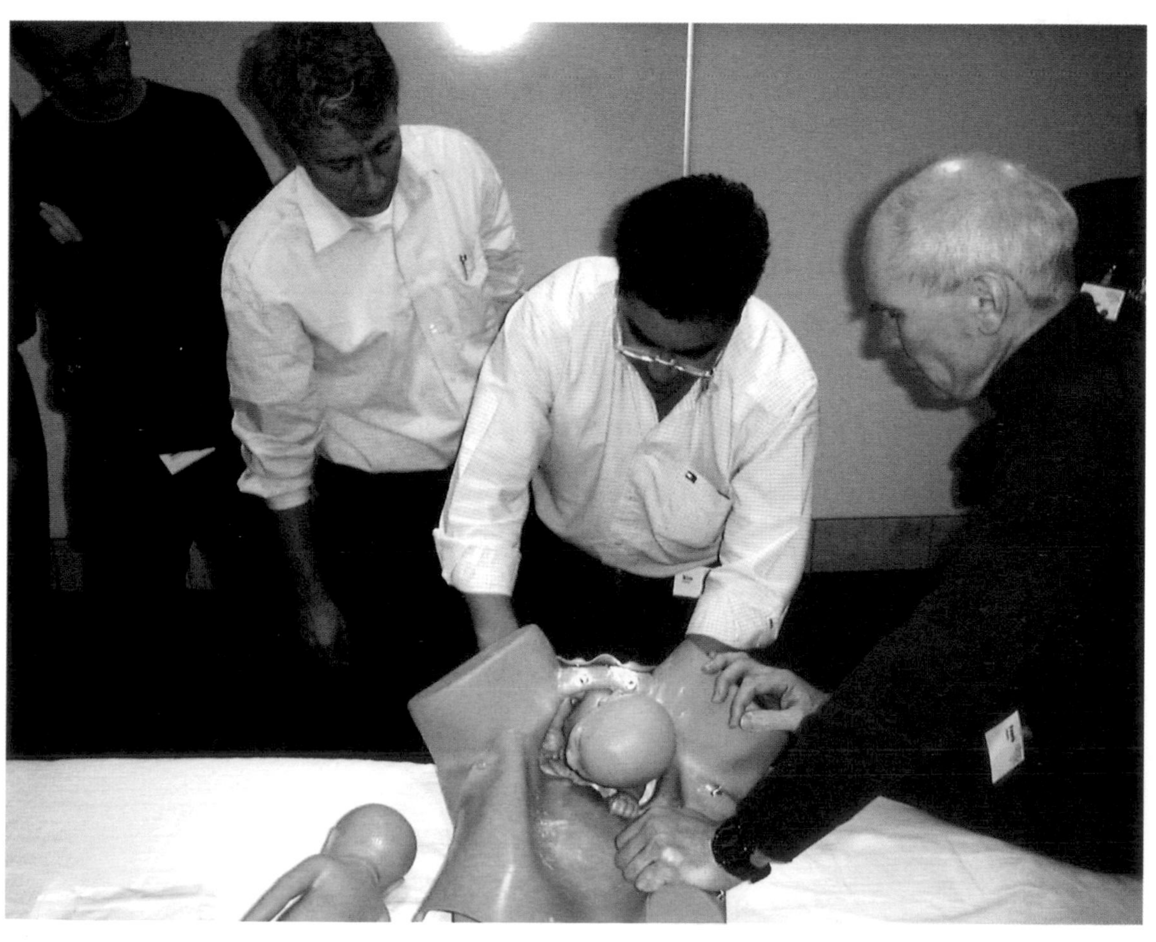

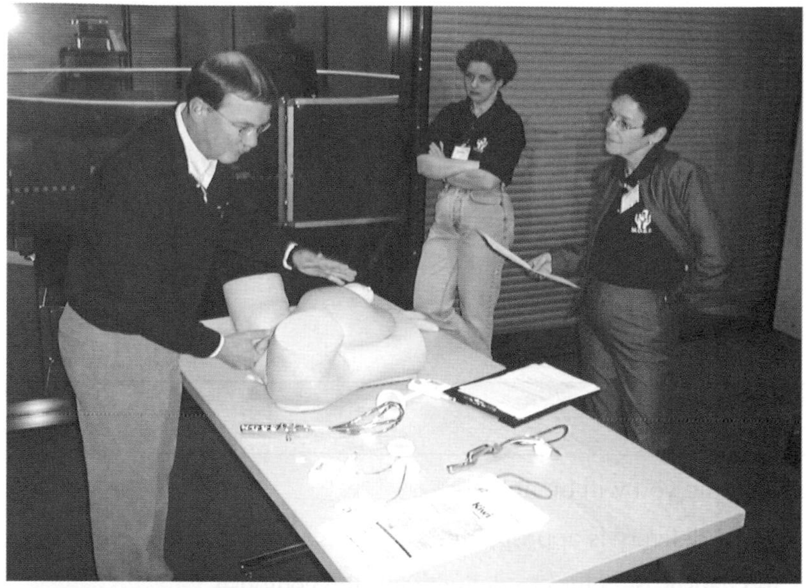

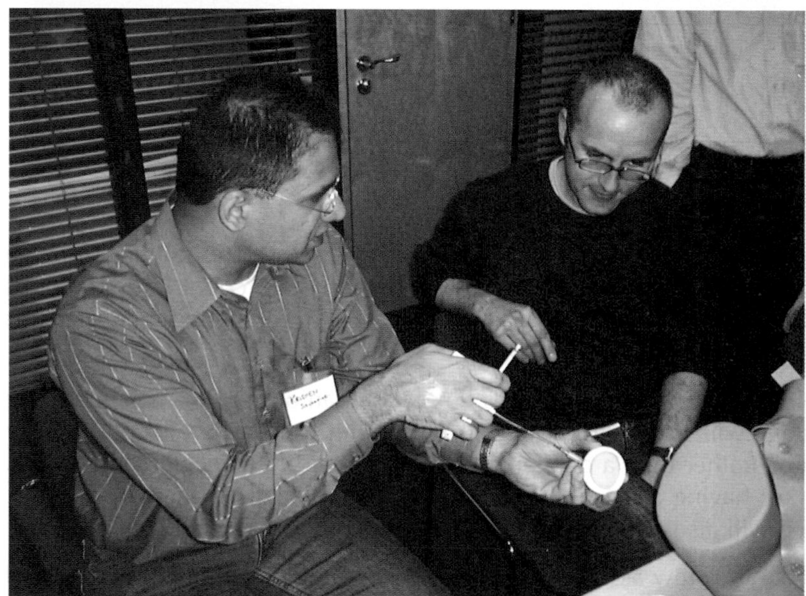

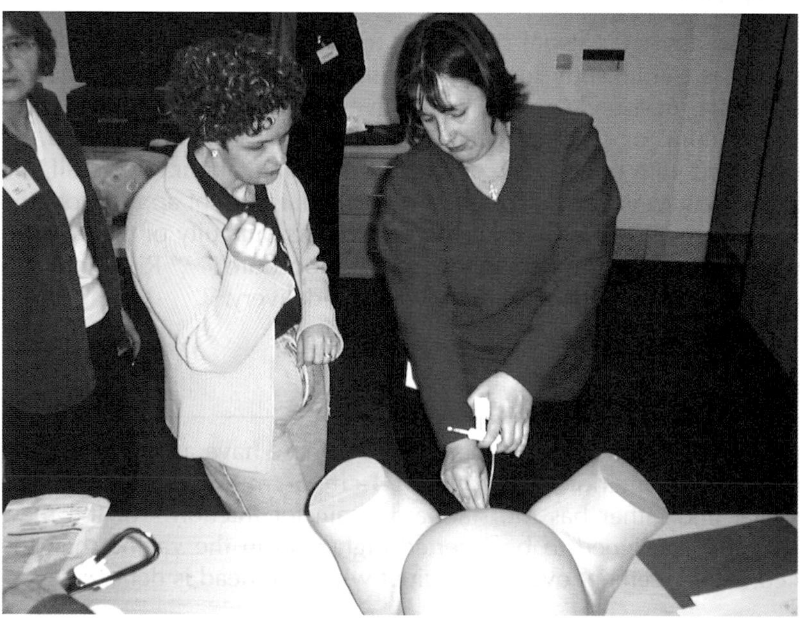

Ventouse delivery

fontanelle. The sagittal suture should point to the centre of the cup. A well-placed cup will result in a well-flexed head, while failure to put the cup far enough back will result in deflexion.[295,297]

A number of soft cups have been developed, one example of which is the silicone-rubber cup (Silc-cup®, Menox-AB). The soft cups are smoothly applied to the contour of the baby's head and do not develop a 'chignon'. The vacuum achieved is particularly poor when soft cups are applied to moderate or severe caput (as adhesion to folds of oedematous skin is poor). In addition, they have limited manoeuvrability and cannot be correctly placed when the head is deflexed. Consequently, the soft cups have a poorer success rate than metal cups. On the other hand, they are less likely to be associated with scalp trauma.[291,299] Being soft, they are easy to apply and unlikely to injure the mother. As they are cleaned and sterilised as one item, they present no problems with assembly or leakage.

Indications and contraindications for use of the ventouse

Indications

- Delay in the second stage.
- Fetal distress in the second stage.
- Maternal conditions requiring a short second stage.

Contraindications

- Face presentation.
- Marked active bleeding from a fetal blood-sampling site.
- Gestation of less than 34 weeks (between 34 and 36 weeks 'relatively' contraindicated).[291]

Delivery with the ventouse

To minimise the chances of any fetal damage the basic rules for delivery with the ventouse should be followed.

Prerequisites

- Full dilatation of the cervix and full engagement of the head.
- Co-operation of the patient.
- Good contractions should be present.

Basic rules

- The delivery should be completed within 15 minutes of application.
  (Fifteen minutes is given as the maximum time allowed for application but the average time from insertion of the cup to delivery in over 400 deliveries was six minutes.)[300,301]
- The head, not just the scalp, should descend with each pull.
- The cup should be reapplied no more than twice (and after one detachment an experienced operator should be summoned).
- If failure with the ventouse occurs despite good traction do not try the forceps as well.

There is no need to catheterise the patient (unless there is another indication, e.g. epidural). No additional anaesthetic is required (perineal infiltration will suffice if an episiotomy is planned). Lithotomy is the most common position used but delivery may be possible in dorsal, lateral or squatting positions.

Method

1. Examine the patient carefully. Estimate the size of the baby per abdomen and ensure that the head is fully engaged (none of the head should be palpable). Determine the position of the vertex and the amount of caput per vaginam. Describe the attitude of the presenting part as 'flexed' or 'deflexed' (in a flexed attitude only the posterior fontanelle can be felt, while any situation where the anterior fontanelle can be felt or where the posterior fontanelle cannot be found should be described as deflexed).
2. The appropriate cup should be chosen.
   The **silicone rubber cup** can be used with any well-flexed cephalic presentation, as long as the baby is average-sized and there is minimal caput (by pressing firmly all details of the cranium should be felt, the skin will not be deep and will feel only slightly spongy). This cup may be used with an occipitolateral position, as long as the cup can be placed over the occiput. Overall, 50% of cases are suitable for this cup.

   The **anterior metal cup** should be chosen if the baby is big, if the second stage is prolonged and if there is a moderate degree or more of caput (the skin may feel deep, may be folded and will definitely be spongy). It may also be used if the head is only slightly deflexed. The 6-cm cup is preferable to the 5-cm cup because it allows greater traction without increasing the risk of scalp trauma. Only where the vagina is narrow should the 5-cm cup be used. The small 4-cm cup is reserved for use with the second twin, particularly if the cervix is no longer fully dilated.

   The most valuable **posterior metal cup**, as its name indicates, is used for posterior positions, particularly those with significant deflexion.
3. Once the correct cup has been chosen it should be connected to the pump (electric or hand) and a check should be made for leakages prior to commencing the delivery. Common problems include suction bottles not tightly screwed in or tubing loosely attached to the metal cups (not locked with the small plastic ring). The metal cups should have a meshed bottom plate, which functions to maintain a clear space between the scalp and the cup so that an effective vacuum can be applied.

Silicone rubber cup

The silicone rubber cup is used in the following manner: it is folded and gently inserted into the vagina with one hand from above downwards, while the other hand parts the labia. A gentle twist may help it to unfold into place in the vagina and thereafter it is essentially not manoeuvrable, being larger in diameter than the metal cup and having a relatively inflexible handle.

Take the pressure up to 0.2 kg/cm^2, check that no maternal tissue is caught under the cup and then continue directly to 0.8 kg/cm^2, beginning traction with the next contraction after this pressure has been achieved.[291] Where gentle to moderate traction is required it is reasonable to take the pressure to 0.6 kg/cm^{2}and in those rare situations where deliveries are undertaken between 34 and 36 weeks it may suffice to stop at 0.4 kg/cm^2.

Traction should be along the pelvic axis for the duration of the contraction. One hand should rest on the bell of the cup while the other applies traction. Malmstrom[302] said 'Vacuum extraction is a matter of cooperation between the traction hand and the backward-pressing hand'. The hand on the cup detects any early detachment and also indicates whether the head moves downwards with each pull. The fingers on the head can promote flexion and can help to guide the head under the arch of the pubis by using the space in front of the sacrum. As the head crowns, the angle of traction changes through an arc of over 90 degrees.

At this point, either an episiotomy is cut or, if the perineum is stretching as normal, it is simply supported with the hand that was on the bell. Occasionally, an edge of the cup might lift off at the introitus (this is more likely to happen if there is caput present). If this occurs, you must be careful not to catch maternal tissue under the cup as it reattaches, and thus this should be rechecked before final delivery of the head.

Anterior metal cup

The metal cup is lightly lubricated and then inserted side-ways into the vagina. To orientate the cup, correctly place the chain over the occiput, which will result in the vacuum pipe lying centrally. Traction can commence once a negative pressure of 0.8kg/cm^2 has been achieved.

The controlled two-handed manner of delivery is similar. Classically a, three-finger grip' has been described for the fingers on the cup and head. As in the use of the silicone rubber cup, this ensures that you know whether the head is descending with each pull (and not just the caput). In addition, the fingers apply a force which opposes the lifting tendency of the upper edge when pulling downwards earlier in the delivery and which oppose the lifting tendency of the lower edge when pulling upwards at the end of the delivery.

Posterior metal cup

When confronted with a deflexed head in an occipitoposterior position, the 'OP' cup should be used. It is applied as far back on the head as possible, again ideally in the mid-line over the occiput. To allow good placement of the cup it sometimes helps to try to flex the head, with two fingers of the left hand pressing on the sinciput, while the right hand inserts the cup behind the head. Occasionally the operator may consider doing an episiotomy before applying the cup, to allow a better application. Once correctly placed the vacuum can be started and taken directly to the required level (because the cup lies parallel to the vagina it is unlikely to catch any maternal tissue). The first pull will be in the direction required to flex the head.

With flexion of the head the presenting diameter immediately becomes smaller. Thereafter, traction will be along the pelvic axis. The delivery may be completed simply by a standard spontaneous rotation with maternal effort and gentle assistance. It is important not to try to twist the cup to rotate the baby. This will only injure the scalp.

Overall, occipitoposterior deliveries are the ones most likely to provide problems.[301] The most difficult are those where the head is markedly deflexed or where there is excessive caput.

Another difficulty sometimes encountered is that the suction pipe tends to kink once the head flexes, making it more likely to detach. If the cup detaches at this point (after flexion and rotation) it may be simplest to change to an anterior cup or, if speed is essential, to perform a lift-out forceps.

The difficult ventouse

Causes and management of failure to deliver with the ventouse

It has been claimed (by an expert) that failure rates of less than 1% should be achieved with well-maintained apparatus and correct technique.[295,303] Johanson *et al.*[301] achieved a vaginal delivery with the first instrument used in 86% of cases. Each of the following factors contributed to the failures.

- Failure to use the correct instrument.
  Failures with the silicone rubber cup will be common if it is used inappropriately when there is deflexion of the head, excess caput, a big baby or a prolonged second stage of labour.
- Inadequate initial assessment of the case:
  - the head being too high.

  A classic mistake is to assume that because caput can be felt below the ischial spines the head must be engaged.

  - misdiagnosis of the position and attitude of the head.

  Attention to simple detail will minimise the occurrence of this problem.
- Either anterior or lateral placements will increase the failure rate.[298]
  Anterior placements are also more likely to be associated with fetal injury.[304] In this respect, preterm infants are more vulnerable (even greater care should be taken to check position before application in these cases). If the cup placement is found to be incorrect, it may be appropriate to begin again with correct placement: mid-line over the occiput.

- Failures due to traction in the wrong direction.
  These may be amenable simply to a change in angle of traction.
- Excessive caput.
  Rarely even with the metal cups adequate traction is not possible because of excessive caput. Careful consideration in these cases must be given to delivery by caesarean section unless the head is well down, in which case forceps can be used.
- Poor maternal effort.
  There is no doubt that maternal effort can contribute substantially to the success of the delivery. Adequate encouragement and instruction should be given to the mother. (This may be a reason for preferring forceps to ventouse if the patient is under general anaesthesia).
- The incidence of cephalopelvic disproportion (true failure) is low.

Special indications

Of particular importance is the use of the ventouse in the first stage of labour. It is commonly believed that the ventouse may be attempted after 7 cm dilatation[305] however, in our series we did not attempt delivery at less than 9 cm.[301] In these circumstances, all the other prerequisites for ventouse delivery should be fulfilled. Delivery before full dilatation should be reserved for acute fetal distress (e.g. abruption), where a straightforward normal delivery would have been expected within the next half hour. Nevertheless, this is a potentially dangerous practice and should only be undertaken by an experienced operator.

Two maternal deaths reviewed in a recent Confidential Enquiry[306] involved junior doctors undertaking ventouse deliveries before full dilatation. In the hands of an experienced operator the ventouse can also be used to expedite delivery complicated by a prolapsed cord at full dilatation and for delivery of the second twin with fetal distress, (thereby avoiding a caesarean section).

The place of trial-of-ventouse

There are few situations where the success of the ventouse should be tested by a 'trial'. Adequate assessment of the case will generally resolve any doubts prior to attempting a ventouse delivery. If the operator is uncertain about the degree of engagement or the position of the head then they should first ensure that adequate analgesia for examination has been provided. If they remain uncertain, someone of greater experience should assist. There is no place for a 'suck-and-see' approach. It has been stated that 'the indications for the use of the vacuum extractor as an alternative to forceps delivery include uncertainty with regard to the position of the sagittal suture and situations where the fetal head is assumed to be too high for application of forceps'.[307] This advice is quite clearly both untrue and potentially dangerous.

Any trial-of-ventouse in theatre must be sanctioned and/or supervised by a consultant or experienced registrar.

The place of forceps after failure to delivery with the ventouse

There is no place for an attempt at forceps delivery if there has been no descent with the ventouse despite adequate traction. However, if traction has been inadequate (due to caput, leaking equipment, no maternal assistance) it may be justified to change to forceps. This decision should be made at an experienced level. The situation may also arise that after good descent and rotation of the head the cup detaches. What might have been a difficult Kielland delivery has now become a straightforward 'lift-out' anterior-cup or forceps delivery.

Audit standard

The RCOG audit standard is: 'the ventouse should be the instrument of first choice for operative vaginal delivery'.

Forceps

Introduction

There are over 700 different makes of forceps.[308] Most authors subscribe to a classification system that divides forceps into classic and specialised subtypes. Classic subtypes include Simpson, Anderson and Neville-Barnes forceps, while specialised forceps include Kielland, Piper and Laufe (of divergent design). Variations in cephalic curvature, fenestration and design of shank allow selection to be made on the basis of individual circumstances.[308] There have been no randomised controlled trials comparing different instruments and it is recognised that the choice is often subjective. One RCT was identified; in this study decreased facial marking was found when soft blade pads were used.[309]

Choice of forceps over ventouse

As discussed above, the current evidence suggests that forceps are more likely to injure the mother and cause pain at time of delivery. In the most recent review,[310] the use of forceps was also found to be associated with increased requirement for epidurals and general anaesthetics, and overall there was a statistically significant increase in requirement for caesarean section if forceps were chosen rather than the ventouse.

Situations where the forceps may be required are, for example, delivery of the after-coming head of a breech, delivery of a mentoanterior face presentation requiring assistance and delivery in other situations where the ventouse is contraindicated for example, a heavily bleeding scalp sample site or with delivery before 34 weeks. It is also important that the practitioner is comfortable with (skilled in the use of) the instrument that is chosen. Adequate supervision should always be available.

Method

1. It is essential to judge that the head is fully engaged. Abdominal palpation must be undertaken and this is particularly true with face presentation.
2. It is generally advised that catheterisation is required for forceps delivery and that an episiotomy is required.
3. It is essential that the position of the head is carefully noted. If occipitotransverse or occipitoposterior, particular expertise is required.[310]
4. It is essential that the operator check the pair of forceps that they have been given. It may be useful to check the maximum diameter between the two blades also (a pair that is not true, will have maximum diameter as little as 7.0 cm or 7.5 cm. The maximum diameter should be at least 9 cm).
5. After repairing the episiotomy, always ensure that the swabs and instruments are correct in number.
6. Do per rectum examination to check rectal sphincter, mucosa for tears.
7. Document every aspect of delivery completely.

Audit standards

The following should be audited routinely (RCOG 2000[310]):

- overall rates and indications for instrumental delivery
- complications, e.g. failed instrumental delivery, neonatal admissions for intensive care
- adequacy of documentation, e.g. level of head assessed abdominally and vaginally
- complaints and medico-legal cases.

Inter-twin delivery interval

Recent studies support the view that no specific time interval needs to be set, provided that there is continuous electronic FHR monitoring of twin two and that it is reassuring.[316–319]

ECV versus internal podalic version

Confusion still exists over whether ECV or internal podalic version (IPV) and breech extraction should be performed. Many investigators report success with attempt at ECV in the first instance.[316,320–322] However, other authors have reported lower success rates with ECV or increased maternal complication rates.[323] Nevertheless, given that ECV is less invasive, it should seem reasonable to consider this in the first place. The experience of the operator is probably the most important factor.

Higher multiples

Even though the incidence of triplets is rising, most obstetricians have relatively little experience of delivering triplets and even less of delivering them vaginally. Although a study from the Netherlands reported improved outcome for triplets with vaginal delivery,[324] when compared with caesarean section, the unit was particularly experienced at this type of delivery. For most obstetricians the safer option would almost certainly be caesarean section.

Previous caesarean section

Although there is little evidence, what there is suggests that a trial of labour is a safe option in the absence of a contraindication to vaginal birth. Scar dehiscence rates were reported to be 0–3%.[325]

Preterm/very-low-birthweight twins

There seems to be little difference in outcome between vaginal and caesarean delivery in very low birthweight gestations. There seemed to be little difference in terms of perinatal outcome.[326,327]

Indications for caesarean section

- Conjoined twins
- Monoamniotic twins
- Placenta praevia
- Certain congenital anomalies
- Possible interlocking twins

The intrapartum management of vaginal twin delivery

Admission to delivery suite

- Intravenous line
- Blood tests – FBC, group and save serum
- **Continuous** CTG on a twin monitor
  - FHR abnormalities twin one – take fetal blood sample
  - FHR abnormalities twin two – perform caesarean section

- If at any stage either twin cannot be monitored then caesarean section may be the only safe option. It is imperative that **both** twins are monitored and the trace should be scrutinised to ensure that this is the case.

Ultrasound assessment

By an appropriately trained practitioner to determine:

- presentation of each fetus
- liquor volume assessment
- placental site
- viability of each fetus
- estimation of fetal weight if not recently performed.

Ultrasound should be used for ECV and may be used to guide the operator undertaking IPV.

Epidural analgesia

The use of an epidural can be justified in terms of analgesia for possible intrauterine manipulations required for the delivery of the second twin.

Inform

- anaesthetist
- paediatrician
- neonatal unit.

Management of stage two

- Top up epidural.
- Prepare oxytocin 10 iu in Hartmann's solution, if not already receiving oxytocin infusion.
- Deliver twin one as if singleton.
- Perform abdominal palpation to determine lie.
- Confirm lie, presentation and fetal heart with ultrasound scan.
- Monitor electronic FHR continuously.
- If transverse lie, perform ECV or IPV.
- When lie longitudinal and presenting part in pelvis, perform amniotomy with contraction.
- If no contractions within 5–10 minutes commence oxytocin infusion.

Management of stage three

- Give Syntometrine® 1 ampoule (or oxytocin 5 iu if Syntometrine contraindicated) with the delivery of the second twin.
- Deliver the placenta.
- Consider commencing oxytocin infusion (40 iu oxytocin in Hartmann's solution), as there is a risk of uterine atony following delivery of multiple gestations.

IPV

The technique used for internal podalic version has been described.[328]

A fetal foot is identified by recognising a heel through intact membranes. The foot is grasped and pulled gently and continuously lowered into the birth canal. The membranes are ruptured as late as possible.

This procedure is easiest when the transverse lie is with the back superior or posterior. If the back is inferior or if the limbs are not immediately palpable, ultrasound may help to identify to the operator where they may be found. This will minimise the risk of bringing down a fetal hand.

Algorithm 26.1 Sepsis key points

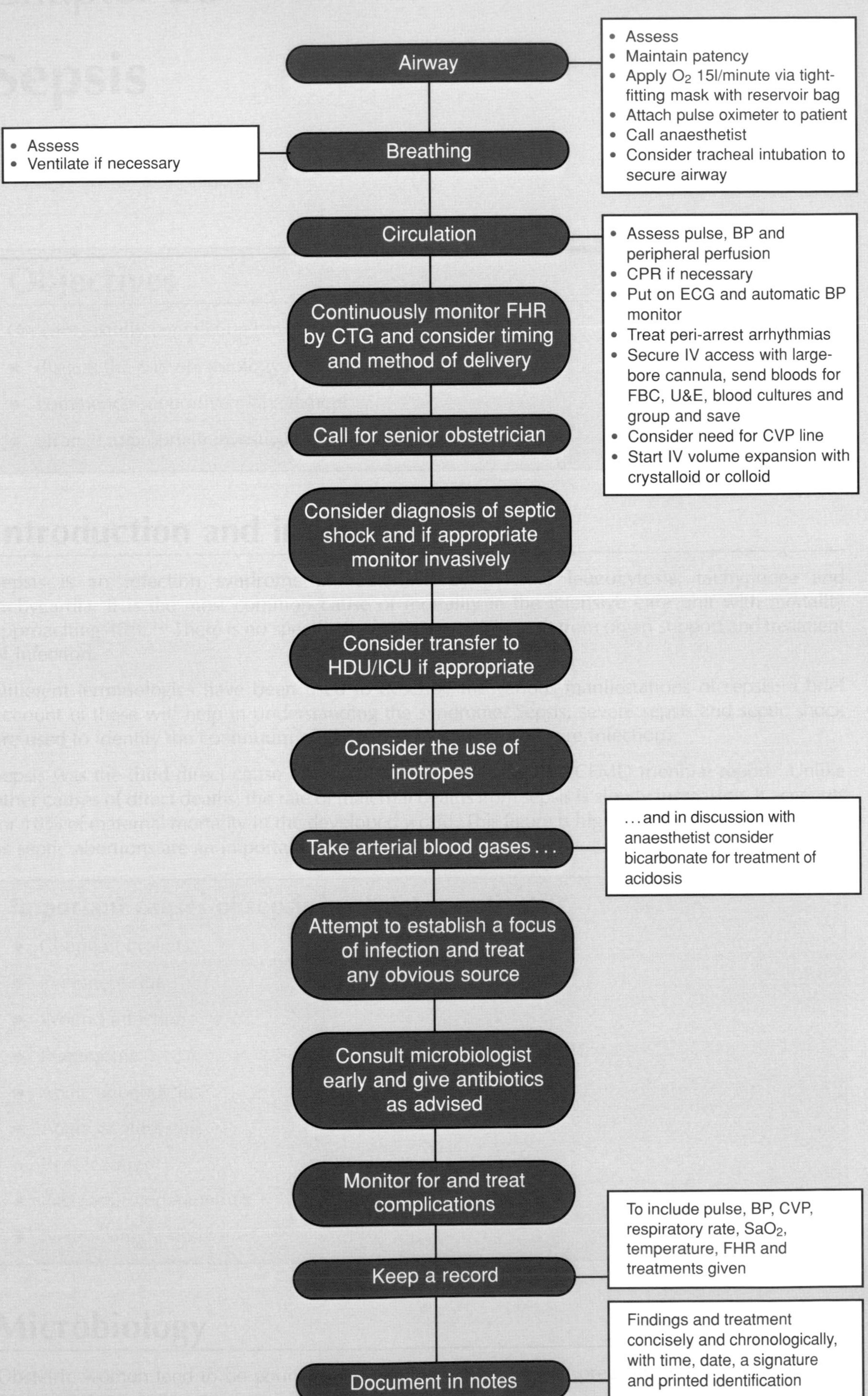

Continuum of the clinical response to severe infection

- Bacteraemia
  Presence of bacteria in blood.
- Septicaemia
  Presence of microbes and their toxins in blood.
- Systemic inflammatory response syndrome (SIRS) (this can be triggered by an infection or a non-infectious cause, e.g. trauma, pancreatitis)

  Presence of any two of the following features:
  - temperature > 38°C or < 36°C
  - tachypnoea respiratory rate > 24 breaths per minute
  - tachycardia > 90 bpm
  - leucocytosis > 11 000 white blood cells/mm^3
  - leucopenia < 4000 white blood cells/mm^3
- Sepsis
  Signs of SIRS and evidence of infection.
- Septic shock
  Clinical diagnosis of sepsis with hypotension.

  Systolic < 90 mmHg or 40 mmHg below baseline.
  - **early**: if duration of hypotension is less than one hour and responds to fluid administration
  - **refractory**: if duration of hypotension is more than one hour and requiring inotropes to treat hypotension
- Multiple organ dysfunction syndrome
  Clinical diagnosis of sepsis and presence of organ dysfunction (severe hypoxemia, oliguria, liver failure, DIC, altered mental state, acidosis)[330]

bacteraemia develop septic shock and, of these, 2–3% die.[331] In the last CEMD triennial report, the mortality reported from sepsis was 6.4 per million maternities.[4] The most common microbes responsible for sepsis in UK include streptococcus groups A and B, followed by *Escherischia coli*. Other organisms that can cause sepsis include obligate anaerobic bacteria, *Listeria monocytogenes*, *Gardnerella vaginalis* and *Staphylococcus aureus*.

Pathophysiology of sepsis

Sepsis represents the body's response to an insult, be it an infection or an injury. The initial response is the release of primary mediators (interleukin-1 and tumour necrosis factor alpha). These cytokines are produced from activated macrophages. These primary mediators in turn stimulate the production of secondary mediators, which in turn activate coagulation and complement cascades.[332] This is followed by the expression of anti-inflammatory mediators, which help to contain the inflammation locally. Consequently, this is the period during which the function of the immune system is compromised. As with many other regulatory processes, there is a fine balance between the pro- and anti-inflammatory mediators.

In situations where the bacterial load is high or there is an imbalance between pro- and anti-inflammatory mediators, inflammation becomes generalised, resulting in severe sepsis. There is growing evidence that this fine balance is controlled genetically.

At a cellular level the inducible form of nitric oxide synthase is stimulated. This causes overproduction of nitric oxide from endothelial cells, macrophages and muscle cells. Nitric oxide is the major mediator of vasodilatation and myocardial dysfunction, which results in hypotension. Superoxide radicals also react with nitric oxide to form peroxynitrate, which causes direct cellular injury.

Haemodynamic alterations

There is a decrease in arteriolar and venous tone. This causes venous pooling of blood and a drop in vascular resistance, resulting in hypotension. In the initial stages of sepsis there is hypotension with reduced cardiac output and low filling pressures. With fluid resuscitation cardiac output increases, resulting in a hyperdynamic circulation, but there is not much change in blood pressure due to a reduced vascular resistance. There is an increase in pulmonary vascular resistance resulting in raised pulmonary arterial pressures. The changes in the vascular tone differ in different vascular beds, resulting in the maldistribution of blood volume and flow. There is evidence to suggest that the ability of tissues to extract oxygen is also impaired. This encourages anaerobic metabolism in tissues, promoting lactic acidosis.

Clinical manifestations

Tachypnoea, tachycardia and altered mental state are early manifestations of sepsis, frequently preceded by fever and hypotension. Some septic patients may not have a fever and, in a state of shock, may even be hypothermic. Isolated thrombocytopenia with no evidence of DIC is seen in more than 50% of patients. The other complications include DIC, ARDS, renal failure and hepatic failure, seen in 30–50% of patients with severe sepsis. One-third of patients who die, die early because of refractory hypotension and the rest who succumb late die due to multiple organ failure.

Treatment

Infection should never be underestimated, as it continues to be an important cause of maternal mortality. Puerperal sepsis can be insidious in onset and progress rapidly to fulminating sepsis and death. Treatment of underlying infection goes hand in hand with supporting failing organ functions. Patients with single organ failure that is not responding to simple measures need to be cared for in a high dependency unit. Two or more organ failures and respiratory failure needs admission to an intensive care unit.

Initial management of patients with sepsis should be aimed at maintaining adequate **A**irway, **B**reathing and **C**irculation. Appropriate monitoring in the early stages of sepsis includes temperature, pulse, respiratory rate, blood pressure, arterial saturation (SaO_2) and hourly urine output. Baseline blood investigations required include full blood count, coagulation profile, urea and electrolytes, liver function tests and blood cultures. Senior clinicians should be involved at an early stage.

Airway and breathing

Maintenance of adequate oxygenation is an important step in the resuscitation of patients with sepsis. This includes a patent airway with adequate breathing and supplemental oxygen. Most patients in shock will ultimately need intubation and ventilation because of increased difficulty in breathing, development of ARDS or for primary underlying disease.

Circulation

Hypovolaemia is present in almost all patients with septic shock and fluid resuscitation is the mainstay of treatment. There is not much to be said about the choice of the fluid for replacement: both crystalloids and colloids are equally effective when administered to similar endpoints.[333]

Should patients not respond to simple measures of resuscitation, CVP monitoring should be instituted to guide further fluid replacement. Use of colloids has a theoretical advantage that it may be associated with lower incidence of pulmonary oedema. In most patients with septic shock, a haemoglobin of 8 g/dl may be appropriate. However, in patients with ischaemic heart disease a haemoglobin of 10 g/dl is more appropriate.[333]

In patients who remain hypotensive despite adequate fluid resuscitation, a pulmonary artery flotation catheter is needed to guide further management. Based on the measurements obtained, which include cardiac output, systemic and pulmonary vascular resistance and wedge pressures, therapy can be fine-tuned to optimise haemodynamics. Evidence suggests that the appropriate vasopressor is norepinephrine and the appropriate inotrope is dobutamine,[334] both of which have no detrimental effects on splanchnic circulation. Other agents used include epinephrine, dopamine and dopexamine, but evidence does not support their use. Sensitivity to catecholamines is significantly altered in septic patients and they require much higher doses than in other clinical situations.

The endpoints with any treatment include a normal or above normal cardiac output and a mean arterial pressure of 70 mmHg.[334] Despite aggressive management of septic shock, mortality is around 40%. During the course of sepsis, it is not uncommon for different organs to fail. The most common include kidneys, haematological, liver and gastrointestinal. These failing organs need support during this critical period; however, predicted mortality increases with increasing number of failed organs, approaching 85–100% with three or more organ failures.

Control of infection

Septic shock carries high morbidity and mortality and it is therefore important to prevent infections. There is strong evidence from Cochrane database for the use of prophylactic antibiotics in preventing postoperative infection following caesarean sections.[335]

In the last CEMD triennial report,[4] substandard care with regards to treating infections was reported in a number of cases. A microbiology consultation must be sought at an early stage to manage patients who are systemically ill. This helps in the collection of appropriate specimens and instituting the correct antibiotic therapy. Choice of antibiotic therapy depends on the clinical suspicion, local flora and culture information if available.

Urgent blood, urine, high vaginal, endocervical and other appropriate cultures must be obtained before starting antibiotics. This should help in identifying the offending microbe. Systemically ill patients require prompt broad spectrum, intravenous antibiotics even before culture reports are available.[4] Empirical treatment should include cover for Gram-negative and anaerobic organism. Gram-positive cover is necessary if the likelihood of this infection is high.

Closed-space infections need surgical drainage including evacuation of retained products of conception. In patients with endometritis not responding to antibiotics, septic pelvic thrombosis should be considered. These patients require heparin, together with antibiotics. Patients not responding appropriately to the above measures are likely to have myometrial necrosis and/or abscess, which continue to seed the bloodstream. In these cases, early surgical intervention with possible recourse to hysterectomy could save lives. Necrotising fasciitis is another condition, which requires early surgical intervention with fasciotomy and aggressive antibiotic therapy.

Recent advances

Recently published data from France by Dr Annane have found better 28-day survival in patients given small steroid supplementation (hydrocortisone 50 mg four times a day with once daily fludrocortisone).[336]

A randomised placebo-controlled PROWESS study[337] showed that use of activated protein C in the management of severe sepsis has shown a 20% relative risk reduction in mortality. For this treatment to be cost effective, further debate continues regarding the subgroup of patients who would derive maximum benefit from this treatment.

Algorithm 27.1 Symphysiotomy key points

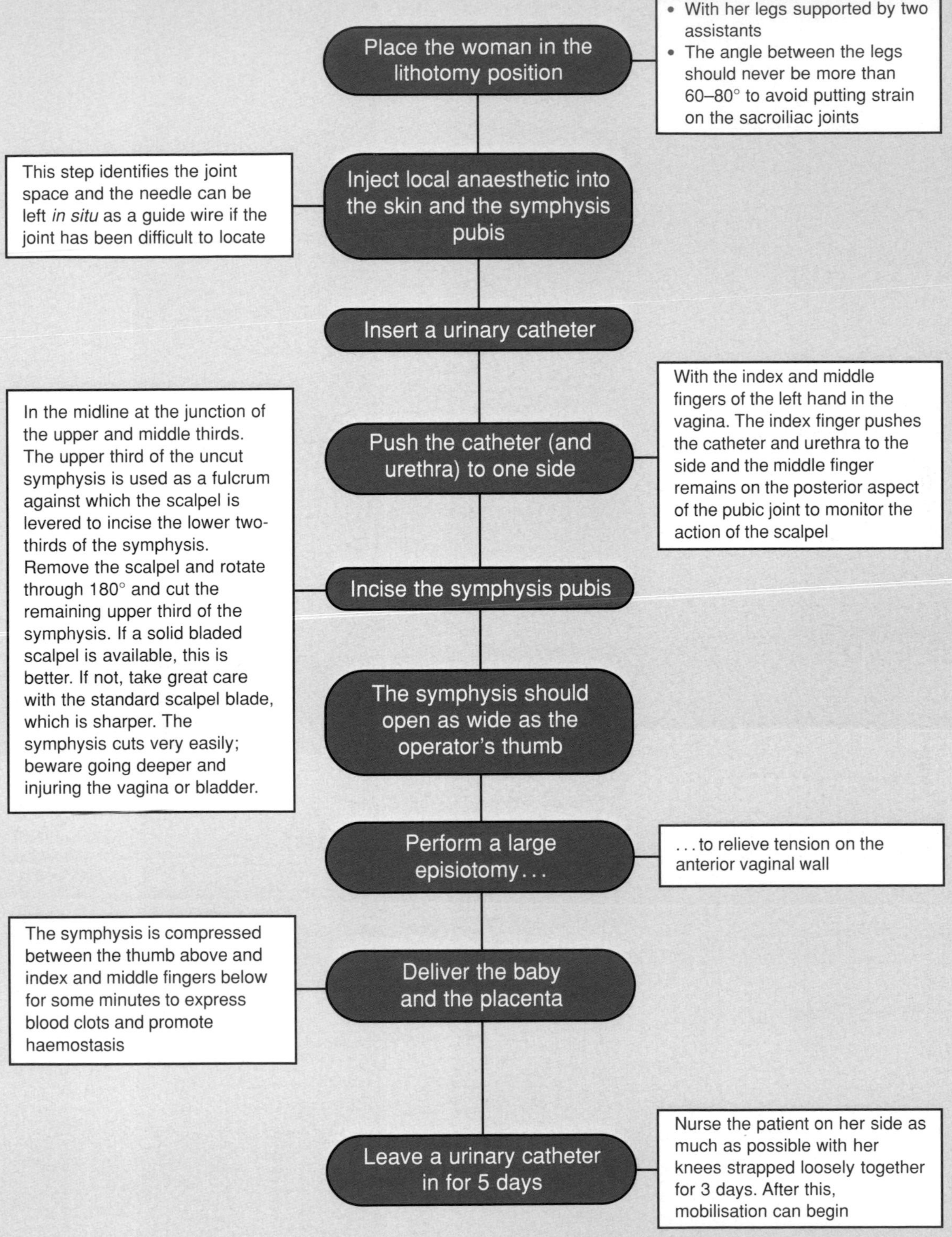

Chapter 27

Symphysiotomy

Objectives

On successfully completing this topic you will be able to:

- discuss the indications for symphysiotomy
- understand the technique.

Introduction

Van Roosmalen[338,339] has outlined the background to symphysiotomy by illustrating the potential morbidity and mortality of caesarean sections carried out in developing nations' rural hospitals. Mortalities of up to 5% have been reported and an incidence of uterine scar rupture in subsequent pregnancies of up to 6.8% has been reported. Symphysiotomy has a low maternal mortality with three deaths reported in a series of 1752 symphysiotomies.[338] All three deaths were unrelated to the procedure.

Hartfield[340] reviewed 138 patients in whom symphysiotomy had been performed. Early and late complications were few and rarely serious if recommended guidelines were adhered to. He also reviewed published series of patients followed up for two years or more after symphysiotomy and concluded that permanent major orthopaedic disability only occurs in 1–2% of cases.[341]

Pape[342] carried out a prospective review of 27 symphysiotomies performed between 1992 and 1994. Five had paraurethral tears needing suturing, nine had oedema of the vulva or haematomas tracking from the symphysiotomy. All patients made a full recovery and severe pelvic pain was not a feature in any patient.

The majority of women (73%) will have an uncomplicated vaginal delivery in a subsequent pregnancy.[4]

In 2001, the question of legal action against obstetricians in Ireland who carried out symphysiotomies was raised.[343] Verkuyl responded in a letter to the *BMJ*,[344] which makes the point that many symphysiotomies were done in Roman Catholic countries because contraception was illegal even for medical reasons and women were spared repeated operative deliveries.

In developing countries, symphysiotomy may be literally life saving, as it avoids the need for caesarean section with all its inherent risks in a future pregnancy while increasing the chance of further vaginal deliveries.

Indications

- Trapped aftercoming head of breech due to cephalopelvic disproportion.[345,346]
- Severe cases of shoulder dystocia that do not resolve with routine manoeuvres.[347]
- In cases of cephalopelvic disproportion with a vertex presentation and a living fetus (in the developing world), when at least one-third of the fetal head has entered the pelvic brim. Note that the use of forceps is contraindicated.[338]

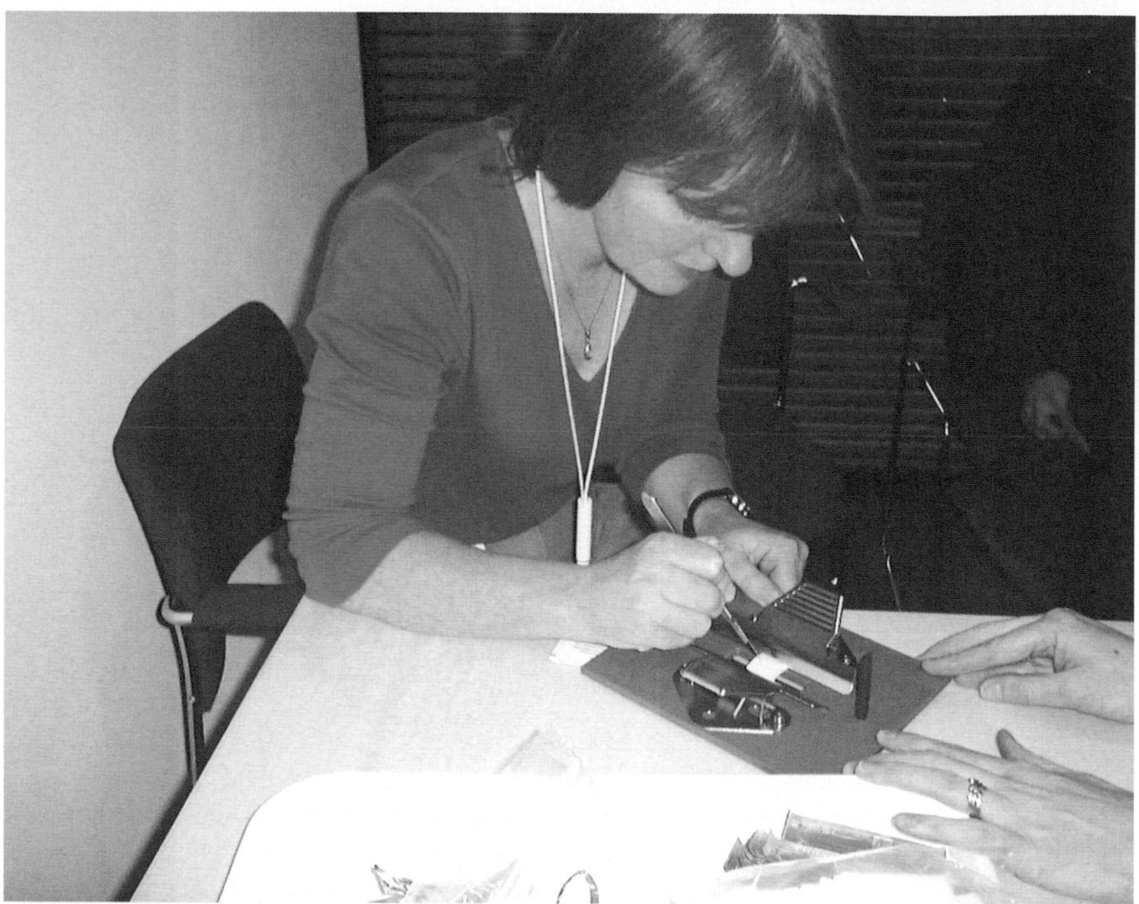

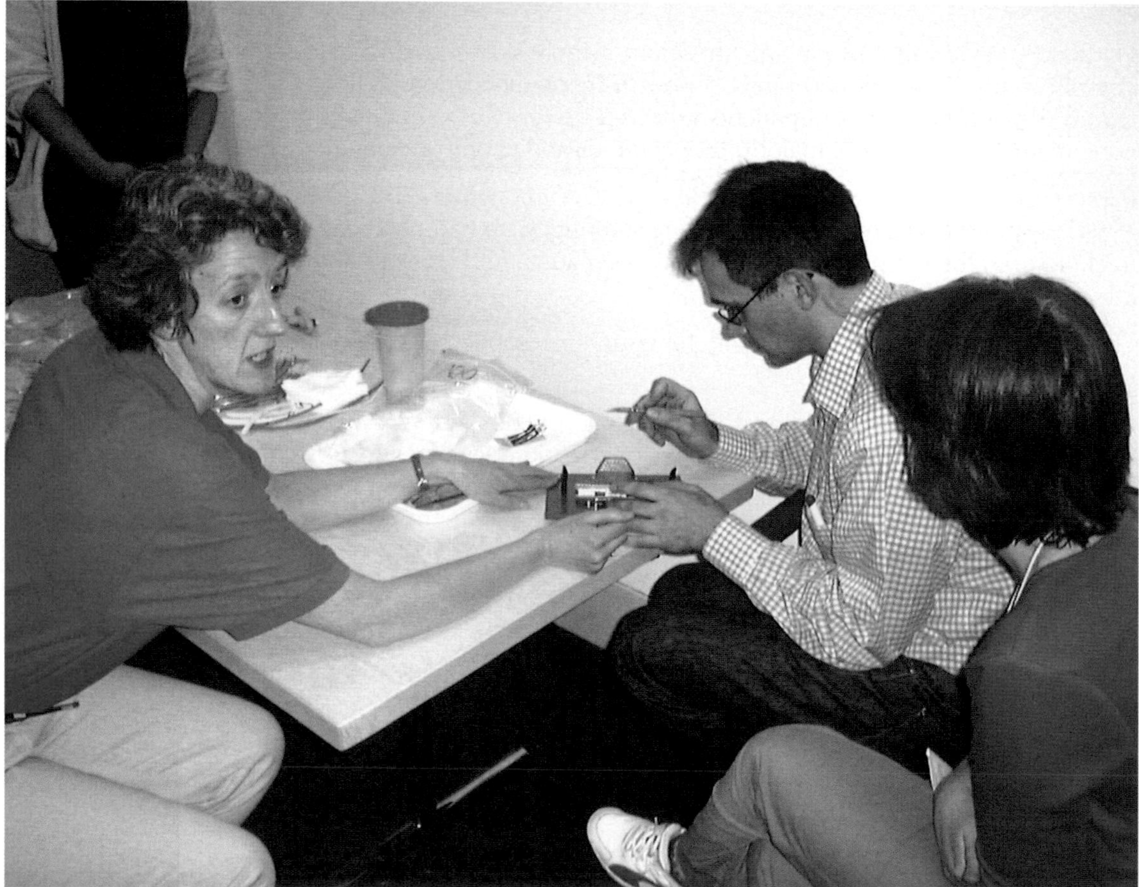

Symphysiotomy practice

Technique[340,345,348]

1. Place the woman in the lithotomy position with her legs supported by two assistants. The angle between the legs should never be more than 60–80° to avoid putting a strain on the sacroiliac joints.
2. Inject local anaesthetic into the skin and symphysis pubis. This step identifies the joint space and the needle can be left *in situ* as a guide wire if the joint has been difficult to locate.
3. Insert a urinary catheter.
4. Push the catheter (and urethra) aside with the index and middle fingers of the left hand in the vagina. The index finger pushes the catheter and urethra to the side and the middle finger remains on the posterior aspect of the pubic joint to monitor the action of the scalpel.
5. Incise the symphysis pubis in the midline at the junction of the upper and middle thirds. Use the upper third of the uncut symphysis as a fulcrum against which to lever the scalpel to incise the lower two-thirds of the symphysis.
6. Remove the scalpel and rotate through 180 degrees and the remaining upper third of the symphysis is cut. If a solid-bladed scalpel is available, this is better. If not, take great care with the standard scalpel blade, which is sharper. The symphysis cuts very easily; beware of going deeper and injuring the vagina or bladder.
7. The symphysis should open as wide as the operator's thumb.
8. Use a large episiotomy to relieve tension on the anterior vaginal wall.
9. After delivery of the baby and placenta, compress the symphysis between the thumb above and index and middle fingers below for some minutes, to express blood clots and promote haemostasis.
10. Leave a urinary catheter in place for five days. The patient needs to be nursed on her side as much as possible with knees strapped loosely together for three days. After this, mobilisation can begin.

Summary

- Symphysiotomy is a useful procedure that can be used in certain emergency situations.
- It must only be performed by trained clinicians.
- Prompt decision is required to avoid fetal morbidity.
- Intrapartum and postpartum management are important to minimise maternal morbidity.

Algorithm 28.1 Patients declining blood and blood products key points

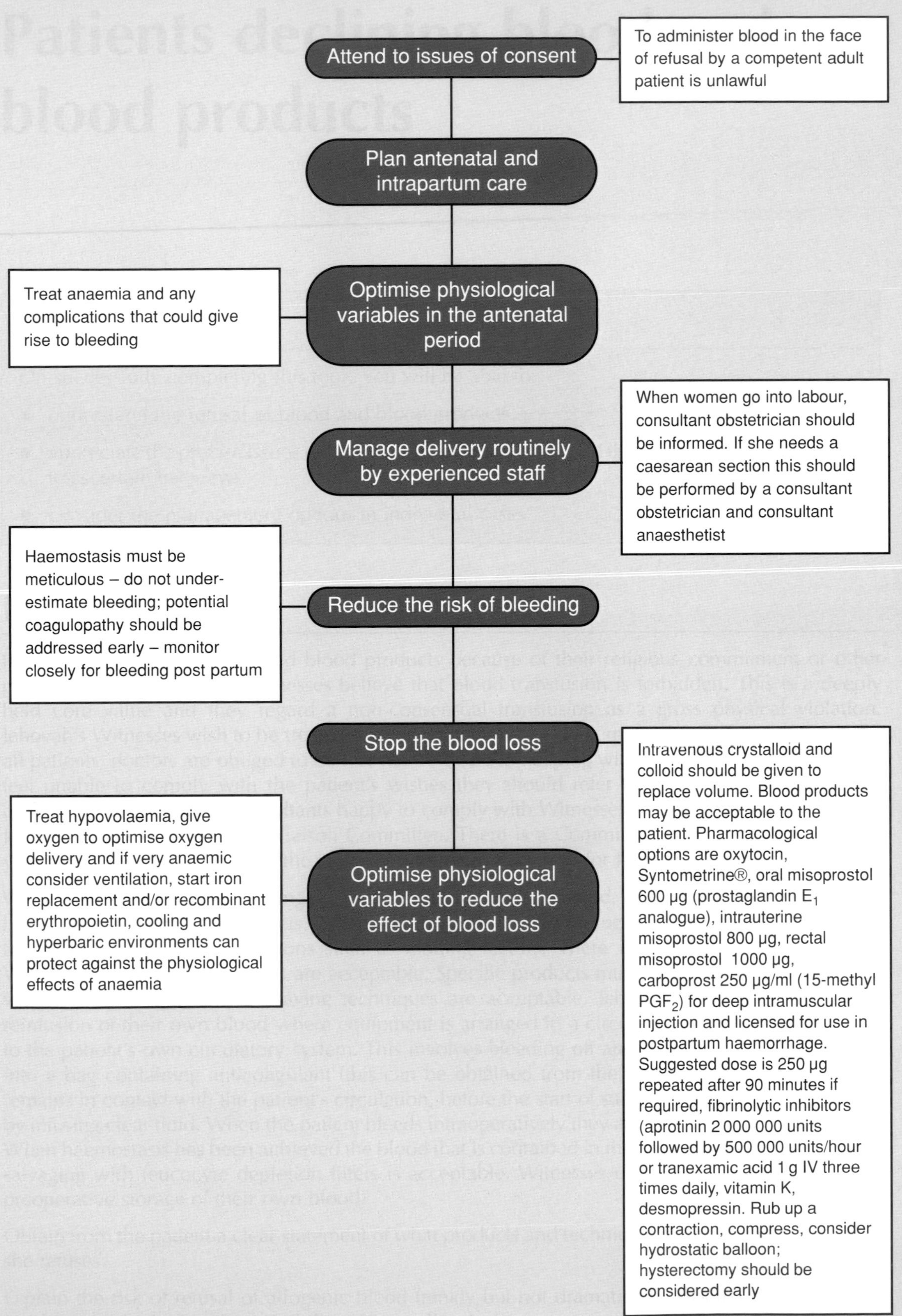

mother. If she continues to refuse blood products in the face of life-threatening haemorrhage, proceed to caesarean section.

If the mother is a minor, parental right to determine whether or not she will have medical treatment terminates if she has sufficient understanding and intelligence to enable her to comprehend fully what is proposed.

The wishes of a competent child may be overruled if, in the opinion of the court, the consequences of refusal are such that it would be inappropriate to comply with the child's wishes.

If the mother is too young to comprehend adequately and the parent refuses to agree to treatment that is, in the opinion of qualified medical practitioners, proper and necessary, the matter can be referred to the High Court and this should be included in any case conferences. The High Court has emergency procedures to arrange for expedited considerations of such applications.

If the child is likely to succumb without the immediate administration of blood and the courts will be too time-consuming, blood should be transfused without consulting the court.

The patient and the parents must be kept informed of proposals.

Most Jehovah's Witnesses will carry with them a clear Advance Directive prohibiting blood transfusions and will have executed a Healthcare Advance Directive, which gives comprehensive personal instructions on a variety of issues. Healthcare Advanced Directives may be lodged with their GP, as well as with family and friends. If the patient is not in a condition to give or withhold consent but has expressed a wish at an earlier date (Advanced Directive or Healthcare Advance Directive), respect the patient's instructions in the Advance Directive or Healthcare Advance Directive.

If such instructions do not specifically apply to the patient's current condition, if the patient's instructions are vague and open to interpretation, or if there is good reason to believe that the patient has had a change of heart since making the declaration, the doctor's duty is to exercise good medical judgement and treat the patient in her best interests as determined by a responsible body of medical opinion.

Allow the patient the opportunity to speak with the Hospital Liaison Committee for Jehovah's Witnesses and, if requested, join their discussion.

Ensure that the patient has had the opportunity to speak with the obstetrician in privacy, without relatives or members of her religious community if she wishes.

Keep a clear record of the discussion and particular aspects of consent. Note precisely which products/treatment she refuses and which she would accept. Complete a Jehovah's Witness consent form. Have discussion and take and document consent in the presence of a witness. The person witnessing the discussion should sign a record of the discussion and consent as made and signed by the doctor.

A verbally expressed change of mind should be honoured. Again, it should be given in the presence of a witness and recorded in the notes.

Plan antenatal and intrapartum care

Massive obstetric haemorrhage is often unpredictable and can become life threatening in a short time. If it is thought likely that a woman may haemorrhage, the management should be considered in advance. Delivery should be planned in a unit that has the facilities to cope with massive obstetric haemorrhage.

An ultrasound scan should be carried out to identify the placental site.

If any complications are noted during the antenatal period, the consultant obstetrician must be informed.

Optimise physiological variables in the antenatal period

The woman's blood group and antibody status should be checked in the usual way and the haemoglobin and serum ferritin should be checked regularly. Haematinics should be given throughout pregnancy to maximise iron stores. Treat any complications that could give rise to bleeding.

Manage delivery routinely by experienced staff

The consultant obstetrician should be informed when a woman who will refuse blood transfusion is admitted in labour. Consultants in other specialties need not be alerted unless complications occur.

The labour should be managed routinely by experienced staff.

Oxytocics should be given when the baby is delivered. The woman should not be left alone for at least an hour after delivery and there should be early intervention to stem postpartum bleeding.

If caesarean section is necessary, it should be carried out by a consultant obstetrician with a consultant anaesthetist.

When the mother is discharged from hospital, she should be advised to report promptly if she has any concerns about bleeding during the puerperium.

Reduce the risk of bleeding

The patient should be monitored closely for bleeding postpartum. Blood loss should not be underestimated, as potential coagulopathy should be addressed early.

Stop the blood loss

Pharmacological and surgical treatment is described in greater detail in Chapter 16 Massive obstetric haemorrhage.

The principle of management of haemorrhage in these cases is to avoid delay. Rapid decision making may be necessary, particularly with regard to surgical intervention.

If unusual bleeding occurs at any time during pregnancy, labour or the puerperium, the consultant obstetrician should be informed and the standard management should be commenced promptly. The threshold for intervention should be lower than in other patients. Extra vigilance should be exercised to quantify any abnormal bleeding and to detect complications, such as clotting abnormalities, as promptly as possible.

Consultants in other specialties, particularly anaesthetics and haematology, are normally involved in the treatment of massive haemorrhage. When the patient is a woman who has refused blood transfusion, the consultant anaesthetist should be informed as soon as possible after abnormal bleeding has been detected. The consultant haematologist should also be informed particularly if the patient is suffering form DIC. Intensive care may need to be warned.

Intravenous crystalloid and colloid should be given to replace volume. Blood products may be acceptable to the patient.

Pharmacological options are:

- oxytocin
- Syntometrine®
- oral misoprostol 600 micrograms (prostaglandin E_1 analogue)
- intrauterine misoprostol 800 micrograms
- rectal misoprostol 1000 micrograms

- carboprost 250 micrograms/ml (15-methyl PGF_2) for deep intramuscular injection and licensed for use in postpartum haemorrhage; can be injected intramyometrially, although not licensed for this. Suggested dose is 250 micrograms repeated after 90 minutes if required
- fibrinolytic inhibitors (aprotinin 2 000 000 units followed by 500 000 units/hour or tranexamic acid 1 g IV x3 daily)
- vitamin K
- desmopressin.

Surgery

See also Chapter 16 Massive obstetric haemorrhage.

Hysterectomy is normally the last resort in the treatment of obstetric haemorrhage but with such women delay may increase the risk. The woman's life may be saved by timely hysterectomy, although even this does not guarantee success.

When hysterectomy is performed, the uterine arteries should be clamped as early as possible in the procedure. Subtotal hysterectomy can be just as effective as total hysterectomy, as well as being quicker and safer. In some cases there may be a place for embolisation or internal iliac artery ligation.

The timing of hysterectomy is a decision for the consultant on the spot. Survival without hysterectomy has been recorded with a haemoglobin concentration of 4.9 g/dl.

The woman should be kept fully informed about what is happening. Information must be given in a professional way, ideally by someone she knows and trusts. If standard treatment is not controlling the bleeding, she should be advised that blood transfusion is strongly recommended. Any patient is entitled to change her mind about a previously agreed treatment plan.

The doctor must be satisfied that the woman is not being subjected to pressure from others. It is reasonable to ask the accompanying persons to leave the room for a while so that the doctor (with a midwife or other colleague) can ask her whether she is making her decision of her own free will.

If she maintains her refusal to accept blood or blood products, her wishes should be respected. The legal position is that any adult patient (i.e. 16 years of age and over) who has the necessary mental capacity to do so is entitled to refuse treatment, even if it is likely that refusal will result in the patient's death. No other person is legally able to consent to treatment for that adult or to refuse treatment on that person's behalf.

The staff must maintain a professional attitude. They must not lose the trust of the patient or her partner as further decisions – for example, about hysterectomy – may have to be made.

If, in spite of all care, the woman dies, her relatives require support like any other bereaved family.

It is very distressing for staff to have to watch a woman bleed to death while refusing effective treatment. Support should be promptly available for staff in these circumstances.

Optimise physiological variables to reduce the effect of blood loss

Treat hypovolaemia with non-blood products and use vasopressors to maintain blood pressure if necessary. Give oxygen to optimise oxygen delivery and, if very anaemic, consider ventilation to deliver oxygen maximally. Start iron replacement and/or recombinant erythropoietin. Cooling and hyperbaric environments can protect against the physiological effects of anaemia

Care plan for women in labour refusing a blood transfusion[350]

This plan was produced by the Hospital Information Services for Jehovah's Witnesses following the publication of the 1994–96 CEMD report,[4] in which there was a finding that, of 147 labour units in the UK, only two had recommendations for the management of women who refuse a blood transfusion.

Actively haemorrhaging

First steps:

- Establish IV colloid infusion
- Give oxygen
- Consider CVP line
- Catheterise and monitor urine output
- Give oxytocic drugs first, then exclude retained products of conception or trauma (this could save time)
- Proceed with bimanual uterine compression
- A useful emergency measure to buy time is aortic compression, using a fist just above the umbilicus directed back against the spine
- Slow but persistent blood loss requires action
- Anticipate coagulation problems
- Involve consultant anaesthetist and haematologist
- Keep patient fully informed.

Proceed with following strategies if bleeding continues:

- Syntometrine is marginally more effective than oxytocin alone. If the patient is hypertensive, use oxytocin.
- Oral Misoprostol 600 μg (prostaglandin E_1 analogue). Use when the patient is unresponsive to oxytocin and ergometrine. Useful while awaiting carboprost. Rectal misoprostol (1000 μg – five tablets) absorption rapid, avoids oral problems, e.g. nausea, faint. Control of haemorrhage with sustained contraction within three minutes of administration reported. Does not appear to cause hypertension.
- Carboprost (Hemabate®, Pharmacia) 250 μg/ml IM, can be repeated after 15 minutes.
- Aprotinin (Trasylol®, Bayer) 2 000 000 units followed by 500 000 units/hour or tranexamic acid (Cyklokapron®, Pharmacia) 1 g IV three times daily. Both agents are fibrinolytic inhibitors, are well established for controlling serious haemorrhage and can be used in combination. Recombinant factor VIIa (NovoSeven®, Novo Nordisk) 90 μg/kg provides site-specific thrombin generation and has been successfully used for haemostasis. Experience with this drug is limited. It should only be used in life-threatening bleeding. Expert advice will be available from the local Haemophilia Comprehensive Care Centre or the Novo Nordisk 24-hour medical advice line. Telephone 0845 600 5055.
- Embolisation or ligation of internal iliac artery or bilateral mass ligation of uterine arteries and veins. Time needed. Radiologist and surgical team required. Uterine packing may avoid hysterectomy, recently re-emergency as an option.
- B-Lynch brace suture. Simple surgical technique to control massive haemorrhage. Could avoid the need for hysterectomy.
- Hysterectomy, subtotal hysterectomy can be just as effective, also quicker and safer. Blood salvage using a cell saver should be considered if surgical blood loss anticipated.

Post-haemorrhage

- For severe anaemia, give oxygen and erythropoietin
- Iron supplementation is essential. Oral iron is slow and unreliable, use IV iron sucrose (Venofer®, Syner-Med) 200mg three times per week Augment with vitamin B12 and folic acid
- Consider elective ventilation on intensive care unit
- Hyperbaric oxygen therapy is an option in life-threatening anaemia. Contact the Hospital Information Services for Jehovah's Witnesses.[349]

Algorithm 29.1 Destructive operations key points

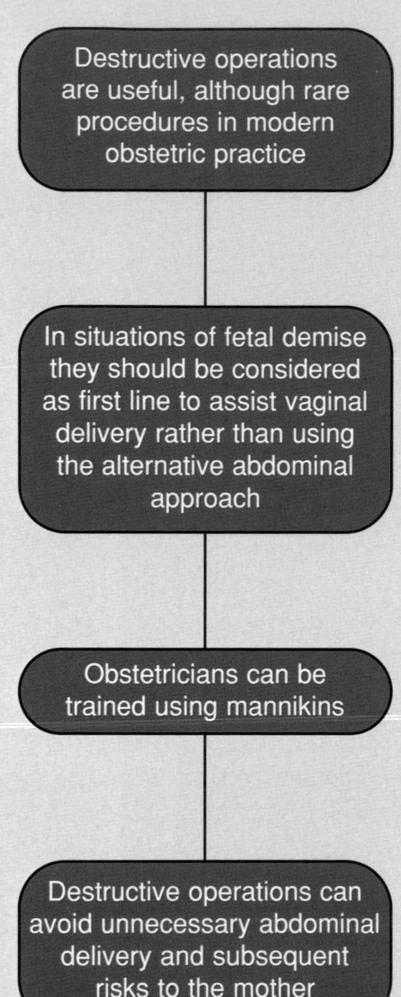

Chapter 29

Destructive operations

Objectives

On successfully completing this topic you will:

- understand the role of destructive operations
- understand the procedures involved in destructive operations.

Introduction

Destructive operations are fairly common in the developing world in cases of obstructed labour, where absent prenatal care and poor intrapartum care at peripheral hospitals are major contributing factors. Reported incidences range between 0.094% and 0.98% of all deliveries.[351–353] With the use of prophylactic antibiotics and thromboprophylaxis, caesarean section has become safer and there is only a limited role in modern practice for destructive procedures in the developed world.

Where there has been prolonged labour and in the presence of anaemia and infection, caesarean section carries significant risks. Potential problems include haemorrhage from uterine extension, generalised peritonitis and the risk of rupture of the scar in a subsequent pregnancy. Gogoi[354] had a much lower morbidity and mortality with craniotomy than with caesarean section in a group of 158 grossly infected patients. Peritonitis occurred in 66% of patients after caesarean section and was nil after destructive operations, 98% of women had fever whereas it occurred in only 40–57% after destructive operations. The maternal mortality in the caesarean section group was 13/107 (12%) compared with 1/37 (2.7%) in the craniotomy group.

Marsden *et al.*[355] described a series of four cases where the Bond-Heidler saw was used in the case of a dead baby in a transverse lie. They had no complications and suggested that in such situations this method of delivery is more appropriate than caesarean section, when a classical incision may often be required, which significantly increases the risk to the patient.

Reports from the developing world of maternal morbidity and mortality following destructive procedures illustrate that most problems encountered can be attributed to obstructed labour, which often necessitate their performance in the first place. It is often not easy to differentiate the complications of one from the other. Ekwempu[356] reported on a series of 112 patients treated by embryotomy between 1974 and 1975. The only complications that he could attribute to the destructive procedure were seven cases of soft-tissue (mainly vaginal and perineal) laceration. The procedures themselves have been shown to be simple with little morbidity.[355,357]

There are several reports from the developing world of postoperative vesicovaginal fistula. These are often attributed to pressure necrosis in obstructed labour. However, it has been suggested that they could be secondary to the use of sharp instruments or from bony spicules exposed during the procedure.[358] This can be avoided by regular training using dummies and appropriate case selection.

Destructive operations, although primarily undertaken in developing countries, have a place in modern obstetric practice. They can provide an optimal method for expediting delivery both in the short and long term. Nevertheless, their need must be minimised by highest standards of education as well as antenatal and intrapartum care for all women.

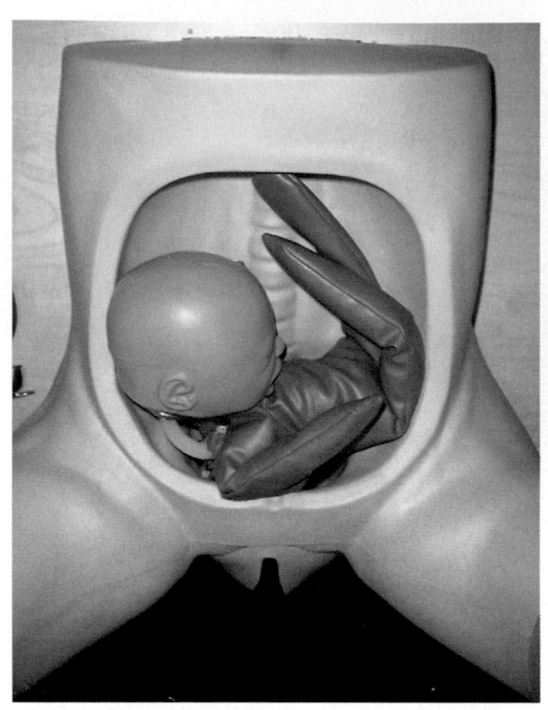

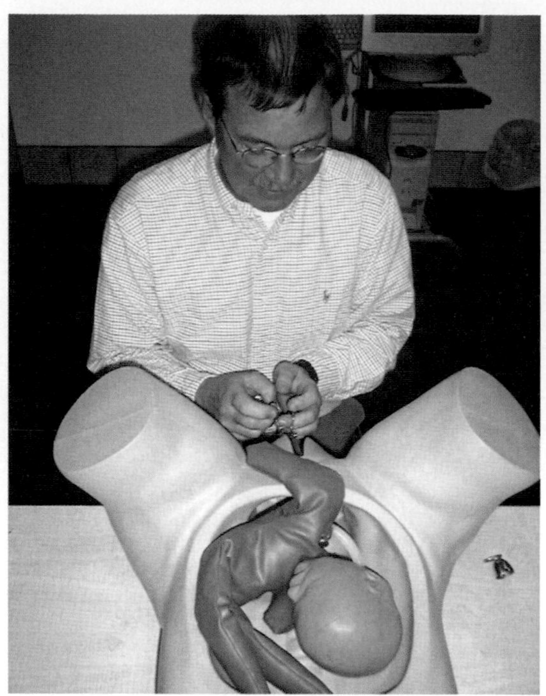

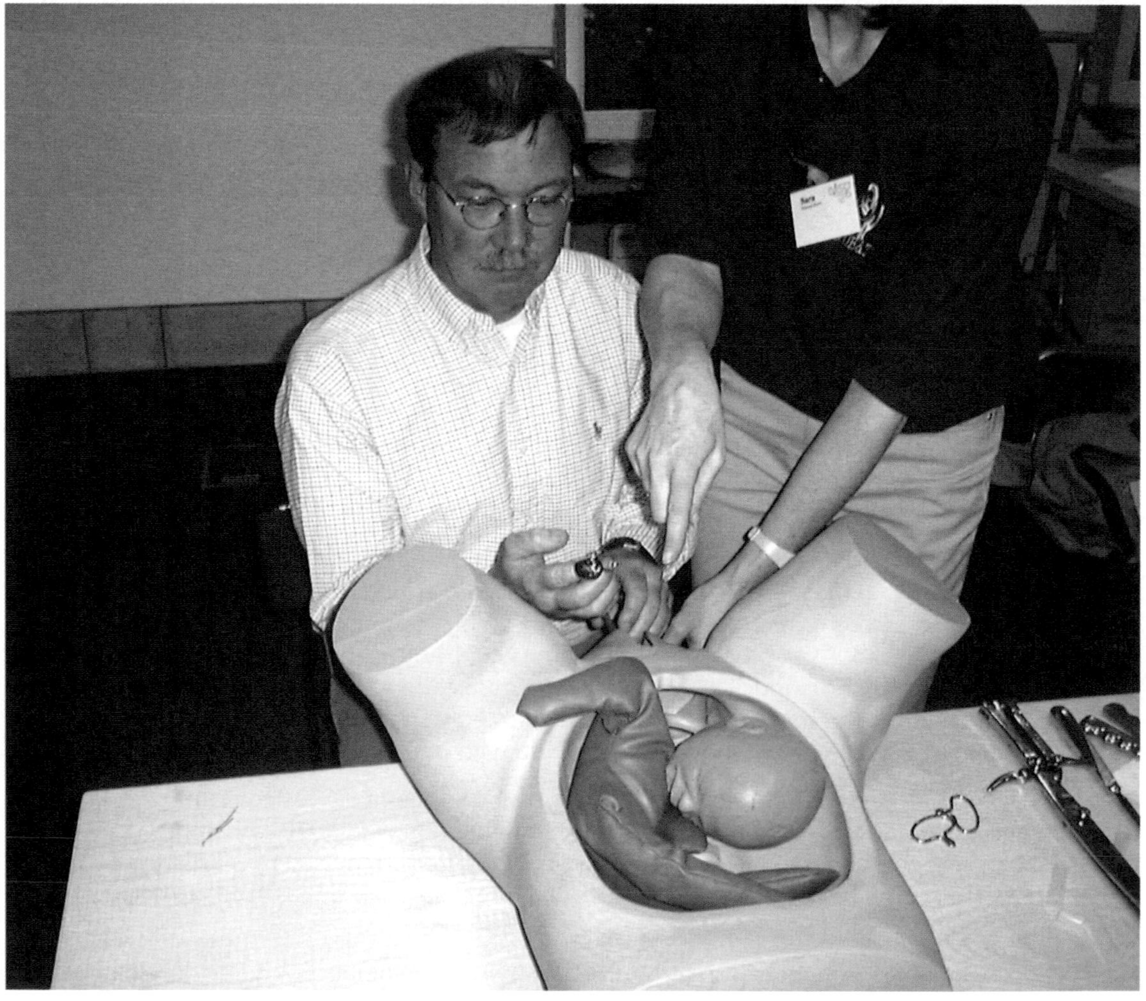

Use of the Blond-Heidler decapitation tool

Destructive procedures

Destructive operations may be required where the fetus is dead and where a vaginal delivery is being attempted. It may be the appropriate method for delivery to minimise maternal risk, or it may be the only route by which the mother wishes to be delivered. Whenever a destructive procedure is being considered it must only be performed with the mother's consent. Initially, basic resuscitation must be carried out quickly to avoid undue delay in delivering a dead fetus. Since urinary and genital tract infections are common, antibiotic prophylaxis should be used and the genital tract and rectum must be carefully examined after the procedure.

The three most common destructive procedures are:

- craniotomy
- perforation of the aftercoming head
- decapitation.[358]

Craniotomy

Indications

Craniotomy is indicated for the delivery of a dead fetus in situations of cephalopelvic disproportion and hydrocephalus.

Method[359]

- Catheterise the mother and administer a suitable analgesic.
- The fetal head should be no more than three-fifths above the pelvic brim, except in cases of hydrocephalus.[357] The cervix should be at least 4 cm dilated.
- Ask an assistant to steady the head from above the pubic symphysis.
- Perforate the skull via the fontanelle using a Simpson's perforator with the instrument at right angles to the surface of the skull, to minimise the risk of slipping. If a fontanelle cannot be palpated, the perforator should be inserted through the bone.
- Push the blades as far as their shoulders and separate first in one direction and then in another direction, at right angles to the first.
- Evacuate the brain and deliver the fetal head by a pull on the skull using vulsellum forceps and counter-traction. It may be gentler to attach the vulsellum to a 1-kg weight (e.g. one-litre bag of fluid) using a bandage. This will allow a slower and possibly more 'normal' delivery.
- If the fetus is very large, reduction in the size of the shoulder girdle by cleidotomy may be required after delivery of the head.

Aftercoming head of the breech

This can be managed similarly by craniotomy, with perforation of the head through the base of the skull, beginning at the nape of the neck, aiming towards the vertex. If the head is deflexed, perforation of the occiput may be achieved in the region of the posterior fontanelle.

Where there is hydrocephalus and accompanying spina bifida, cerebrospinal fluid can either be withdrawn by exposing the spinal canal and passing a catheter into the canal and up into the cranium. The hydrocephalic head can be decompressed transabdominally under ultrasound control using a spinal needle.

Decapitation

Indications

Decapitation is indicated in cases of neglected, obstructed labour with shoulder presentation and a dead fetus. In an already emotionally fraught situation, the prospect of explaining the options to parents may be distressing for all. Nevertheless, in terms of minimising harm to the mother, a very early delivery remains optimal.

Method

- If the fetus is small and the neck can easily be felt, it may be severed with stout scissors.[360] However, for the larger fetus, and especially where the neck is not easily accessible, the Blond-Heidler decapitation tool[361] is the safest instrument.
- The cervix should be at least 7 cm dilated and the fetal neck should be accessible per vaginam.
- If possible, an arm is brought down and firmly pulled on by an assistant, which brings the neck lower to make it more accessible.
- Thread the saw around the fetal neck and keep the handles attached to the ends of the saw close together. This prevents injury to the vagina and the neck is soon severed after a few firm strokes.
- Deliver the trunk by traction on the arm, with the operator's hand protecting the vagina from laceration by spicules of bone.
- Deliver the aftercoming head by grasping the stump with a heavy vulsellum and performing the Mauriceau-Smellie-Veit manoeuvre. It is easy to restore anatomic continuity with skin sutures to the neck.
- The baby should be wrapped nicely before showing the parents.

Chapter 30

Domestic violence

Objectives

On successfully completing this topic you will be able to:

- appreciate the incidence of domestic violence
- understand the implications for the woman and the fetus in the perinatal period
- plan to identify cases and familiarise yourself with local support services.

Key point

- All women should be seen at least once on their own during the antenatal period, to allow for disclosure of information about domestic violence.

Domestic violence is a major public health issue, which threatens the health, emotional wellbeing and lives of women and their families.

Definition

Domestic violence is defined as the intentional abuse inflicted on one partner by another in an intimate relationship. The abuse can be physical, psychological or sexual. It can occur within the context of a heterosexual or homosexual relationship and need not occur in the home. Women are more likely to be victims in heterosexual relationships (90%).[363] Domestic violence affects all social classes, all ethnic groups, occurs in any part of the world and affects all age groups.

Scale

- One in three women experiences domestic violence at some point in their lives.[4]
- One in ten women will have experienced domestic violence in the past year.[4]
- Over one million domestic violence incidents are recorded by the police each year.[4]
- 30% of domestic violence starts in pregnancy.[4]
- 40% of women who are murdered are killed by a current or ex-partner.[4]
- Domestic violence is more common than violence in the street or in a pub.[364]
- In the latest report of the CEMD, six women were murdered by their partners, three during pregnancy.[4]

What keeps women in violent relationships?

To outsiders, it seems almost bizarre that anyone would stay within a violent relationship. However, women all too often do. The reasons for staying are often multiple.[365]

Reasons why women stay in violent relationships

Fear	If she leaves she or her family will experience more violence or possibly be killed
Financial	Control of her resources by her abuser
Family	Pressures to stay with the abuser
Father	Wanting a father figure for her children
Faith	That she places in a religious doctrine
Forgiveness	Because the abuser is often contrite
Fatigue	From living under high and constant stress and erosion of self-esteem

Domestic violence and pregnancy

The incidence of domestic violence in pregnancy is reported as being 0.9–20.1%.[366,367] Domestic violence often begins or escalates during pregnancy. In some cases, domestic violence commences in the puerperium.[368] The risk of moderate to severe violence appears to be greatest in the postpartum period.[369] Battered women are at increased risk for miscarriage, premature labour, placental abruption, low-birthweight infants, fetal injury and intrauterine fetal death.[370] Often, as a result of the violence, women are 15 times more likely to abuse alcohol, nine times more likely to abuse drugs, three times more likely to be clinically depressed and five times more likely to attempt suicide.[371] These all obviously have implications for both the mother and fetus.

Classically, injuries toward the pregnant abdomen, genitals and breasts are seen in pregnancy. However, the injuries can be multiple affecting any part of the woman's body. Campbell[372] reported that 9.5% of women reported sexual abuse and 13.9% were raped by their partners.

Recognising domestic violence in pregnancy

Women who are being abused often book late and may be poor attenders. Their partners may not give them enough money to get to the hospital. Alternatively, they may attend repeatedly with trivial symptoms and appear reluctant to be discharged home. If the partner accompanies the woman, he may be constantly present not allowing for private discussion. The woman may seem reluctant to speak in front of or contradict her partner.

Any signs of violence on the woman's body will be minimised. As with child abuse, the mechanism of injury often does not fit with the apparent injury. There may be untended injuries of different ages or the late presentation of injuries. A history of behavioural problems or abuse in the children may be indicative. Often the patient will give a history of psychiatric illness.

Diagnosing domestic violence

As domestic violence often begins or escalates during pregnancy it is essential that we, as obstetricians and midwives, **routinely** ask women whether they are subject to domestic violence. Violent pregnancies are high risk and much more prevalent than most other complications of pregnancy, such as pre-eclampsia or gestational diabetes mellitus. Standard questions should therefore be included, in the same way as we would ask about medical disorders, smoking or alcohol use. Systematic multiple assessment protocols lead to increased detection and reporting of violence during pregnancy.[372]

Health professionals should be given appropriate training and education to improve awareness.[373–375] Questions should be asked in a non-judgemental, respectful, supportive manner. Obstetricians and midwives should be aware of what help is available should a woman request help.

Questions to ask that may allow the woman to disclose that she is subject to violence:

- I have noticed you have a number of bruises. Did someone hit you?
- You seemed frightened by your partner. Has he ever hurt you?
- You mention that your partner loses his temper with the children. Does he ever with you?
- How does your partner act when drinking or on drugs?

If routine questioning is to be introduced, it is important that local guidelines are developed for referral to appropriate agencies.[373–375] Other strategies, such as questionnaires in the women's toilets, may help those women whose husbands are constantly by their sides. Community midwives visiting women at home may have the privacy to discuss such sensitive issues. The provision of interpreters is essential. It is not acceptable to rely on family members to act as interpreters, as this does not allow free dialogue to occur.

Audit standard

All women should be seen on their own at least once during the antenatal period to enable the disclosure of such information.[373]

Conclusion

Domestic violence is a major health and social problem in pregnancy. It represents a serious threat to the physical and emotional health of women and their children. All health professionals have an obligation to identify cases of domestic violence and provide support and help to the victims.

SECTION 5
Triage and Transfer

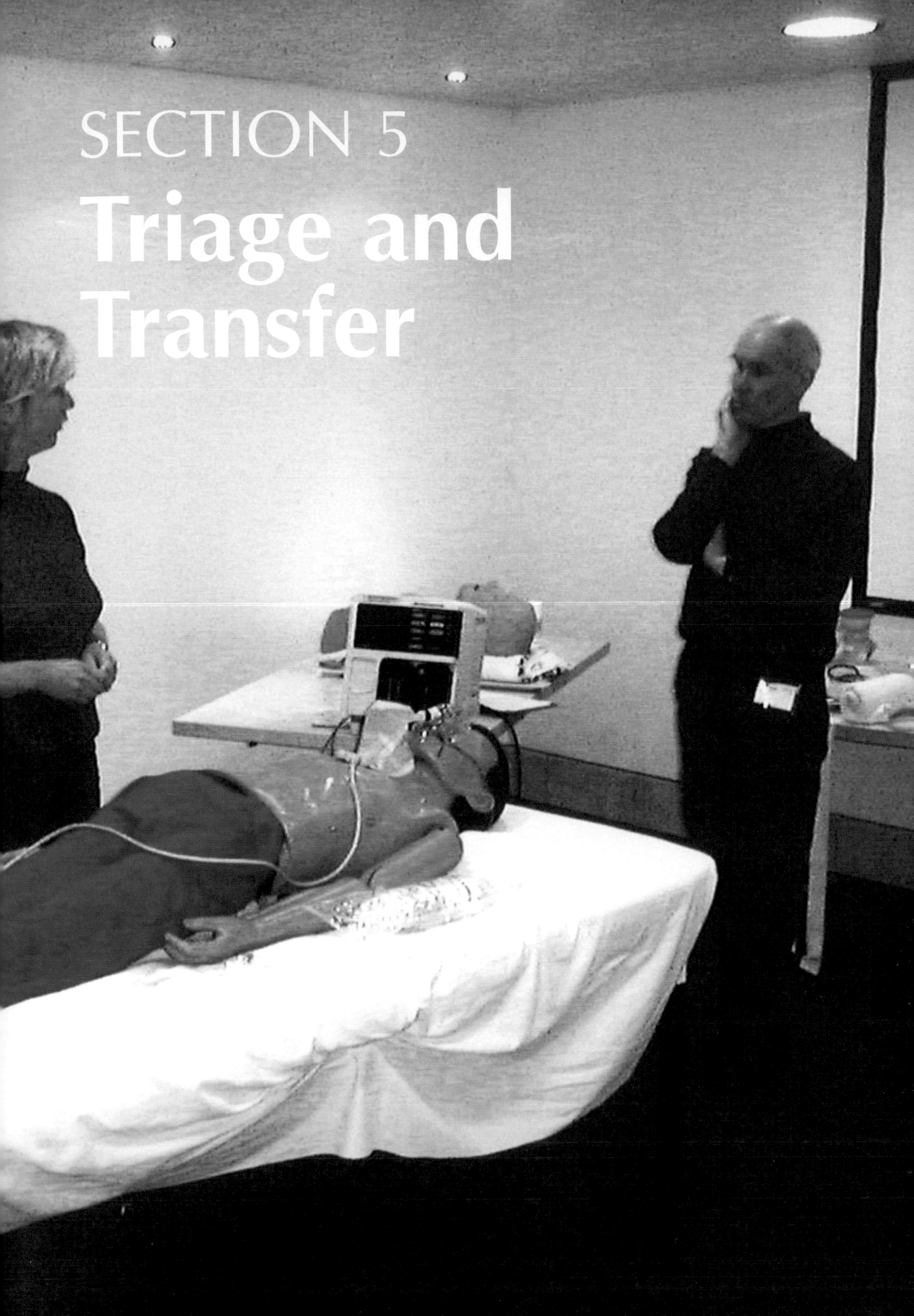

Algorithm 32.1 Triage

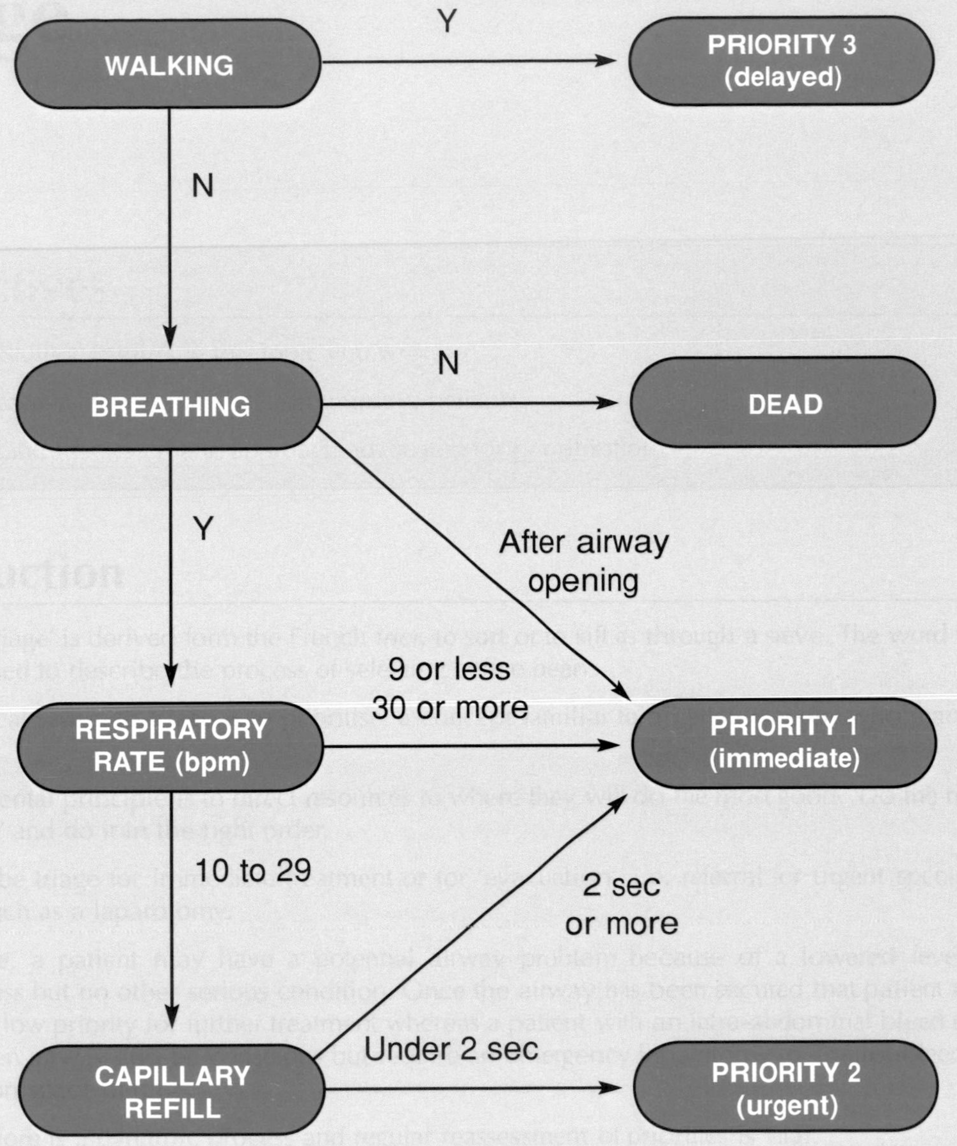

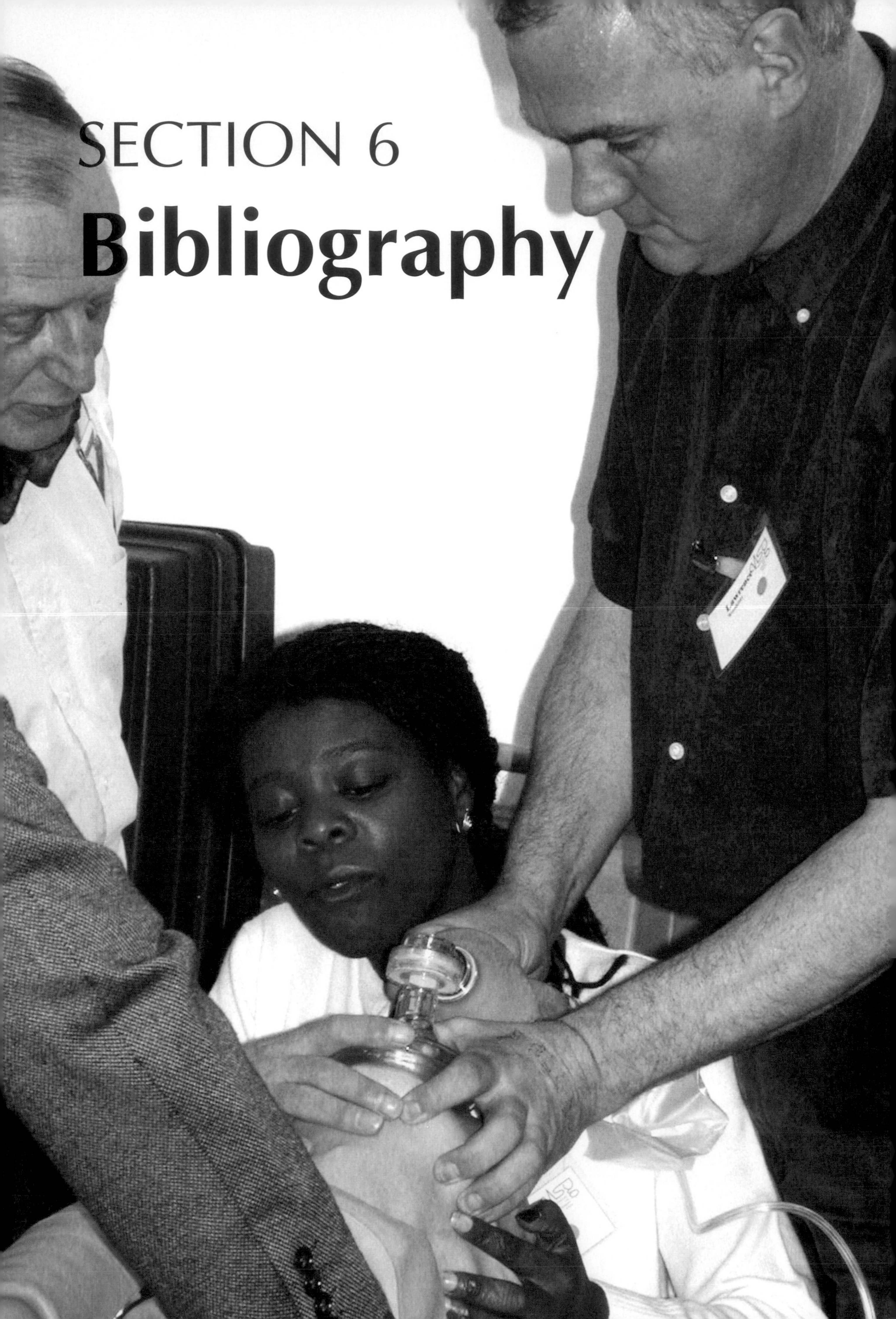

SECTION 6
Bibliography

References

1. Johanson RB, Hinshaw K. Better life-saving skills are needed for safer childbirth. *Br J Midwifery* 2001;9:199–202.
2. Jyothi NK, Cox C, Johanson RB. Management of obstetric emergencies and trauma (MOET): Regional questionnaire survey of obstetric practice amongst career obstetricians in the UK. *J Obstet Gynecol* 2001;21:107–11.
3. Johanson RB, Cox C, O'Donnell E, Grady K, Howell C, Jones P. Managing obstetric emergencies and trauma (MOET): structured skills training using models and reality-based scenarios. *The Obstetrician & Gynaecologist* 1999;1(2):46–52.
4. Lewis G, Drife J, editors. *Why Mothers Die 1997–1999. 5th Report on Confidential Enquiries into Maternal Deaths in the United Kingdom 1997–1999.* London: RCOG Press; 2001.
5. Graja AC, Zacarios E, Bergströ. S. Violent deaths: the hidden face of maternal mortality. *BJOG* 2000;109:5–8.
6. Kloeck W, Cummins RO, Chamberlain D, Bossaert L, Callanan V, Carli P, *et al.* Special resuscitation situations. An Advisory Statement from the International Liaison Committee on Resuscitation. *Circulation* 1997;95:2196–2210.
7. Kerr MG. The mechanical effects of gravid uterus in late pregnancy. *J Obstet Gynaecol Br Cwlth* 1965;72:513–29.
8. Ueland K, Novy MJ, Peterson EN. Maternal cardiopulmonary dynamics IV: The influence of gestational age on the maternal cardiovascular response to posture and exercise. *Am J Obstet Gynecol* 1969;43:856–64.
9. Zakowski MI, Ramanathan S. CPR in pregnancy. *Current Reviews in Clinical Anesthesia* 1990;10:106.
10. Katz VL, Dotters DJ, Droegemuller W. Perimortem caesarean delivery. *Obstet Gynecol* 1986;86:571–6.
11. Rees GAD, Wills BA. Resuscitation in late pregnancy. *Anaesthesia* 1988;43:347–9.
12. Oates S, Williams GL, Rees GAD. Cardiopulmonary resuscitation in late pregnancy *BMJ* 1988;297:404–5.
13. Marx GF. Cardiopulmonary resuscitation of late-pregnant women. *Anaesthesiology* 1982;56:156.
14. Emergency Cardiac Care Committee and Subcommittees, American Heart Association. Guidelines for cardiopulmonary resuscitation and emergency cardiac care. Part IV. Special resuscitation situations. *JAMA* 1992;268:2242–50.

11. Depace NL, Beetesh SS, Kolter MN. 'Postmortem' caesarean section with recovery of both mother and offspring. *JAMA* 1982;248:971–97.
12. Loopez-Zeno JA, Carlo WA, O'Grady JP, Fanaroff AA. Infant survival following delayed postmortem caesarean delivery. *Obstet Gynaecol* 1990;76:991–2.
13. Selden BS, Burke TJ. Compete maternal and fetal recovery after prolonged cardiac arrest. *Annals of Emergency Medicine* 1988;17:346–9.
14. Whitten M, Montgomery L. Postmortem and perimortem caesarean section: what are the indications. *J R Soc Med* 2000;93:6–9.
15. Clark SL, Hankins GD, Dudley DA, Dildy GA, Porter TF. Amniotic fluid embolism: analysis of the national registry. *Am J Obstet Gynecol* 1995;**172**:1158–69.
16. Gilbert WM, Danielsen B. Amniotic fluid embolism: decreased mortality in a population-based study. *Obstet Gynecol* 1999;**93**:973–7.
17. Clark SL. Amniotic fluid embolism. *Clin Perinatol* 1986;**13**:801–11.
18. Morgan M. Amniotic fluid embolism. *Anaesthesia* 1979;**34**:20–32.
19. Benson MD, Lindberg RE. Amniotic fluid embolism, anaphylaxis and tryptase. *Am J Obstet Gynecol* 1996;**175**:737.

20. Benson MD. Anaphylactoid syndrome of pregnancy. *Am J Obstet Gynecol* 1996;175:749.
21. Hankins GDV, Snyder RR, Clark SL, Schwartk L, Patterson WR, Butzin CA. Acute hemodynamic and respiratory effects of amniotic fluid embolism in the pregnant goat model. *Am J Obstet Gynecol* 1993;**168**:1113–30.
22. Lumley J, Owen R, Morgan M. Amniotic fluid embolism. A report of three cases. *Anaesthesia* 1979;**34**:33–6.
23. Schaerf RH, DeCampo T, Civetta JM. Hemodynamic alterations and rapid diagnosis in a case of amniotic fluid embolus. *Anesthesiology* 1977;**46**:155–7.
24. Schaerf RH, de Campo T, Civetta JM. Hemodynamic alterations and rapid diagnosis in a case of amniotic-fluid embolus. *Anesthesiology* 1977;46:155–7.
25. Johanson R, Kumar M, Obhrai M, Young P. Management of massive postpartum haemorrhage: use of a hydrostatic balloon catheter to avoid laparotomy. *BJOG* 2001;108:420–2.
26. Esposito RA, Grossi EA, Coppa G, Giangola G, Ferri DP, Angelides EM, *et al.* Successful treatment of postpartum shock caused by amniotic fluid embolism with cardiopulmonary bypass and pulmonary artery thromboembolectomy. *Am J Obstet Gynecol* 1991;**164**:572–4.
27. Clark SL. Successful pregnancy outcomes after amniotic fluid embolism. *Am J Obstet Gynecol* 1992;**167**:511–12.
28. De Swiet M. Management of pulmonary embolus in pregnancy. *Eur Heart J* 1999;20:1378–85.
29. American College of Obstetrics and Gynecology. Educational bulletin. Thromboembolism in pregnancy. *Int J Gynecol Obstet* 1997;57:209–18.
30. De Swiet M. Thromboembolism. In: de Swiet M, editor. *Medical Disorders in Obstetric Practice*, 3rd ed. Oxford: Blackwell Scientific; 1995. p. 116–42.
31. PIOPED Investigators. Value of the ventilation/perfusion scan in acute PE. Results of the prospective investigation of pulmonary embolism diagnosis. *JAMA* 1990;263:2753–9.
32. Thomson AJ. Greer IA. Non-haemorrhagic obstetric shock. *Balliere's Best Pract Res Clin Obstet Gynaecol* 2000;14(1):19–41.
33. Toglia MR, Nolan TE. Venous thromboembolism during pregnancy: a current review of diagnosis and management. *Obstet Gynecol Surv* 1997;52:60–72.
34. Ginsberg JS, Hirsh J, Rainbow AJ, Coates G. Risks to the fetus of radiological procedures used in the diagnosis of maternal venous thromboembolic disease. *Thromb Haemost* 1989;61:189–96.
35. Greer IA. Thrombosis in pregnancy: maternal and fetal issues. *Lancet* 1999;353:1258–65.
36. Macklon NS. Diagnosis of deep venous thrombosis and pulmonary embolism in pregnancy. *Curr Opin Pulm Med* 1999;5:233–7.
37. Thompson AJ, Walker ID, Greer IA. Low molecular weight heparin for the immediate management of thromboembolic disease in pregnancy. *Lancet* 1998;**352**:1904.
38. Heffner JE. Airway management in the critically ill patient. *Crit Care Clin* 1990;6:533–50.
39. Palme-Kilander C. Methods of resuscitation in low Apgar score in newborn infants – a national survey. *Acta Paediatr* 1992;81:739–44.
40. Figure 14.1. The correct and incorrect use of a seat belt in pregnancy. In: Lewis G, Drife J, editors. *Why Mothers Die 1997–1999. Fifth Report of the Confidential Enquiries into Maternal Deaths in the United Kingdom.* London: RCOG Press; 2001. p. 228.
41. Douglas KA, Redman CWG. Eclampsia in the United Kingdom. *BMJ* 1994;309:1395–400.
42. Clinical Resource Efficiency Support Team. *Management of Severe Pre-eclampsia and Eclampsia.* Belfast: CREST Secretariat; 2001. [Copies available from: The CREST Secretariat, Room 517, Dundonald house, Upper Newtownards Road, Belfast BT4 3SF; or online at: www.n-i.nhs.uk/crest]
43. Waisman GD, Mayorga LM, Camera MI, Vignolo CA, Martinotti A. Magnesium plus nifedipine: potentiation of hypotensive effect in preeclampsia. *Am J Obstet Gynecol* 1988;159:308–9.
44. Ben-Ami M, Giladi Y, Shaley E. The combination of magnesium sulphate and nifedipine: a cause of neuromuscular blockade. *Br J Obstet Gynaecol* 1994;101:262–3.
45. Scott W, Snyder SW, Cardwell MS. Neuromuscular blockade with magnesium sulfate and nifedipine. *Am J Obstet Gynecol* 1989;161:35–36.
46. Royal College of Obstetricians and Gynaecologists. *Antenatal Corticosteroids to Prevent Respiratory Distress Syndrome. Guideline No. 7.* London: Royal College of Obstetricians and Gynaecologists; 1996. [Superseded by reference 64.]

47. Royal College of Obstetricians and Gynaecologists. *Management of Eclampsia. Guideline No. 10.* London: Royal College of Obstetricians and Gynaecologists; 1996 (reviewed July 1999).
48. Young PF, Johanson RB. Haemodynamic, invasive and echocardiographic monitoring in the hypertensive parturient. *Balliere's Best Pract Res Clin Obstet Gynaecol* 2001;15:605–22.
49. Department of Health and Social Security. *Delivering the Future: Report of the High Risk Pregnancy Group.* London: HMSO; 1996.
50. Enkin M, Keirse MJNC, Chalmers I. *A Guide to Effective Care in Pregnancy and Childbirth.* Oxford: Oxford University Press; 1989.
51. Royal College of Obstetricians and Gynaecologists. *Report of the RCOG Working Party on Prophylaxis Against Thromboembolism in Gynaecology and Obstetrics.* London: RCOG; 1995.
52. Clinical Resource Efficiency Support Team. *Review of Adult Intensive Care Services in Northern Ireland.* Belfast: CREST Secretariat; 1998.
53. Hunt BJ, Scully M, Nelson-Piercy C, Bewley S, Khamashta M. Antiphospholipid antibodies and pregnancy. *Reproductive Vascular Medicine* 2000;1:8–13.
54. Walker JJ. The case for early recognition and intervention in pregnancy induced hypertension. In: Sharp F, Symonds EM, editors. *Hypertension in Pregnancy: Proceedings Sixteenth Study Group of the Royal College of Obstetricians and Gynaecologists.* New York: Perinatology Press, 1987. p. 289-99.
55. Steer P. The definition of pre-eclampsia. *Br J Obstet Gynaecol* 1999;106:753–5.
56. Halligan AWF, Bell S, Taylor DJ. Commentary: Dipstick proteinuria: caveat emptor. *Br J Obstet Gynaecol* 1999;106:1113–15.
57. Redman CW, Beilin LJ, Wilkinson BH. Plasma urate. Measurements in predicting fetal death in hypertensive pregnancy. *Lancet* 1976;i:1370–4.
58. Metz J, Cincotta R, Francis M, De Roas L, Balloch A. Screening for consumptive coagulopathy in pre-eclampsia. *Int J Gynaecol Obstet* 1994;46:3–9.
59. Weinstein L. Syndrome of hemolysis, elevated liver enzymes and low platelet count: a severe consequence of hypertension in pregnancy. *Am J Obstet Gynecol* 1982;142:159–67.
60. Roberts WE, Perry KG, Woods JB. The intrapartum platelet count in patients with HELLP (haemolysis, elevated liver-enzymes, and low platelets) syndrome: is it predictive of later hemorrhagic complications. *Am J Obstet Gynecol* 1994;175:799–804.
61. Redman CW. Controlled trials of anti-hypertensive drugs in pregnancy. *American Journal of Kidney Diseases* 1991;171:149–53.
62. Ramanathan J, Sibai BM, Mabie WC. The use of labetolol for attenuation of the hypertensive response to endotracheal intubation in pre-eclampsia. *Am J Obstet Gynecol* 1988;159:650–4.
63. Royal College of Obstetricians and Gynaecologists. *Antenatal Corticosteroids to Prevent Respiratory Distress Syndrome. Guideline No. 7.* London: Royal College of Obstetricians and Gynaecologists; 1999.
64. Thornton JG. Prophylactic anticonvulsants for pre-eclampsia? *Br J Obstet Gynaecol* 2000;107:839–40.
65. Duley L, Neilson JP. Magnesium sulphate and pre-eclampsia. *BMJ* 1999;319:3–4.
66. Leitch CR, Cameron AD, Walker JJ. The changing pattern of eclampsia over a 60-year period. *Br J Obstet Gynaecol* 1997;104:917–922.
67. Ventura JE, Villa M, Mizraji R, Ferreiros R. Acute renal failure in pregnancy. *Renal Failure* 1997;19:217–20.
68. Cotton DB, Gonik B, Dorman K, Harrist R. Cardiovascular alterations in severe pregnancy-induced hypertension: relationship of central venous pressure to pulmonary capillary wedge pressure. *Am J Obstet Gynecol* 1985;151:762–4.
69. Sibai BM. Hypertension. In: Gabbe SG, Simpson JL, editors. *Obstetrics: Normal and Problem Pregnancies.* New York: Churchill Livingstone; 1995. p. 969–71.
70. Duley L, Carroli G, Belizan J. Which anticonvulsant for women with eclampsia: evidence from the collaborative eclampsia trial. *Lancet* 1995;345:1455–63.
71. Geary M. Review: The HELLP syndrome. *Br J Obstet Gynaecol* 1997;104:887–91.
72. Walker ID, Walker JJ, Colvin BT, Letsky EA, Rivers R, Stevens R. Investigation and management of haemorrhagic disorders in pregnancy. *J Clin Pathol* 1994;47:100–8.
73. Sherman SJ, Greenspoon JS, Nelson JM, Paul RH. Identifying the obstetric patient at high risk of multiple-unit blood transfusions. *J Reprod Med* 1992;37:649–52.

74. Kamani AA, McMorland G, Wadsworth LD. Utilization of red blood cell transfusion in an obstetric setting. *Am J Obstet Gynecol* 1988;159:1177–81.
75. Hayashi RH, Castillo MS, Noah ML. Management of severe postpartum haemorrhage with a prostaglandin F2 analogue. *Obstet Gynecol* 1984;63:806–8.
76. Maresh M, James D, Neales K. Critical care of the obstetric patient. In: James DK, Steer P, Gonik B, editors. *High Risk Pregnancy.* 2nd ed. London: WB Saunders; 2001. p. 1129–321.
77. Nolan TE, Gallup DG. Massive transfusion: A current review. *Obstet Gynecol Surv* 1991;46:289–95.
78. Jones JA. Recent changes in transfusion practice. In: Kaufman L, editor. *Anaesthesia Review.* London: Churchill Livingstone; 1989. p. 177-91.
79. Kruskall MS. Controversies in transfusion medicine. The safety and utility of autologous transfusions in pregnant patients: pro. *Transfusion* 1990;30:168–71.
80. Sayers MH. Controversies in transfusion medicine. The safety and utility of autologous transfusions in pregnant patients: con. *Transfusion* 1990;30:172–4.
81. Zichella L, Gramolini R. Autotransfusion during cesarean section. *Am J Obstet Gynecol* 1990;162:295.
82. Letsky EA. *Coagulation Problems in Pregnancy. Current Reviews in Obstetrics and Gynaecology No. 10.* London: Churchill Livingstone; 1985. p. 62–87.
83. Sander-Jensen K, Secher NH, Bie P, Warberg J, Schwartz TW. Vagal slowing of the heart during haemorrhage: observations from 20 consecutive hypotensive patients. *BMJ* 1986;292:364–6.
84. Anthony JA, Johanson RB, Dommisse J. Critical care management of severe pre-eclampsia. *Fetal and Maternal Medicine Review* 1994;6:219–29.
85. Crane S, Chun B, Acker D. Treatment of obstetrical hemorrhagic emergencies. *Curr Opin Obstet Gynecol* 1993;5:675–82.
86. Yamashita Y, Harada M, Yamamoto H, Miyazaki T, Takahashi M, Miyazaki K, *et al.* Transcatheter arterial embolization of obstetric and gynaecological bleeding: efficacy and clinical outcome. *Br J Radiol* 1994;67:530–4.
87. Oleen MA, Mariano JP. Controlling refractory atonic postpartum haemorrhage with hemabate sterile solution. *Am J Obstet Gynecol* 1990;162:205–8.
88. Maier RC. Control of postpartum haemorrhage with uterine packing. *Am J Obstet Gynecol* 1993;169:317–23.
89. Pelage JP, Le Dref O, Mateo J, Soyer P, Jacob D, Kardache M, *et al.* Life threatening primary postpartum haemorrhage: treatment with emergency selective arterial embolization. *Radiology* 1998;208:359–62.
90. O'Leary JA. Stoppage of hemorrhage with uterine artery ligation. *Contemporary Ob/Gyn* 1986;28:13–16.
91. Likeman RK. The boldest procedure possible for checking the bleeding: a look at an old operation and a series of 13 cases from an Australian hospital. *Aust N Z J Obstet Gynaecol* 1992;32:256–262.
92. B-Lynch C. Coker A, Lawah AH, Abu J, Cowen MJ. The B-Lynch surgical technique for the control of massive postpartum haemorrhage: an alternative to hysterectomy? Five cases reported. *Br J Obstet Gynaecol* 1997;104:372–5.
93. Bannon L. The high risk parturient. In: Ostheimer GW, editor. *Manual of Obstetric Anaesthesia.* 2nd ed. London: Churchill Livingstone; 1992. p. 228–35.
94. Gilstrap LC, Hauth JC, Hankins GDV, Patterson AR. Effect of type of anaesthesia on blood loss at cesarean section. *Obstet Gynecol* 1987;69:328–32.
95. Combs CA, Murphy EL, Laros RK. Factors associated with hemorrhage in cesarean deliveries. *Obstet Gynecol* 1991;77:77–82.
96. Redick LF, Livingston E. A new preparation of nitroglycerin for uterine relaxation. *International Journal of Obstetric Anesthesia* 1995;4:14–16.
97. Clark SL, Koonings PP, Phelan JP. Placenta previa/accreta and prior cesarean section. *Obstet Gynecol* 1985;66:89–92.
98. Chestnut DH, Eden RD, Gall SA, Parker RT. Peripartum hysterectomy: a review of cesarean and postpartum hysterectomy. *Obstet Gynecol* 1985;65:365–70.
99. Oakley PA, Morrison PJ. Resuscitation and monitoring of hypovolaemic shock. *Curr Opinion Anesthesiol* 1994;7:177–83.
100. Louca O, Johanson RB. Shoulder dystocia. In: O'Brien PMS, editor. *Yearbook of Obstetrics and Gynaecology Volume 6.* London: RCOG Press; 1998. p. 73–84.

101. Spong CY, Beall M, Rodrigues D. An objective definition of shoulder dystocia: prolonged head to body delivery intervals and/or the use of ancillary obstetric manoeuvres. *Obstet Gynecol* 1995;86:433–6.
102. Resnik R. Management of shoulder girdle dystocia. *Clin Obstet Gynecol* 1980;23:559–64.
103. Benedetti T. Added complications of shoulder dystocia. *Contemporary Ob/Gyn* 1989;33(6):150–61.
104. Gibb D. Clinical focus: shoulder dystocia. The obstetrics. *Clinical Risk* 1995;1:49–54.
105. Sandmire HF, O'Halloin TJ. Shoulder dystocia. Its incidence and associated risk factors. *Int J Gynaecol Obstet* 1988;95:26–73.
106. Confidential Enquiry into Stillbirths and Deaths in Infancy. *Annual Report from 1 January to 31 December 1993*. London; HMSO; 1993.
107. Roberts L. Shoulder dystocia. In: Studd JWW, editor. *Progress in Obstetrics and Gynaecology Volume 11*. Edinburgh: Churchill Livingstone; 1994. p. 201–16.
108. Confidential Enquiries into Stillbirths and Deaths in Infancy. *5th Annual Report 1998*. London: Maternal and Child Health Research Consortium; 1999.
109. Wood C, Ng K, Hounslow D, Benning H. Time: an important variable in normal delivery. *J Obstet Gynaecol Br Cwlth* 1973;80:295–300.
110. Boyd M, Usher R, McLean FH. Fetal macrosomia: prediction, risks, proposed management. *Obstet Gynecol* 1983;61:715–22.
111. Patterson C, Graves W, Bugg G, Sasso S, Brann A. Antenatal and intrapartum factors associated with the occurrence of seizures in the term infant. *Obstet Gynecol* 1989;74:361–5.
112. Johnson S, Kolberg B, Varner M, Railsback LD. Maternal obesity and pregnancy. *Surg Gynecol Obstet* 1987;164:431–7.
113. Tan K. Brachial Palsy. *J Obstet Gynaecol Br Cwlth* 1973;80:60–2.
114. Baskett T F. Letter. *Obstet Gynecol* 1996;87:639.
115. Rubin A. Management of shoulder dystocia. *JAMA* 1964;189:835–5.
116. Gordon M, Rich HDJR. The immediate and long term outcome of obstetric birth trauma. *Am J Obstet Gynecol* 1973;117:51–4.
117. Baksett TF, Allen AC. Perinatal implications of shoulder dystocia. *Obstet Gynecol* 1995;86:14–17.
118. Nocon J, McKenzie, Thomas L, Hansell R. Shoulder dystocia: an analysis of risks and obstetric manoeuvres. *Am J Obstet Gynecol* 1993;168:1732–7.
119. Jennett R, Tarby T, Kreinick C. Brachial plexus palsy: an old problem revisited. *Am J Obstet Gynecol* 1992;166:1673–7.
120. Johnstone FD, Myerscough PR. Shoulder dystocia. *Br J Obstet Gynaecol* 1998;105:811–15.
121. Hankins GDV, Clark SL. Brachial plexus palsy involving the posterior shoulder at spontaneous delivery. *Am J Perinatol* 1995;12:44–5.
122. Graham EM, Forouzon I, Morgan MA. A retrospective analysis of Erb's palsy cases and their relation to birthweight and trauma at delivery. *J Matern Fetal Med* 1997;6:1–5.
123. Sandmire HF, DeMott RK. Erb's palsy: concepts of causation. *Obstet Gynecol* 2000;95:941–2.
124. Gherman RB, Ouzounian JG, Goodwin TM. Obstetric manouevres for shoulder dystocia and associated fcetal morbidity. *Am J Obstet Gynecol* 1998;178:1126–30.
125. Wolf H, Hoeksma AF, Oei SL, Bleker OP. Obstetric brachial plexus injury: risk factors related to recovery. *Eur J Obstet Gynecol Reprod Biol* 2000;88:133–8.
126. Benedetti TJ, Gabbe S. Shoulder dystocia. A complication of fetal macrosomia and prolonged second stage of labor with midpelvic delivery. *Obstet Gynecol* 1978;52:526–9.
127. Moller-Bek K, Laurberg S. Intervention during labor: risk factors associated with complete tear of the anal sphincter. *Acta Obstet Gynecol Scand* 1992;175:515–22.
128. Acker D, Sachs B, Friedman E. Risk factors for shoulder dystocia in the average weight infant. *Obstet Gynecol* 1986;67:614–18.
129. Khatree MH. Features predictive of brachial plexus injury during labour. *JAMA* 1982;61:232–3.
130. McFarland M, Hod M, Piper JM, Xenakis EMJ, Langer O. Are labor abnormalities more common in shoulder dystocia? *Am J Obstet Gynecol* 1995;173:1211–14.
131. Acker D, Sachs B, Friedman E. Risk factors for shoulder dystocia. *Obstet Gynecol* 1985;66:762–8.
132. Langer O, Berkhus M, Huff R, Saueloff A. Shoulder dystocia: should the fetus weighing

greater than or equal to 4000 grams be delivered by cesarean section? *Am J Obstet Gynecol* 1991;165:831–8.

133. Boekhuizen F, Washington J, Johnson F, Hamilton P. Vacuum extraction versus forceps delivery: indications and complications, 1979 to 1984. *Obstet Gynecol* 1987;69:338–42.
134. Keller J, Lopex-Zeno J, Dooley S, Socol M. Shoulder dystocia and birth trauma in gestational diabetes: a five year experience. *Am J Obstet Gynecol* 1991;165:928–30.
135. Gross T, Sokol R, Williams T, Thompson K. Shoulder dystocia, a fetal-physician risk. *Am J Obstet Gynecol* 1987;156:882–4.
136. Diani F, Moscatelli C, Toppano B, Turinetto A. [Fetal macrosomia and mode of delivery. Italian.] *Minerva Ginecol* 1995;47:77–82.
137. O'Leary J, Gunn D. Cephalic replacement for shoulder dystocia. *Am J Obstet Gynecol* 1985;153:479–84.
138. Naef R, Morrison J. Guidelines for management of shoulder dystocia. *J Perinatol* 1994;14:435–41.
139. Spellacy W, Miller S, Winegar A, Peterson P. Macrosomia: maternal characteristics and infant complications. *Obstet Gynecol* 1985;66:158–61.
140. Jackovits A. Medicolegal aspects of brachial plexus injury: the obstetrician's point of view. *Med Law* 1996;15:175–82.
141. Friesen CD, Miller AM, Rayburn WF. Influence of spontaneous labor on delivering macrosomic fetus. *Am J Perinatol* 1995;12:63–6.
142. Weeks JW, Pitman T, Spinnato J. Fetal macrosomia: does antenatal prediction affect delivery route and birth outcome? *Am J Obstet Gynecol* 1995;173:1215–19.
143. Combs CA, Singh NB, Khoury JC. Elective induction versus spontaneous labor after sonographc diagnosis of fetal macrosomia. *Obstet Gynecol* 1993;81:492–6.
144. Kjos S, Henry O, Montoro M, Buchanan TA, Mestman JH. Insulin-requiring diabetes in pregnancy: a randomised trial of active induction of labor and expectant management. *Am J Obstet Gynecol* 1993;169:611–15.
145. Dignan W. Difficulties in delivery including shoulder dystocia and malpresentation of the fetus. *Clin Obstet Gynecol* 1976;19:577–85.
146. Lurie S, Ben-Arie A, Hagay Z. The ABC of shoulder dystocia management. *Asia Oceania J Obstet Gynaecol* 1994;20:195–7.
147. Hernandez C, Wendel G. Shoulder dystocia. *Clin Obstet Gynecol* 1990;33:3.
148. Gonik B, Stringer CA, Held B. An alternative maneuver for management of shoulder dystocia. *Am J Obstet Gynecol* 1983;145:882–4.
149. Gonik B, Allen R, Sorab J. Objective evaluation of the shoulder dystocia phenomenon; effect of maternal pelvic orientation on force reduction. *Obstet Gynecol* 1989;74:44–7.
150. Allen RH, Bankoski BR, Butzin CA, Nagey DA. Comparing clinician-applied loads for routine, difficult and shoulder dystocia deliveries. *Am J Obstet Gynecol* 1994;171:1621–7.
151. Woods CE, Westbury NYA. A principle of physics as applicable to shoulder delivery. *Am J Obstet Gynecol* 1943;45:796–804.
152. Glynn M, Olah KS. The management of shoulder dystocia. *Br J Midwifery* 1994;2:108–12.
153. Gobbo R, Baxley E. Shoulder dystocia. In: Damos JR, Eisinger SH, Murphy N, Baxley E, editors. ALSO Course Manual. 4th ed. Leawood, KS: American Association of Family Physicians; 2000. p. 1–13.
154. Gaskin IM. Shoulder dystocia: controversies in management. *Birth Gazette* 1988;5:14.
155. Bruner JP, Drummond SB, Meenan AL. All four maneuvers for reducing shoulder dystocia. *J Reprod Med* 1998;43:439–43.
156. Meenan AL, Gaskin IM, Hunt P, Ball CA. A new (old) maneuver for the management of shoulder dystocia. *J Fam Pract* 1991;32:625–9.
157. O'Leary J. Cephalic replacement for shoulder dystocia: present status and future role of Zavanelli manoeuvre. *Obstet Gynecol* 1993;82:847–55.
158. Graham JM, Blanco JD, Wen T, Magee KP. The Zavanelli manoeuvre: a different perspective. *Obstet Gynecol* 1992;79:883–4.
159. Spellacy W. The Zavanelli manoeuvre for fetal shoulder dystocia. Three cases with poor outcomes. *J Reprod Med* 1995;40:543–4.
160. Hartfield VJ. Symphysiotomy for shoulder dystocia. *Am J Obstet Gynecol* 1986;155:228.
161. Reid PC, Osuagwu FI. Symmphysiotomy in shoulder dystocia. *J Obstet Gynaecol* 1999;19:664–6.
162. Magowan B. Shoulder dystocia. In: Magowan B. *Churchill's Pocketbook of Obstetrics and Gynaecology*. 2nd ed. Edinburgh: Churchill Livingstone; 2000. p. 92–5.

163. Neill AM, Thornton S. Shoulder dystocia. *The Obstetrician & Gynaecologist* 2000;2(4):45–7.
164. Johanson RB, Wykes C. Shoulder dystocia (letter). *The Obstetrician & Gynaecologist* 2001;3:101–2.
165. Leigh TH, James CE. Medicolegal commentary: shoulder dystocia. *Br J Obstet Gynaecol* 1998;105:815–17.
166. Johanson RB, Hinshaw K. Better life-saving skills are needed for safer childbirth. *Br J Midwifery* 2001;9:199–202.
167. Taylor HA, Kiser WR. Reported comfort with obstetrical emergencies before and after participation in the advanced life support in obstetrics course. *Fam Med* 1998;30:103–7.
168. Critchlow CW, Leet TL, Benedetti TJ, Daling JR. Risk factors and infant outcomes associated with umbilical cord prolapse: a population-based case–control study among births in Washington State. *Am J Obstet Gynecol* 1994;170:613–18.
169. Murphy DJ, MacKenzie IZ. The mortality and morbidity associated with umbilical cord prolapse. *Br J Obstet Gynaecol* 1995;102:826–30.
170. Panter KR, Hannah ME. Umbilical cord prolapse: so far so good? *Lancet* 1996;347:74.
171. Fenton AN, d'Esopo DA. Prolapse of the cord during labor. *Am J Obstet Gynecol* 1951;62:52–64.
172. Mesleh T, Sultan M, Sabagh T, Algwiser A. Umbilical cord prolapse. *J Obstet Gynaecol* 1993;13:24–8.
173. Koonings PP, Paul RH, Campbell K. Umbilical cord prolapse: a contemporary look. *J Reprod Med* 1990;35:690–2.
174. Yla-Outinen A, Heinonen PK, Tuimala R. Predisposing and risk factors of umbilical cord prolapse. *Acta Obstet Gynecol Scand* 1985;64:567–70.
175. Ferrara TB, Hoekstra RE, Gaziano E, Knox GE, Couser RJ, Fangman JJ. Changing outcome of extremely premature infants (< 26 weeks' gestation and < 750 gm): survival and follow-up at a tertiary center. *Am J Obstet Gynecol* 1989;161:1114–18.
176. Usta IM, Mercer BM, Sibai BM. Current obstetrical practice and umbilical cord prolapse. *Am J Perinatol* 1999;16:479–84.
177. Raga F, Osborne N, Ballister MJ. Color flow Doppler: a useful instrument in the diagnosis of funic presentation. *J Natl Med Assoc* 1996;88(2):94–6.
178. Goldthorp WO. A decade in the management of prolapse and presentation of the umbilical cord. *Br J Clin Pract* 1967;21:21–6.
179. Prabulos AM, Philpson EH. Umbilical cord prolapse: so far so good. *J Reprod Med* 1998;43:129–132.
180. Tchabo JG. The use of the contact hysteroscope in the diagnosis of cord prolapse. *Int Surg* 1988;73:57–58.
181. Dare FO, Owolabi AT, Fasubaa OB, Ezechi OC. Umbilical cord prolapse: a clinical study of 60 cases seen at Obafemi Awolowo university teaching hospital. *East Afr Med J* 1998;75:308–10.
182. Katz Z, Shoham Z, Lancet M, Blickstein I, Mogilner BM, Zalel Y. Management of labor with umbilical cord prolapse: A 5 year study. *Obstet Gynecol* 1994;94:278–81.
183. Driscoll JA, Sadan O, Van Gelderen CJ, Holloway GA. Cord prolapse: can we save more babies? Case reports. *Br J Obstet Gynaecol* 1987;94:594–5.
184. Barrett JM. Funic reduction for the management of umbilical cord prolapse. *Am J Obstet Gynecol* 1991;165:654–7.
185. Vago T. Prolapse of the umbilical cord. A method of management. *Am J Obstet Gynecol* 1970;107:967–9.
186. Caspi E, Lotan Y, Schreyer P. Prolapse of the cord: reduction of perinatal mortality by bladder insilation and cesarean section. *Isr J Med Sci* 1983;19:541–5.
187. Chetty RM, Moodley J. Umbilical cord prolapse. *S Afr Med J* 1980;57:128–9.
188. Griese ME, Prickett SA. Nursing management of umbilical cord prolapse. *J Obstet Gynecol Neonatal Nurs* 1993;311–15.
189. Loeffler F. Postpartum haemorrhage and abnormalities of the third stage of labour. In: Chamberlain G, editor. *Turnbull's Obstetrics.* 2nd ed. Edinburgh: Churchill Livingstone; 1995. p. 729–34.
190. Manassiev N, Shaw G. Uterine inversion. *Modern Midwife* 1996;6(5):32–4.
191. Stirrat G. *Aids to Obstetrics and Gynaecology for MRCOG.* 4th ed. Edinburgh: Churchill Livingstone; 1997. p. 162.
192. Watson P, Besch N, Bowes WA. Management of acute and subacute puerperal inversion of the uterus. *Obstet Gynecol* 1980;55:12–16.

365. Grunfeld A, MacKay K. Diagnosing domestic violence. *Canadian Journal of Diagnosis* 1997;14:61–9.
366. Ballard TJ, Salzman LE, Gazmararian JA, Spitz AM, Lazorick S, Marks JS. Violence during pregnancy: measurement issues. *Am J Public Health* 1998;88:274–6.
367. Abbasi K. Obstetricians must ask about domestic violence. *BMJ* 1998;316:9.
368. Widding Hedin L. Postpartum, also a risk period for domestic violence. *Eur J Obstet Gynecol Reprod Biol* 2000;89:41–5.
369. Gielen AC, O'Campo PJ, Faden RR, Kass NE, Xue X. Interpersonal conflict and physical violence during the childbearing year. *Soc Sci Med* 1994;39:781–7.
370. Mezey GC, Bewley S. Domestic violence and pregnancy. *Br J Obstet Gynaecol* 1997;104:528–31.
371. Stark E Flitcraft A. *Women at Risk.* London: Sage; 1996.
372. Campbell JC. Nursing assessment for risk of homicide with battered women. *Adv Nurs Sci* 1986;8:36–51.
373. Covington DL, Diehl SJ, Wright BD, Piner M. Assessing for violence during pregnancy using a systematic approach. *Matern Child Health J* 1997;1(2):129.
374. Bewley S, Friend J, Mezey G, editors. *Violence Against Women.* London: RCOG Press; 1997.
375. Royal College of Midwives. *Domestic Abuse in Pregnancy. Position Paper no.19.* London: RCM; 1997.
376. Howell CJ, Dean T, Lucking L, Dziedzic K, Jones PW, Johanson RB. Randomised study of long-term outcome after epidural versus non-epidural analgesia during labour. *BMJ* 2002;325:357–9.

Further reading

General

Clark SL, Cotton DB, Hankins GDV, Phelan JP. *Handbook of Critical Care Obstetrics*. Boston, PA: Blackwell Scientific; 1994.

Chapter 8

Del Rossi AJ, editor. Blunt thoracic trauma. *Trauma Quarterly* 1990;6:1–74.

Graham JG, Mattox KL, Beall AC Jr. Penetrating trauma of the lung. *J Trauma* 1979;19:665–9.

Symbas PN. Cardiothoracic trauma. *Curr Probl Surg* 1991;28:741–97.

Chapter 9

Clark SL, Cotton DD, Lee W, Bishop C, Hill T, Southwick J, *et al.* Central haemodynamic assessment of normal term pregnancy. *Am J Obstet Gynecol* 1989;161:1439–42.

Clark SL. Shock in the pregnant patient. *Semin Perinatol* 1990;14:52–8.

Chapter 11

American Association of Neurological Surgeons. Brain Trauma Foundation. *Guidelines for Severe Head Injury Management*. 2nd ed. *Journal of Neurotrauma* 2000;17:449–554.

Chapter 12

Narayan RK, Wilberger JE, Povlishock JT, editors. *Neurotrauma*. New York: McGraw Hill; 1996.

Wilberger JE. Diagnosis and management of spinal cord trauma. *Journal of Neurotrauma* 1991;8:75–86.

Chapter 14

Deitch EA, Rightmire DA, Clothier J, Blass N. Management of burns in pregnant women. *Surg Gynecol Obstet* 1985;161:1–4.

Matthews RN. Obstetric implications of burns in pregnancy. *Br J Obstet Gynaecol* 1982;89:603–9.

Polko LE, McMahon MJ. Burns in pregnancy. *Obstet Gynecol Surv* 1998;53:50–6.

Schmitz JT. Pregnant patients with burns. *Am J Obst Gynecol* 1971;110:57.

Chapter 28

El-Refaey H, O'Brien P, Morafa W, Walder J, Rodeck C. Use of oral misoprostol in the prevention of postpartum haemorrhage. *Br J Obstet Gynaecol* 1997;104:336–9.

Surbek DV, Fehr PM, Hosli I, Holzgreve W. Oral misoprostol for third stage of labour: a randomised placebo-controlled trial. *Obstet Gynaecol* 1999;94:255–8.

O'Brien P, El-Refaey H, Gordon A, Geary M, Rodeck CH. Rectally administered misoprostol for the treatment of postpartum hemorrhage unresponsive to oxytocin and ergometrine. A descriptive study. *Obstet Gynaecol* 1998;92:212–14.

Drife J. Management of primary postpartum haemorrhage. *Br J Obstet Gynaecol* 1997;104:275–7.

Alok KA, Hagen P, Webb JB. Tranexamic acid in the management of postpartum haemorrhage. *Br J Obstet Gynaecol* 1996;103:1250–1.

Maier RC. Control of postpartum hemorrhage with uterine packing. *Am J Obstet Gynecol* 1993;169:317–23.

B-Lynch C, Coker A, Lawal AH, Abu J, Cowen MJ. The B-Lynch surgical technique for the control of massive postpartum haemorrhage: an alternative to hysterectomy? Five cases reported. *Br J Obstet Gynaecol* 1997;104:372–5.

Ferguson JEI, Bourgeois FJ, Underwood PB. B-Lynch suture for postpartum hemorrhage. *Obstet Gynaecol* 2000;95:1020–2.

Buscuttil D, Copplestone A. Management of blood loss in Jehovah's Witnesses. *BMJ* 1995;311:1115–16.

Breymann C, Richter C, Huttner C, Huch R, Huch A. Effectiveness of recombinant erythropoietin and iron sucrose vs iron therapy only, in patients with postpartum anaemia and blunted erythropoiesis. *Eur J Clin Invest* 2000;30:154–61.

McLoughlin PL, Cope TM, Harrison JC. Hyperbaric oxygen therapy in the management of severe acute anaemia in a Jehovah's Witness. *Anesthesia* 1999;54:891–5.

The Hospital Liaison Committee for Jehovah's Witnesses. Treating Jehovah's Witnesses in Obstetric and Gynaecology Departments. [In-house unpublished document available from: Hospital Information Services for Jehovah's Witnesses, IBSA House, The Ridgeway, London NW7 1RN, UK. Telephone: +44 (0) 20 8906 2211; email: his@wtbts.org.uk.]

Association of Anaesthetists of Great Britain and Ireland. *Management of Anaesthesia for Jehovah's Witnesses.* London: Association of Anaesthetists of Great Britain and Ireland; 1999.

Reid MF, Nohr K, Birks RJS. Eclampsia and haemorrhage in a Jehovah's Witness. *Anesthesia* 1986;41:324–5.

Bonakdar MI, Eckhous AW, Bacher BJ, Tabbilos RH, Peisner DB. Major gynaecologic and obstetric surgery in Jehovah's Witnesses. *Obstet Gynaecol* 1982;60:587–90.

Boyd ME. The obstetrician and gynaecologists and the Jehovah's Witness. *Journal of the Society of Obstetricians and Gynaecologists of Canada* 1992;14:7–9.

Thomas JM. Management of the severely anaemic patient who refuses transfusion: lessons learnt during the care of a Jehovah's Witness. *Ann Intern Med* 1994;117:1042–8.

Thomas. JM. The worldwide need for education in nonblood management in obstetrics and gynaecology. *Journal of the Society of Obstetricians and Gynaecologists of Canada* 1994;16:1483–7.

Hart GB. Exceptional blood loss anaemia, treatment with hyperbaric oxygen. *JAMA* 1974;228:1028–9.

Kafer ER, Collins ML. Acute intraoperative hemodilution and perioperative blood salvage. *Anesthesiol Clin North America* 1990;8:543–67.

Jackson SH, Lonser RE. Safety and effectiveness of intracesarean blood salvage. *Transfusion* 1993;33:181.

Neff TA, Stocker R, Wight E, Spahn DR. Extreme intraoperative blood loss and hemodilution in a Jehovah's Witness: new aspects in postoperative management. *Anesthesiology* 1999;91:1949–51.

Chapter 31

Howell CJ. Epidural versus non epidural analgesia for pain relief. *Cochrane Database Syst Rev* 2000; Issue 2.

Index

6 BIBLIOGRAPHY